LIVER TUMORS:
Multidisciplinary Management

To Jean

LIVER TUMORS:
Multidisciplinary Management

Compiled and edited by

W. John B. Hodgson, M.D.

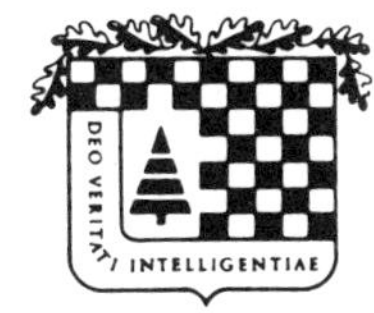

WARREN H. GREEN, INC.
St. Louis, Missouri, U.S.A.

Published by

WARREN H. GREEN, INC.
8356 Olive Boulevard
St. Louis, Missouri 63132, U.S.A.

ISBN No. 0-87527-351-3

Contributors

W. JOHN B. HODGSON, M.D.
Associate Professor of Surgery
New York Medical College
Chief of G.I. Surgery
Westchester County Medical Center

LOUIS R.M. DELGUERCIO, M.D.
Chairman and Professor
Department of Surgery
New York Medical College
Westchester County Medical Center

NORMAN B. ACKERMAN, M.D.
Chief of Surgery
Metropolitan Hospital Medical Center
Professor of Surgery
New York Medical College

HOWARD BERMAN, M.D.
Associate Professor of Radiology and
    Surgery
New York Medical College
Director, Angiography and Special
    Procedures
Westchester County Medical Center

STUART KATZ, M.D.
Assistant Professor of Radiology
New York Medical College
Associate Director of Angiography
    and Special Procedures
Westchester County Medical Center

TAUSEEF AHMED, M.D.
Associate Professor of Medicine
New York Medical College
Director, Bone Marrow Transplanta-
    tion Services
Westchester County Medical Center

JOHN A. SAVINO, M.D.
Associate Professor of Surgery
New York Medical College
Chief of Trauma and Critical Care
Westchester County Medical Center

MICHAEL FRIEDLAND, M.D.
Professor of Clinical Medicine
Sr. Assoc. Dean for Clinical Affairs
New York Medical College

JOSEPH McCARTHY, M.D.
Assistant Professor of Radiology
New York Medical College

MARVIN WEINGARTEN, M.D.
Assistant Professor of Radiology
New York Medical College
Assistant Attending–Director CT
Westchester County Medical Center

FADI F. ATTIYEH, M.D.
Assistant Professor of Surgery
New York Medical College
Attending Surgeon
St. Luke's/Roosevelt Hospital
    Medical Center

RAMON KAUL, M.D.
Assistant Professor of Radiology
New York Medical College
Assist. Attending, Radiation Therapy
Westchester County Medical Center

CHITTI MOORTHY, M.D.
Associate Professor of Radiology
New York Medical College
Director, Radiation Oncoloby
Westchester County Medical Center

DATTATREUYUDU NORI, M.D.
Assistant Professor of Radiology
Cornell University Medical College
Attending Physician, Radiation
    Therapy
Memorial Sloan-Kettering Medical
    Center

Foreword

The idea for this book came out of the rapid expansion of our programs at New York Medical College of an aggressive approach toward patients with liver tumors. We felt that as there are 30,000 new cases a year of metastases to the liver from colorectal cancer alone in the United States, and the literature covers no more than a few hundred such cases, that perhaps a major reason for this disparity was simply lack of coherent information. Such information that is available leads to the perception in practice that there are only two alternatives open to patients with these diseases. Either intermittent systemic chemotherapy is given, or a few highly selected cases have massive hepatic resections in a very few major medical centers. Further, the perception has been clouded by a combination of high surgical mortality and poor results obtainable with conventional systemic chemotherapy which were the rule in the 1950s and perhaps early 1960s. Consequently, many physicians have believed that nothing could or should be done.

We feel that there is a rising interest in the aggressive management of liver tumors and a greater range of therapeutic management is becoming recognized. Thus, there is a clear alternative to therapeutic nihilism as it is known that hepatic metastases have been shown to exert an over-riding influence upon the future course of the patient despite concurrent pulmonary, peritoneal and/or lymph node involvement. The median survival time for all patients with liver tumors is in the region of 4–5 months and in the more fortunate group, those with colorectal metastases, it is in the region of 6–7 months.

It is a major objective of this book to show that is it possible to obtain superior results by presenting a range of options. The book is dedicated to the interested physician and is written in such a way that less difficult modes of management are first described and when mastered, the reader is ready to progress further. It is hoped that practice of the principles described herein will become more widespread and that this book will have helped our patient population.

It is recognized that frequently liver metastases are widespread and unresectable. But in these cases there are alternatives which are described. Significant palliation is obtained by hepatic artery ligation since both primary and metastatic tumors receive their blood supply almost exclusively from the hepatic artery with portal venous input occurring at later stages.

Many of the complications of intra-arterial infusional chemotherapy have recently been solved, especially with the use of the new silastic catheters currently available on the market. Continuous intra-arterial chemotherapy seems to have at least a 2:1 superiority over systemic chemotherapy. Response rates vary between 35–85% with a two or three-fold prolongation in survival in responders as compared to non-responders. Furthermore, non-responders to systemic chemotherapy sometimes respond to intra-arterial infusion.

It is possible to combine intra-arterial chemotherapy, given by continuous infusion with hepatic resection and obtain an improved survival time. Preferably, the tumor should be excised completely but recent literature seems to indicate that local resection can have as good long-term survival times as hepatic lobectomy. For single metastases, the 5-year survival rate has been reported to be as high as 50%.

There are also more esoteric methods dealing with patients with advanced disease or in patients with anatomically difficult disease. These include embolization by the interventional radiologist and radiotherapy. All of these methods are described in this book.

I wish to thank Dr. Louis R.M. DelGuercio, Chairman of the Department of Surgery, New York Medical College for his major support of the hepatic tumor program based at the primary campus of New York Medical College, the Westchester Medical Center in Valhalla, New York. I also wish to thank my secretary, Nancy Pesce for her invaluable assistance and the Publisher, Warren H. Green, for taking on this project.

W. John B. Hodgson, M.D.

Introduction

The title of this book indicates that adequate management of liver tumors involves more than one individual, including the primary physician who is first approached by the patient, the diagnostician and finally the group of individuals who actually try to treat the disease. To understand the rationale for our aggressive multidisciplinary approach, a basic description of the physiopathology of this disease was included. Clinically an accurate method of staging such as the Percent Hepatic Replacement by tumor or PHR (1, 2) Systems is useful, but with the following modifications:

Stage I   Less than 25% involvement in the liver

Stage Ia   As I but tumor involving major drainage veins in the liver

Stage II   25–75% involvement of liver

Stage IIa   As II but tumor involving major draining veins of the liver

Stage III   More than 75% involvement of the liver

Stage IIIa   As III but tumor involving major draining veins of the liver

Stage IV   Extra-hepatic disease including nodes at porta hepatis.

Poor performance is an important clinical diagnostic factor and is usually associated with Stage III or Stage IV disease. In order to adequately treat the various groups, a range of approaches must be available. The general philosophy of the New York Medical College Liver Group has been to reduce tumor size by resection, embolization and sometimes radiotherapy and then to continue management of the patients by means of intrahepatic chemotherapy, usually given via an Infusaid pump with its catheter directed at the liver or when complications such as chemical hepatitis supervene, or in Stage IV disease, the catheter is directed so that systemic treatment may be given. Also, in patients with more advanced disease where survival is expected to be limited, continuous chemotherapy has been given by means of an external pump.

Louis R.M. Del Guercio, M.D.

REFERENCES

1. Pettaval, J., Leyvraz, S., Douglas, P.: The necessity for staging liver metastases and standardizing treatment response criteria. The case of secondaries of colorectal origin. IN: Van de Velde, C.J.H., and Sugarbaker, P.H. (Eds.), *Liver Metastases.* Amsterdam: Martinus Nijhoff, 1984, pp. 358-367.

2. Taylor, I.: Colorectal liver metastases — to treat or not to treat? *Br J Surg*, 72:511-516, 1985.

Cover photographs used with permission from SGO.

Contents

LIVER TUMORS:
Multidisciplinary Management

NORMAN B. ACKERMAN, M.D., Ph.D.

CHAPTER 1
Liver Tumor Vascularity: Morphology and Dynamics

The vascularity of hepatic tumors is more complicated than most tumors because of the dual blood supply of the liver. In addition to possible contributions of both systems to the vasculature of the tumor, there may be shunting, both arterioportal and arteriovenous, especially in very massive tumors and also after arterial or portal occlusion. The neovasculature which constitutes part of the tumor circulation is often rapidly growing, adapting to the changes in tumor size and to eventual compression.

The study of tumor vascularity has included development, growth and morphology of the vessels, as well as identification of angiogenesis factors. In addition, the histological and ultrastructural appearance of these vessels as compared to normal host vessels has also received attention. Finally, there have been investigations of the responses of tumor vessels to vasoactive chemical and physical changes, particularly in regard to alterations in blood pressure, flow, perfusion and permeability.

Knowledge has been gained from both experimental animal and patient studies. In animals, tumors can be induced by chemical agents or produced by injection of tumor cells via intraportal or intra-arterial injection or by direct introduction into the liver. It has been shown that tumors implanted into the liver by all of these methods develop morphologically similar vasculatures (1). Studies in patients have been performed mostly during the course of diagnostic angiography, but some valuable information has been gained as result of autopsy studies on patients with liver tumors.

VASCULAR MORPHOLOGY

Development of Vascularity

There is evidence that substantial changes occur in the vasculature of tumors as result of development and growth of the tumors. The actual development of neovascularity is initiated as the earliest tumors begin to grow. More advanced, larger tumors cause changes in the tumor vasculature by compression and destruction of the pre–existing liver vessels as well as, perhaps, the tumor vessels themselves. Obliteration may occur as result of direct invasion, particularly of portal vessels, as well as collapse of other vessels as a result of rising interstitial pressure in the tumor.

It is believed that in the earliest stages tumor cells are nourished by diffusion from the surrounding normal liver vessels. Studies have been performed with pigmented silicone rubber (Microfil) injected into arterial and portal circulations in rats with Walker carcinosarcoma tumors implanted in the liver (2). No tumor vascularity was identified in the very earliest implanted tumors, those less than 1 mm in diameter. With early tumor growth, single vessels began to encircle the tumor implants (Figure 1.1) and with further growth multiple vessels became involved. The derivation of these vessels appeared to be either arteriolar or portal, in a random fashion. In some instances both arteriolar and portal vessels contributed to this neovascularity with free mixing of the two circulations (Figure 1.2). With increasing growth of tumors, this encircling plexus became more developed and extensive. While either arteriolar or portal vessels perfused the smallest tumors, eventually the arterial circulation became predominant.

This changing pattern of early tumor vascularity was also identified by angiography in rats with implanted interhepatic Walker tumors (3). No vascularity was evident for the first three days after implantation. By the fourth day, some arteriolar involvement was seen near the implanted tumors. In some tumors, a small encircling vessel was identified as an early phase of neovascularity.

Studies with radioactive tracers have confirmed the presence of both arteriolar and portal circulations in the vicinity of small liver tumors. Injections of radioiodinated human albumin (RISA) into either arterial or portal circulations demonstrated increased radioactivity in the tumors as compared to surrounding circulations (4).

Study of the earliest vascularity in small human tumors has been limited by the difficulty in identifying tumors at this stage. In studies of autopsy specimens some of the liver metastatic tumors were only a few millimeters in diameter (5). There was evidence of portal perfusion in several of these specimens where the primary tumors were from breast, colon or rectum. There is

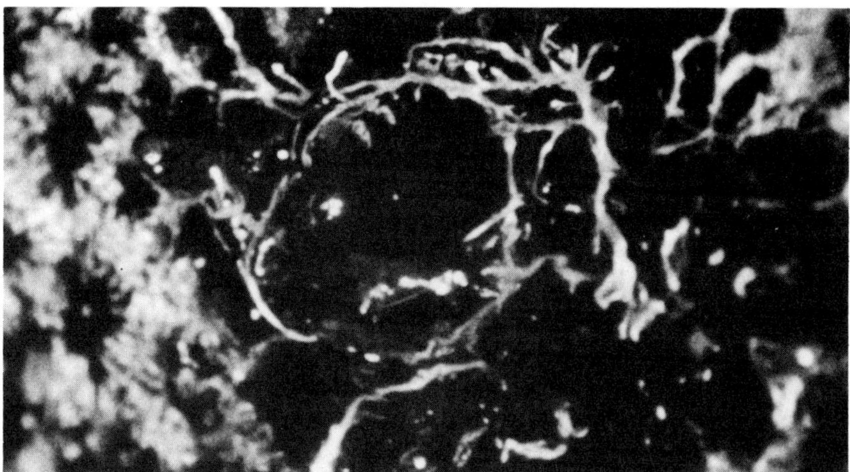

Figure 1.1. Implanted Walker carcinoma in liver of rat studied by perfused Microfil. Encircling vascularity of early tumor (1 mm in diameter) derived from portal circulation.

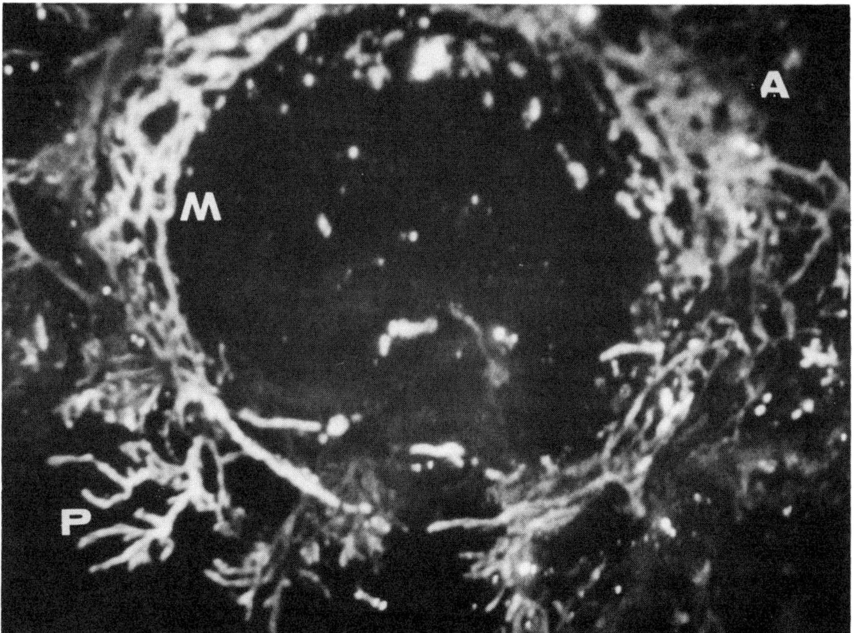

Figure 1.2. Encircling vascularity of early tumor (2 mm in diameter) derived from both arterial and portal circulations. A = arterial, P = portal, M = mixed.

also indirect evidence of the contribution of the portal circulation in small human tumors; chemotherapy delivered into the portal circulation by the umbilical vein appeared to be effective only when administered to very small tumors (6).

Vascularity of Mature Tumors

As the liver tumors grow larger, vascularity eventually becomes well developed. It is at this point that we have labelled the tumors as mature. This is before the tumors begin to outgrow their blood supply and develop avascular or necrotic centers. In experimental animals (rats) these tumors range in diameter from approximately 4 to 10 mm.

There has been considerable study of this type of tumor using injected Microfil into hepatic arterial and portal circulations in rats with intra–hepatic Walker tumors (7). A well developed encircling plexus (EP) was identified around the tumors (Figure 1.3 and 1.4). These vessels were considerably different from the

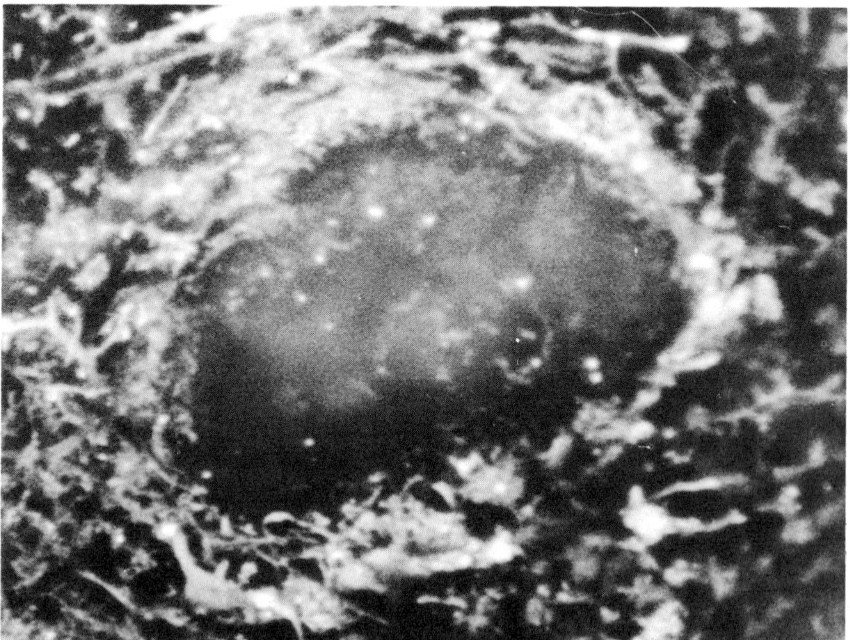

Figure 1.3. Encircling plexus of vessels derived from arterial circulation. (Tumor size 4 x 5 mm.)

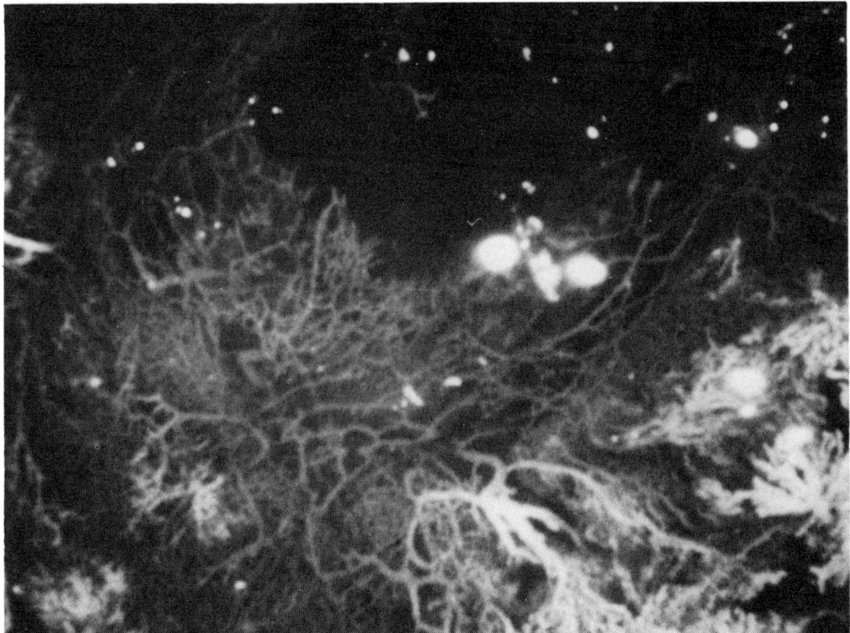

Figure 1.4. Well developed encircling plexus of vessels derived from arterial circulation. (Tumor 4 mm in diameter.)

sinusoid vasculature of the surrounding liver. The EP was perfused mostly by arterial circulation, but randomly there was a minor portal component to the circulation. This was sometimes observed in one small area of the EP. Usually, portal vessels were compressed or displaced by the tumor. The vessels of the EP were irregular in diameter and markedly tortuous and convoluted. The central portions of the tumors were usually avascular but occasionally there were a few small, irregular vessels perfused via the arterial circulation. Other investigators using colored gelatin solutins injected into the arterial and portal circulation have reported similar findings (8).

In the same type of animal preparation angiographic studies have demonstrated new vessel formation surrounding the tumors (3). These vessels were described as tortuous, with areas of dilatation, and irregular with a totally bizarre arrangement. In some specimens pooling of the contrast material was noted.

Experiments on the circulation in rabbits with VX2 carcinomas implanted in the livers have confirmed the predominantly arterial source of tumor perfusion (5). This was also seen on angiographic studies in these animals.

In humans, studies on autopsy specimens have shown a predominance of arterial perfusion in these mature tumors similar to that seen in the animal studies (5). This was also seen in studies on livers with metastatic tumors where vinyl acetate was injected into the circulation (9). In this technique only relatively large vessels can be identified. Either relatively normal arterial architecture or avascularity was seen, and there was a total absence of portal vascularity in these tumors.

Arteriography has been the major technique for the investigation of tumor vascularity in patients. With experience, it has been learned that the major branches of hepatic artery may arise from other than the usual source. The right hepatic artery originates from the superior mesenteric artery in about 16% of patients and the left hepatic artery arises from the left gastric artery in about 18%.

When human liver tumors are relatively vascular, the vessels are generally irregular with localized areas of both saccular and fusiform dilatation. There is a tendency toward disorganization and randomized branching. The vessels do not taper as normal vessels do. Within the tumors themselves, contrast material may form small collections of pooled material. As multiple x-rays are taken, it is noted that circulation through the tumor is slower than in surrounding liver and there is a tendency toward retention of contrast material within the tumor after the surrounding liver vessels have been emptied. During the capillary phase of angiography, a tumor blush is often seen. Because of abnormal arteriovenous shunting there may be earlier venous filling at the same time. Finally, surrounding hepatic vessels may be stretched as the tumor grows or they may be narrowed and obstructed. In more avascular tumors, the stretching and compression of the surrounding arterial circulation may be the major findings indicating the presence of tumors. Further on, when the portal-hepatogram phase is present in the normal liver, a radiolucent defect may be present in the area of the tumor.

There is a great variability in the degree of vascularity of intrahepatic tumors in patients. Some generalizations may be helpful. Primary hepatomas usually are relatively vascular. Metastatic tumors show more variation. Renal cell carcinomas, leiomyosarcomas, carcinoid tumors, islet cell and papillary cell tumors of the pancreas and transitional cell tumors generally tend to be more hypervascular. In contrast, adenocarcinomas of the stomach, pancreas, breast and adrenal, as well as tumors of the lungs and melanomas are usually relatively avascular.

Changes in Vascularity of Massive Tumors

There is good experimental evidence that significant changes in vascularity occur as tumors continue to grow to more massive dimensions. These changes were identifiable in Walker tumors implanted in the livers of rats studied by Microfil perfusion (2). In tumors as large as 33 x 33 mm in size, vascularity was generally significantly decreased. In these tumors, a great diversity of patterns was seen. Some of these extensive tumors appeared to have little or no arterial circulation and portal vascularity around the tumors varied from sparse to fairly dense (Figure 1.5). With other tumors, the arterial circulation remained well developed. In some, there was a mixture of arterial and portal elements (Figure 1.6). With most of these tumors there were areas that were relatively

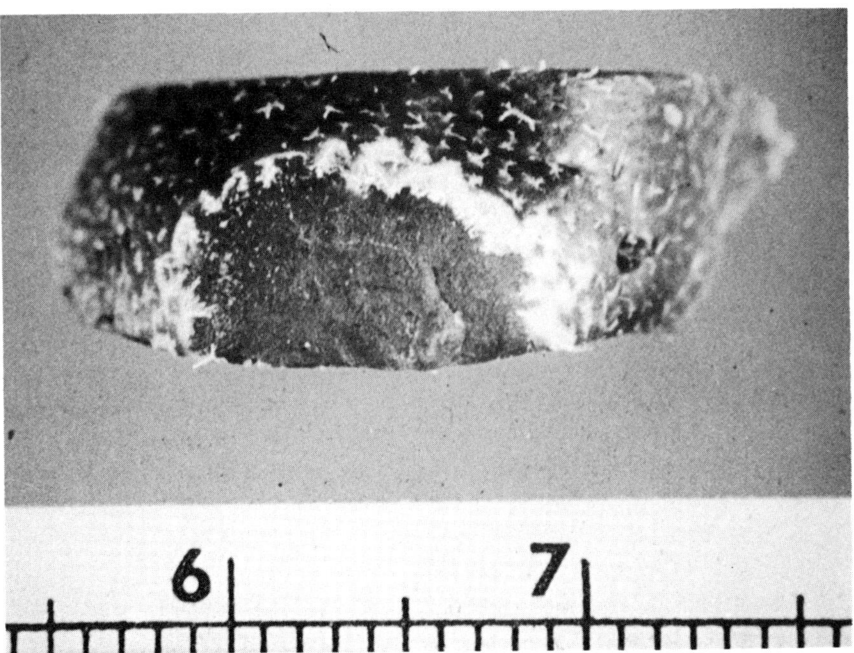

Figure 1.5. Plexus of vessels derived from portal circulation surrounding massive sized tumor. (Tumor size 12 x 13 mm.)

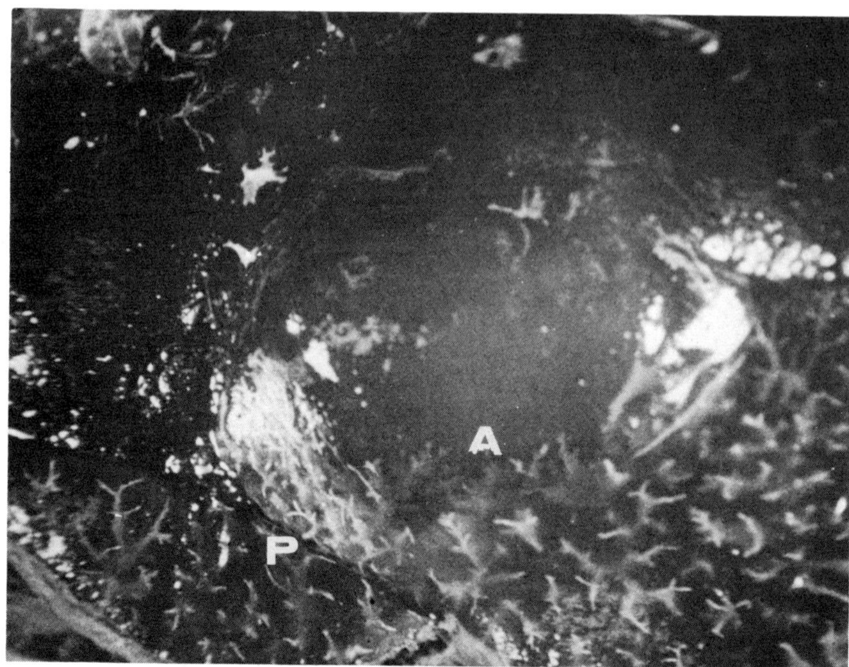

Figure 1.6. Sparse vascularity of both arterial and portal derivation surrounding massive sized tumor. (Tumor size 17 x 17 mm.) A = arterial, P = portal.

avascular, particularly in the centers. One could infer that as growth continued to a massive size, invasion, destruction and displacement of vessels occurred. While some new vessels continued to develop, the destructive aspects of growth seemed to predominate. As will be discussed later, some of these avascular areas may consist of collapsed vessels that are not well perfused under ordinary circumstances.

In angiographic studies on experimental animals, decreased vascularity was also noted as the tumors became massive (3). The angiographic pattern became more confused, and the vascularity seen with small tumors was absent. Vascular patterns indicating adhesions between peritoneum and tumors were seen.

Although there have been few human studies documenting the changes in circulation in larger liver tumors, excessively large human liver tumors are often described as avascular on angiography.

VASCULAR DYNAMICS

Perfusion and Flow

Perfusion and blood flow of vessels feeding liver tumors have been studied in several experimental laboratories using radio active tracers. In rats with Walker tumors implanted in the livers, distribution of radioactivity was measured after injection of radioiodinated human serum albumin (RISA) in either portal or arterial circulations (4). Significantly greater quantities of radioactivity were measured in the tumor as compared to that in the surrounding liver after arterial injection. This suggested that arterial perfusion of the tumor was greater than arterial perfusion of the liver. After portal injection, equivalent amounts of radioactivity were found in the tumors and liver. This may reflect the shunting of portal blood into the arterially perfused tumor plexus. In similar animal preparations distribution of radioactivity was measured after injection of yttrium–90 tagged microspheres measuring less than 55 microns in diameter into either arterial or portal circulations. After arterial injection, radioactivity was greater in the tumor than in the surrounding liver indicating an increase in arteriolar sized vessels in and around the tumor. After intraportal injection of these microspheres, there was a decreased radioactivity in the tumors compared to the livers indicating less perfusion of portal venules in and around the tumors.

Other investigators have found similar results in studies on Walker tumors in rats (10) and in liver implants in rabbits (11) after intra–arterial injections of tagged microspheres 15 microns in diameter. Tumor radioactivity after portal injection was low but some radioactivity was detected in these tumors. There have been some studies on similar preparations that have suggested that tumor flow was not any greater than in the surrounding liver (12). Findings may be different depending on the specific type of tumor. Greater blood flow may occur in smaller tumors. The greatest blood flow probably occurs in the periphery of the tumor rather than in the center.

There have been few studies on tumor blood flow in human livers. In one study where liver blood flow was investigated by use of colloidal radioiodinated human albumin and hepatic vein catheterization, flow through normal liver was unaffected. However, total hepatic blood flow was increased, presumably due to an increased flow through the tumors. It was speculated that increased shunting between arterial and venous circulations in the areas of the tumors could account for the increase in flow.

There is still much confusion about the relationship of vascularity and blood flow in these intrahepatic tumors. While some tumors may appear to have an extensive blood supply, actual tumor blood flow may be relatively slow. Factors such as pressure and red cell velocity have not been measured. Differences in flow in various parts of tumors are probably significant and add to the confusion. More specifically, it is felt that blood flow to the central parts of tumors is probably decreased as compared to that in the periphery. The degree of shunting is another complicating factor. There also may be differences in both vascularity and blood flow in different types of metastatic and primary tumors in the liver. Obviously, additional study is needed to clarify these points. A better understanding of these relationships would aid in the design of more effective intravascular chemotherapy.

Effects of Hepatic Artery Ligation

Interest in studying the effect of hepatic artery ligation stems from the fact that in most instances, the arterial system is the predominant source of vascularity of intrahepatic tumors. Considerable experimental and clinical studies have attempted to determine whether arterial ligation alone or in conjunction with other therapeutic measures might have a beneficial effect on reducing viability and growth of these tumors. In very early experimental studies, dye injected into the portal system after hepatic artery ligation was identified only in the liver surrounding the tumors but not within the tumors themselves (13).

More recent qualitative and quantitative studies have shown that flow of blood between the two circulations may occur after vessels are ligated (7, 14). With injection of RISA into the portal system after acute hepatic artery ligation, perfusion of the tumor appeared to decrease below control levels. This result was in conflict with studies where Microfil was injected intraportally in the same tumors after hepatic artery ligation (7). In these latter studies filling of the encircling plexus (EP) of the tumors via portal vein injection occurred in half the studies (Figure 1.7). There has not been total resolution of these conflicting data but experimental design and timing may be important factors. It does appear that the portal system may be able to assume an important role in the nourishment of tumors after hepatic artery ligation in some

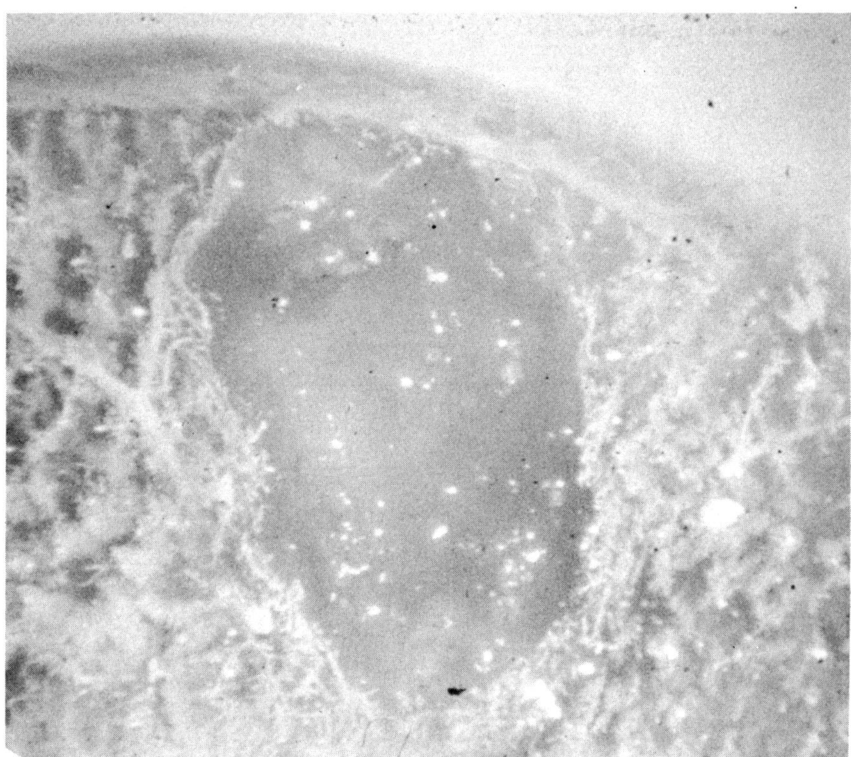

Figure 1.7. Encircling plexus of tumors (5 x 7 mm) filled by portal perfusion after acute ligation of hepatic artery.

instances. It is of interest that shunting from the portal circulation into the arterial does not usually occur in the normal liver although shunting from the arterial to the portal circulation does occur.

By four days after hepatic artery ligation, some changes in vascular dynamics occurred (14). Perfusion with RISA via the portal circulation returned to normal. This may be related to hemodynamic changes occurring as a result of development of collateral arterial circulation. It is known that collateral circulation develops rapidly even in humans.

Some experimental studies have measured survival time of rats with liver tumors after hepatic artery ligation. In one study, tumor growth was slowed at first and in some instances, necrosis appeared to occur in the tumors (15). However, after several days new tumor growth was noted around the necrotic area. With several different types of experimental tumors, survival time doubled. Results from other laboratories have been less impressive. When the hepatic artery was ligated at the time of tumor implantation, tumors appeared to grow normally. Sufficient arterial collaterals developed so that vascularity appeared normal at three and seven days after implantation. When arterial ligation was carried out acutely on the third or fourth day after implantation, arterial flow to the EP or to the internal tumor circulation (ITC) was deficient. Growth, however, was not affected since portal perfusion of the tumors was seen at three days, and arterial collateral flow from adhesions and other sources was seen at seven days. Thus, the effect of acute hepatic artery ligation in experimental animals appeared transient at best in most studies.

Hepatic artery ligation, with or without additional chemotherapy, has been used in patients to decrease tumor growth. In some of these operative procedures, blood flow in normal liver and in tumors was measured after intrahepatic injection of radioactive xenon–133 (16). Blood flow was calculated from the disappearance rate of the isotope. Liver blood flow was acutely decreased after hepatic artery ligation to 66% of controls and tumor blood flow decreased to 8% of controls. Others have verified these results reporting a decrease in arterial perfusion in tumors to 5% of control values (17). In similar studies, portal perfusion of liver tumors increased after hepatic artery ligation.

The development of collateral arterial circulation of the liver has been studied in patients after hepatic artery ligation. In some patients total dearterialization was performed, which included division of the falciform ligament and all attachments between the liver and surrounding tissues except for the common bile duct, portal vein, hepatic veins, and vena cava (18). These investigators identified collateral arterial flow by four days. Hepatic arterial vessels were filled by collaterals from the pancreaticoduodenal, phrenicoabdominal and intercostal arteries. These findings in patients were similar to those in animals and the conclusion was that hepatic artery ligation has only a short term effect.

Effect of Portal Vein Ligation

The effect of portal vein ligation on intrahepatic tumors has received less attention because of the relatively small role played by the portal system in tumor nutrition. There have been some experimental studies where the portal branch leading to the lobe with a Walker tumor implant was ligated (19). Atrophy of the hepatic lobe generally developed and in about one third of animals, the tumor implant appeared to regress. If in addition to portal vein ligation, the artery and bile duct of the involved lobe were also ligated, 73% of animals survived with infarction of the hepatic lobe and elimination of the tumor. In experiments where the portal circulation alone was ligated and regression of tumors resulted, it was postulated that arterial inflow may also have decreased (20).

With RISA injected into the arterial system after acute portal ligation in animals with intrahepatic Walker tumors, measured arterial perfusion of the tumors dropped significantly. Shunting of arterial blood away from the tumor to the liver could be due to increased flow into the normal hepatic arterial circulation or into the intrahepatic portal circulation. These shunts were relatively small, less than 55 microns in diameter, since the distribution of microspheres of this size after portal ligation was unaffected.

There have been some patients treated by ligation of a branch of the portal system (21, 22). Care was taken to spare the circulation to at least one hepatic lobe, and morbidity and mortality were reported as minimal. This was used for both primary and metastatic liver tumors and reports of palliation were documented. Atrophy of the ligated lobe including the malignant tissue occurred and compensatory hypertrophy of the remaining lobes resulted.

Effects of Vasoactive Drugs

Certain vasoactive drugs have been used in attempts to alter the dynamics of tumor circulation. In part, this has been directed toward improving visualization of liver tumors by angiography. The possiblity of improving delivery of antineoplastic drugs to liver tumors by use of vasoactive drugs has also been a major goal.

In preliminary studies on rats with intrahepatic Walker tumors, penetration of lissamine green dye into the central portions of the tumors occurred after administration of epinephrine. Confirmatory studies were performed with injection of pigmented silicone rubber (Microfil) into arterial and portal circulations. Epinephrine, in doses of 10 and 100 μg, administered intra-arterially immediately before administration of Microfil caused an increased perfusion of vessels in the encircling plexus. In addition, a very dramatic increase in vascularity was noted in the central portions of the tumors which are usually considered as avascular (Figure 1.8) (23). Similar findings were seen after injections of epinephrine into the portal system. This suggested that epinephrine penetrated into the arterial circulation by the portal route. Intra-arterial epinephrine also increased vascularity of very large, massive sized tumors averaging 14 x 18 mm in size (Figure 1.9). Without epinephrine, these large tumors had variable vascularity with virtually no perfusion of central areas. With epinephrine, these tumors appeared to have a well developed circulation. The dense central network of vessels seen after epinephrine administration consisted of small, irregular, capillary sized vessels measuring six to eight microns in diameter. In some of the larger tumor specimens, a small central avascular area was present and in some there was a large structureless area of silicone rubber present. These "lakes" of silicone rubber may have represented areas of actual necrosis.

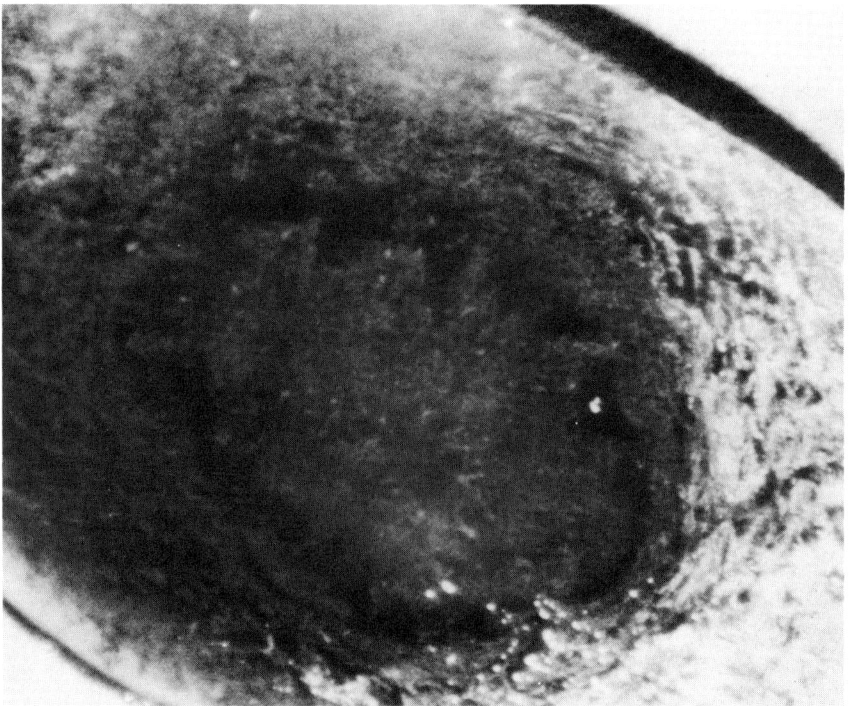

Figure 1.8. Increased arterial vascularity of central portion of tumor after intra-arterial administration of epinephrine. (Tumor size 6 x 9 mm.)

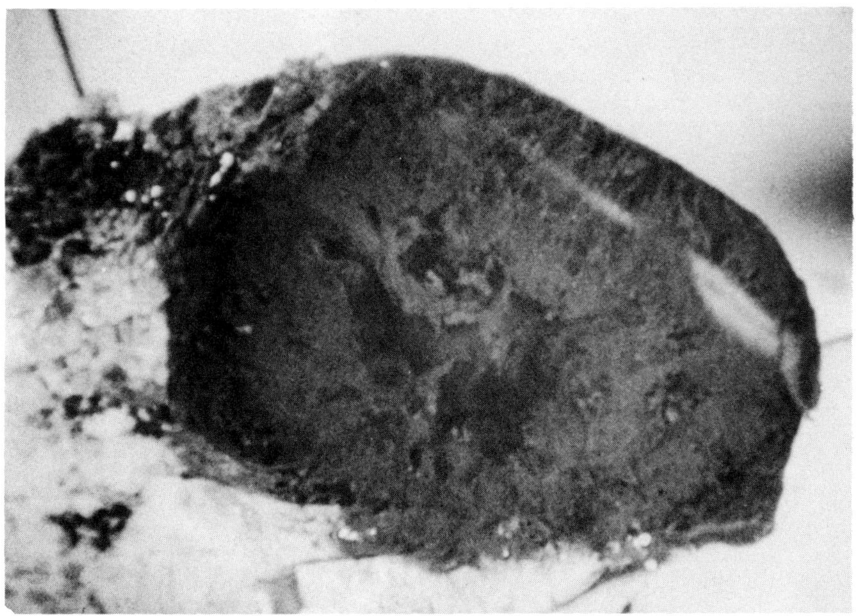

Figure 1.9. Increased arterial vascularity of central portion of massive sized tumor after intra-arterial administration of epinephrine. (Tumor size 16 x 23 mm.) Compare with Figures 1.5 and 1.6.

The exact mechanism produced by epinephrine is not totally understood. The appearance of increased vascularity in the tumor was not affected by prior administration of propranolol, but phenoxybenzamine did appear to block this effect. Additional study will be necessary to understand fully the physiological changes occurring with epinephrine. Although alterations in blood pressure and flow may occur, these have not been specifically measured. Similarly, decreases in arterioportal shunting around the tumor resulting in an increased internal flow, while possible, have not been studied. The possibility of an acute decrease in interstitial pressure resulting in less external compression of pre-existing central vessels will also have to be studied.

Similar increases in vascularity with epinephrine have been found in studies on induced liver tumors in rats (Figure 1.10). Other studies have been more variable. Differences may be due to types of investigative techniques, specific tumors used, time relationships, and dose ranges of the drugs. Experiments on VX2 carcinomas in the liver of rabbits showed, with epinephrine, an in-

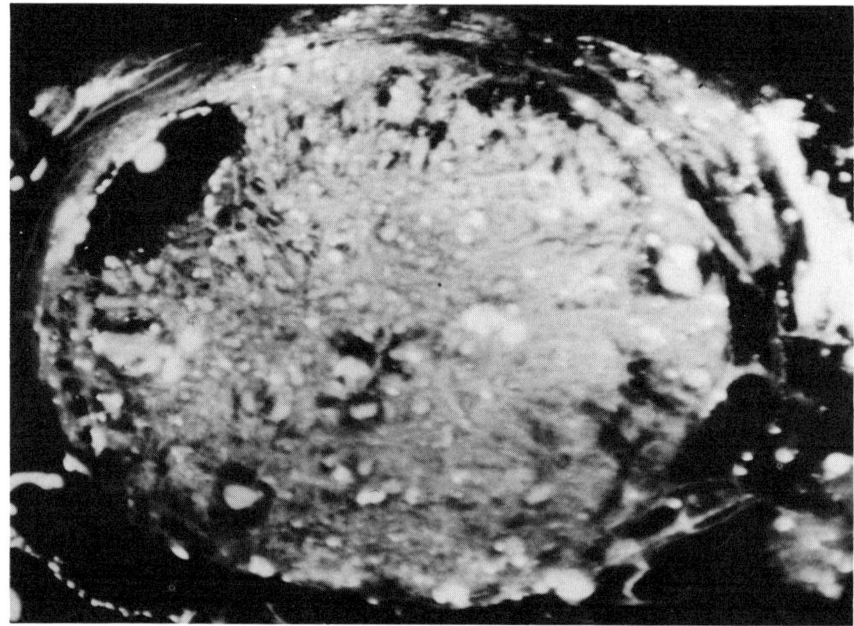

Figure 1.10. Liver tumor induced with 1% orotic acid, cholesterol and cholic acid. Increased arterial vascularity of central portion of tumor after intra-arterial administration of epihephrine. (Tumor size 9 x 10 mm.)

creased opacification of the tumors on arteriography (24). In these same studies, however, administration of mitomycin C through the hepatic arterial system after infusion of epinephrine did not result in an increase of drug in the liver tumors although the concentration of mytomycin C in the liver was decreased. In other studies, no increase in perfusion was seen in adenocarcinomas in the livers of rats after epinephrine, but the doses of epinephrine were relatively low (25).

To summarize the effect of epinephrine in experimental animals with liver tumors, there have been some promising studies demonstrating an increased vascularity of tumors as result of the vasoactive drug, but results have not been uniform in all studies and in all tumors investigated. Possible mechanisms involved are still speculative and further study is necessary.

Epinephrine has been used in patients during hepatic angiography in order to improve the diagnosis of suspected liver tumors (26). As result of the epinephrine, there was an intense vasoconstriction of the liver for about 15 seconds and then gradually a hyperemia occurred with an increased diameter of arteries, an increase in flow and a greater opacification of the veins. Vessels leading to the tumors appeared to be less responsive. However, relatively vascular tumors were more easily diagnosed because of an increased blood flow and opacification. Relatively avascular tumors may be less easily identified after epinephrine. In the experience of some radiologists, improvement in diagnostic accuracy occurred in 45% of patients with the use of epinephrine.

There have been some experiments with other vasoactive drugs. Several studies with norepinephrine in both rabbits and rats using radioactive tracers indicated a decrease in tumor perfusion (10). In other studies using a different tumor line, blood flow appeared to increase in the tumors with norepinephrine (25). Angiographic studies with norepinephrine in experimental animals have also given contradictory results. With Microfil perfused intra-arterially after norepinephrine, central vascularity of the tumors appeared to be markedly decreased (Figure 1.11) (27). Norepinephrine is probably less promising than epinephrine as a means of

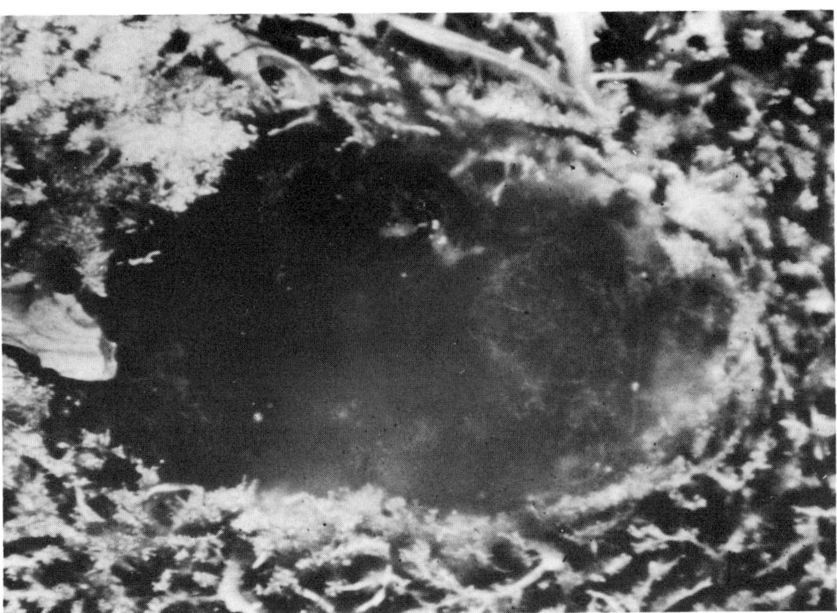

Figure 1.11. Decreased vascularity of tumor after intra-arterial administration of norepinephrine. (Tumor size 4 x 7 mm.)

increasing tumor vascularity, although additional studies with a
full dose range should be performed.

Other vasoactive drugs have been studied in experiments with
intra–arterial Microfil perfusion. Varying degrees of changes in perfusion were noted, but these appeared to be unrelated to effects of
vasoconstriction or vasodilatation per se (28). However, all of
these drugs have various other effects on the circulation including
changes in cardiac output, blood pressure, resistance and flow. The
greatest increase in tumor vascularity was seen with epinephrine.

With some of these drugs, attempts have been made to
improve diagnostic accuracy of hepatic angiography. However,
results have similarly been inconsistent and there can be few conclusions from these studies.

Effects of Physical Changes

Except for the responses to the extremes of temperature,
there have been few studies on the effects of changing physical
conditions on liver tumor vascularity. In studies with Microfil
perfusion, tumor vascularity appeared to decrease markedly when
tumors were cooled to 5° C (29). In contrast, freezing with liquid
nitrogen followed by thawing produced major increases in vascularity, both in the encircling plexus and internal circulation
(Figure 1.12). These specimens appeared similar in vascularity to
those observed after administration of epinephrine. No changes
were seen in tumor vascularity following low grade hyperthermia.
Studies on other tumor systems have indicated that vascular occlusion occurs in tumors when hyperthermia reaches levels of 43.5° C
(30).

Physical changes following bile duct ligation, heparinization,
or administration of hypertonic glucose do not appear to affect
tumor vascularity, in studies using Microfil perfusion. Apparent
small increases in vascularity were seen as a result of partial occlusion of hepatic outflow and of hepatic lymph vessel ligation.

Changes in Vascular Permeability

There is evidence that newly formed tumor vessels are more
permeable than vessels in most normal organs. The tumor vessels
appear to lack a definite smooth muscle layer and have only an
endothelial lining. Electron microscope studies indicate that the
endothelial cell lining in some tumor vessels is defective. Fenestra-

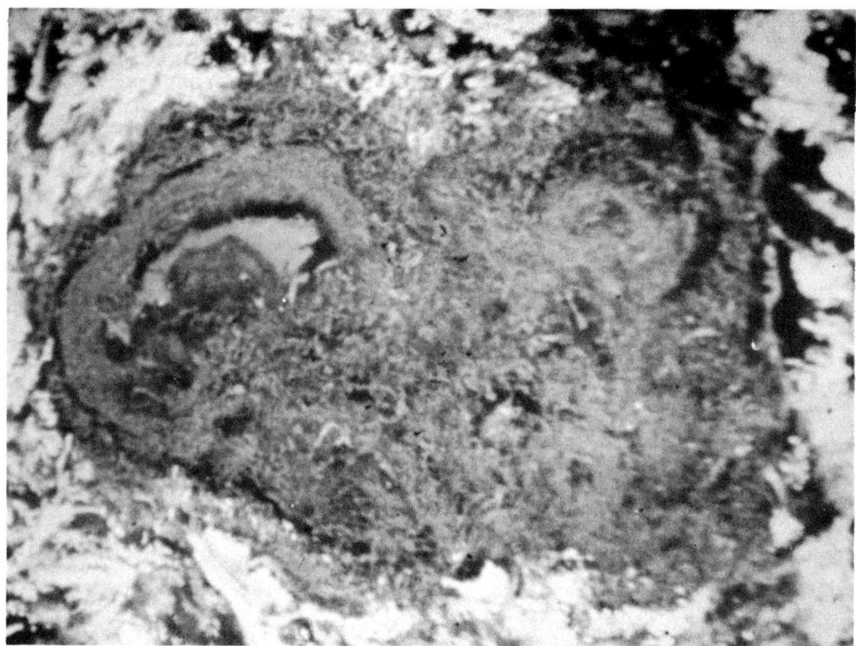

Figure 1.12. Increased arterial vascularity of central portion of tumor after freezing with liquid nitrogen and thawing. (Tumor size 4 x 6 mm.)

tions are present and appear similar to those seen in the wall of vessels with high levels of transport such as in intestinal villi, endocrine organs and kidneys, as well as inflamed tissues. There is also an absence of nerve fibers in these tumor vessels. Although the structural deficiencies would explain increases in permeability, there is also some evidence of permeability promoting factors elaborated by the tumors themselves.

Quantitative measurements of permeability have been performed with various test substances. Studies on implanted Walker carcinosarcomas in the liver were carried out measuring vascular permeability by the extraction of administered Evans blue. The extracted dye is then measured spectrophotometrically. During the first five minutes after injection of the dye, there was less Evans blue recovered from the tumors than from the normal liver (31). This may actually have reflected a slower blood flow and distribution of dye in the tumors than in the normal liver rather than decreased vascular permeability. Between 15 and 60 minutes after administration of Evans blue, concentration of dye was equal in liver and in tumors. However, from two hours to 72 hours after dye administration measured permeability was significantly higher in the tumor. At 18 hours the recovery of dye in the tumor was at a maximum. At 6 to 18 hours the greatest difference in permeability between the two tissues was seen.

These findings may be important since an increase in passage of diagnostic and therapeutic agents into the tumors may depend on the increased tumor vessel permeability. Attempts to increase tumor vessel permeability further have been made with the use of various chemical agents and changing physical conditions. Histamine type mediators, including histamine, bradykinin and serotonin are known to have a direct effect on blood vessels, increasing permeability rapidly but for only a relatively short period of time. This effect occurs predominantly in the post–capillary venules and is due to direct action on the endothelial lining. The endothelial cells contract producing increased intercellular gaps. When these drugs were administered to experimental animals with Walker carcinosarcoma tumors in the liver permeability increased, as expected, in the normal liver. Tumor vessels, however, did not respond with an increase in permeability, and in some instances actually decreased (32). This decrease may have been due to other vasoactive effects of the drugs. It is possible that fenestrations may be maximally spread in these tumor vessels and may not respond further to histamine.

Thus far, no drugs tested have caused an increase in permeability in the tumor vessels. On the other hand, various anti–inflammatory drugs including antagonists to histamine and serotonin have caused a decrease in tumor vessel permeability (33). Similarly, steroids and non–steroidal anti–inflammatory drugs have also decreased tumor vessel permeability. These drugs included indomethacin, phenylbutazone, ibuprofen, and naproxan.

Tumor vessel permeability was increased by other means. Significant increases in the tumors were produced by reactive hyperemia (32). This was produced by clamping the aorta above the celiac artery for two minutes and then releasing. This was a relatively short lasting increase, apparent at five minutes after unclamping but not at 30 minutes or 6 hours. This effect may be either directly on permeability or may be related to an increase in tumor blood flow.

Changes in temperature also had a major effect on vascular permeability of intrahepatic tumors. After freezing the tumors with liquid nitrogen and rapid thawing, marked increases of permeability occurred (30). This effect was produced rapidly and persisted for as long as 24 hours after freezing and thawing. The freezing and thawing probably produced direct damage to the endothelial lining of the vessels. Electron microscopic studies of vessels after freezing have demonstrated injury to cellular membranes, endothelial cell swelling and destruction, as well as enlargement of the endothelial gaps.

Recent interest in the therapeutic effects of extreme hyperthermia prompted study of vascular changes during these treatments. Intrahepatic tumor vessel permeability was studied with the Evans blue technique. Increased temperatures to $40°$ C appeared to have no effect on vascular permeability in the tumors (34). However, at $43°$ C marked increases in permeability occurred in the tumor vessels, and was apparent at both 30 minutes and 6 hours after heating. This is of some significance since $40°$ C is not an effective dose therapeutically, but $43°$ C is well within the therapeutic range. It has been speculated that an increase in permeability associated with the development of vascular stasis and ultimate cessation of flow to the tumors may be partly responsible for the favorable therapeutic effect of hyperthermia.

IMPORTANCE OF LIVER TUMOR VASCULARITY
IN THERAPY

Several established and experimental therapeutic techniques have been devised that depend directly on tumor vascularity. These techniques have included regional therapy to the liver by hepatic artery infusion and hepatic artery ligation or dearterialization. The possibility of combining ligation of the hepatic artery with later liver resection has also been proposed. More recently, ligation of the hepatic artery with simultaneous infusion of tumor therapy distal to the ligation has been described. Attempts to decrease arterial feeding of these tumors by embolization are still being studied. There have also been some attempts to irradiate the liver tumor by injection of radioactive particles via the hepatic artery. Finally, administration of chemotherapy by the portal system or via the obliterated umbilical vein has been described. Future techniques may include better control of perfusion by vasoactive drugs (35) and changing physical conditions and better delivery of antineoplastic agents to the tumor by altering vascular permeability.

REFERENCES

1. Burgener, FA, and Violante, MR: Comparison of hepatic VX2-carcinomas after intra-arterial, intraportal and intraparenchymal tumor cell injection. An angiographic and computed tomographic study in the rabbit. *Invest Radiol, 14:*410-414, 1979.

2. Ackerman, NB: The blood supply of experimental liver metastases. IV. Changes in vascularity with increasing tumor growth. *Surgery, 75:*589-596, 1974.

3. Kido, C: Hepatic angiography of experimental transplantable tumor. *Invest Radiol, 5:*341-347, 1970.

4. Ackerman, NB, Lien, WM, Kondi, ES, and Silverman, NA: The blood supply of experimental liver metastases, I. The distribution of hepatic artery and portal vein blood to "small" and "large" tumors. *Surgery, 66:*1067-1072, 1969.

5. Breedis, C, and Young, G: The blood supply of neoplasms in the liver. *Am J Path, 30:*969-985, 1954.

6. Kessler, RE and Ramos-Yordan, F: Evaluation of anticancer drugs by umbilical vein hepatography. *Cancer, 20:*319-322, 1967.

7. Lien, WM and Ackerman, NB: The blood supply of experimental liver metastases. II. A microcirculatory study of the normal and tumor vessels of the liver with the use of perfused silicone rubber. *Surgery, 68:*334-340, 1970.

8. Honjo, I, and Matsumura, H: Vascular distribution of hepatic tumors. Experimental study. *Rev Internat Hepatol, 15:*681-690, 1965.

9. Healey, JE, Jr.: Vascular patterns in human metastatic liver tumors. *Surg Gynec & Obstet, 120:*1187-1193, 1965.

10. Young, SW, *et al.*: Resting host and tumor perfusion as determinants of tumor vascular responses to norepinephrine. *Cancer Res, 39:*1898-1903, 1979.

11. Blanchard, RJW, *et al.*: Blood supply to hepatic VX2 carcinoma implants as measured by radioactive microspheres. *Proc Soc Exp Biol Med, 118:*465-468, 1965.

12. Lundqvist, K, Hafstrom, L, and Persson, B: Management of total and regional tumor blood flow and organ blood flow using 99Tc^{m} labelled microspheres. *Europ Surg Res, 10:*433-443, 1978.

13. Fisher, B, Fisher, ER, and Lee, SH: The effect of alteration of liver blood flow upon experimental hepatic metastases. *Surg Gynec & Obstet, 112:*11-18, 1961.

14. Ackerman, NB; Lien, WM, and Silverman, NA: The blood supply of experimental liver metastases. III. The effects of acute ligation of the hepatic artery or portal vein. *Surgery, 71:*636-641, 1972.

15. Nilsson, LAV: Therapeutic hepatic artery ligation in patients with secondary liver tumors. *Rev Surg, 23:*374-376, 1966.

16. Gelin, LE, Lewis, DH, and Nilsson, L: Liver blood flow in man during abdominal surgery. II. The effect of hepatic artery occlusion on the blood flow through metastatic tumor nodules. *Acta Hepatosplen, 15:*21-24, 1968.

17. Taylor, I, Bennett, R, and Sherriff, S: The blood supply of colorectal liver metastases. *Brit J Cancer, 39:*749-756, 1979.

18. Bengmark, S, and Rosengren, K: Angiographic study of the collateral circulation to the liver after ligation of the hepatic artery in man. *Am J Surg, 119:*620-624, 1970.

19. Kraus, GE, and Beltran, A: Effect of induced infarction on rat liver implanted with Walker carcinoma 256. *Arch Surg, 79:*769-774, 1959.

20. Honjo, I, *et al.*: Evaluation of ligation of a branch of the portal vein for unresectable hepatic tumor. *Bull Soc Internat Chir, 3:*207-210, 1974.

21. Honjo, I, *et al.*: Ligation of a branch of the portal vein for carcinoma of the liver. *Am J Surg, 130:*296-302, 1975.

22. Yoshida, K, *et al.*: Portal branch ligation as a palliative procedure for unresectable hepatoma. *Chir Gastroent, 11:*343-345, 1977.

23. Ackerman, NB, and Hechmer, PA: The blood supply of experimental liver metastases. V. Increased tumor perfusion with epinephrine. *Am J Surg, 140:*625-631, 1980.

24. Iwaki, A, *et al.*: Intra-arterial chemotherapy with comcomitant use of vasoconstrictors for liver cancer. *Cancer Treatment Rep, 62:*145-146, 1878.

25. Hafstrom, L, *et al.*: Effects of catecholamines on cardiovascular response and blood flow distribution to normal tissue and liver tumors in rats. *Cancer Res, 40:*481-485, 1980.

26. Kahn, PC, Frates, WJ, and Paul, RE, Jr.: The epinephrine effect in angiography of gastrointestinal tract tumors. *Radiol, 88:*686-690, 1967.

27. Ackerman, NB: Experimental studies on the circulatory dynamics of intrahepatic tumor blood supply. *Cancer, 29:*435-439, 1972.

28. Ackerman, NB, Hechmer, PA, and Makahon, S: The blood supply of experimental liver metastases. VI. Comparison of the effects of epinephrine and other catecholamines on tumor vascularity. *Microcirculation 2:*111-125, 1982.

29. Ackerman, NB and Makohon, S: The effects of cooling, freezing and thawing on vascular permeability and perfusion in experimental liver metastases. *Surg Gynec & Obstet, 152:*262-267, 1981.

30. Kang, MS, Song, CW, and Levitt, SH: Role of vascular function in response of tumors in vivo to hyperthermia. *Cancer Res, 40:*1130-1135, 1980.

31. Ackerman, NB, and Hechmer, PA: Studies on the capillary permeability of experimental liver metastases. *Surg Gynec & Obstet, 146:*884-888, 1978.

32. Ackerman, NB, Hechmer, PA, and Makohon, S: Failure of histamin-type mediators to enhance vascular permeability in experimental liver metastases. *Surg Gynec & Obstet, 151:*647-651, 1980.

33. Ackerman, NB, and Makohon, S: The effects of steroidal and non-steroidal anti-inflammatory agents on vascular permeability in intrahepatic tumors. *Internat J Microcirc, 1:*254, 1982.

34. LeFor, AT, Makohon, S, and Ackerman, NB: The effects of hyperthermia on vascular permeability in experimental liver metastases. *J Surg Oncology,* *28:*279–300, 1985.

35. Peterson, HI, Altsten, M, Skolnik, G, and Karlsson, L: Influence of a prostaglandin synthesis inhibitor and of thrombocytopenia on tumor blood flow and tumor vascular permeability. Experimental studies in the rat. *Anticancer Res,* *5:*253–257, 1985.

FADI F. ATTIYEH, M.D.

CHAPTER 2
Early Detection
in Asymptomatic Patients

Liver involvement by neoplastic lesions, whether primary or secondary, has until recently been considered incurable, and that nothing could be done to alter the rapidly fatal outcome in such patients. Unfortunately, many physicians, including surgeons, still ascribe to the defeatest notions that aggressive efforts at treating liver tumors are an exercise in futility. Several reports in the literature (2, 4, 9, 10, 33) clearly demonstrate that long–term survival, and definite cures, are achievable with surgical resections of primary or metastatic liver tumors. The purpose of this chapter is not to review the details of those studies, but rather to outline methods for early detection in populations at high risk, and the current methods of follow--up, especially in patients with colo-rectal cancer, in the hope of detecting small, and preferably solitary liver tumors that have the best chance of being cured with surgery.

INCIDENCE

Primary liver malignancies are rare, and hepatomas constitute the majority of such tumors, the rest being cholangiocarcinomas, angiosarcomas, etc. It is estimated that in 1986 (26), there will be 13,600 new cases of cancers of the liver and biliary passages in the United States alone, an incidence of 1.5% of all cancers. However, in Africa and parts of Asia, the incidence of primary liver cancer is much increased to about 20% of all cancers (26).

Secondary liver malignancies, on the other hand, constitute the majority of hepatic neoplasms. These are a common occurrence in a major proportion of patients with neoplastic diseases; about 50% of patients who die from cancer have metastases to the liver, and the commonest cancers causing liver metastasis are adenocarcinomas of the alimentary tract, primarily the large bowel.

Of the 140,000 estimated new cases of adenocarcinoma of the colon and rectum in the U.S. in 1986, roughly 50% will develop recurrence or metastases, and about half of these will have hepatic metastases either as a single organ involvement, or part of widespread disease. About 15–20% of patients with liver metastases are resectable and the rest have bilobar disease, or extrahepatic metastases.

A relatively small number of patients with either primary or secondary hepatic tumors are suitable for surgical resection with the potential for cure. The vast majority of patients with liver tumors on the other hand, being unresectable, are treated by an ever–evolving variety of methods, both surgical and medical. These approaches will be covered in detail in other chapters of this book.

TUMOR MARKERS

Primary Liver Tumors

Screening for primary tumors of the liver is rather difficult because they are uncommon and usually asymptomatic, at least in the early stages of disease. However, there are some efforts being directed towards the screening of patients at high risk, such as those who are HBsAg positive and patients with some forms of cirrhosis, especially the macronodular variety (11).

Hsu, *et al.* (16), Blumberg, and London (7), and Beasley, *et al.* (5), have demonstrated a strong association between persistent hepatitis B virus infection and the development of hepatocellular carcinoma. According to Beasley (5), the relative risk for developing hepatomas is more than 250 times greater in carriers than in non–carriers. Since Abelev, *et al.* (1) reported that alpha–fetoprotein (AFP) was produced by hepatocellular carcinoma, serum AFP determination has been considered valuable for the diagnosis of hepatoma. The serum AFP is abnormal in a high percentage of patients with hepatoma, but may be elevated in other malignant tumors; however, levels above 500 ng/ml strongly suggest hepatoma (24). Periodic determinations of the serum alpha–fetoprotein is thus an attractive and easy way for the detection of hepatomas, hopefully at an early and resectable stage. This is very important considering the fact that long–term survival is achievable in 50–75% of patients with resectable hepatomas (9, 29). It is of interest, that in a study in Taiwan, Sheu *et al.* noted that the median doubling time of hepatocellular carcinoma was 117 days with a geometric mean of 110 days. This doubling time appeared to be independent of all factors but in half the cases, doubling was exponential and in these, the increase in alpha-fetoprotein was exponential as well. He used ultrasound to measure growth rates and calculated that hepatocellular carcinoma remained undetected for over three years. He also calculated that a suitable screening window for early detection was only 4–5 months, after which the tumor became too large for resection (25).

In 1980, a pilot alpha-fetoprotein screening program was begun among 20 HBsAG-positive Alaskan natives from three families at high risk for primary hepatocellular carcinoma. Each family had a high rate of HBV infection and had two family members die of hepatoma. In 1982, semiannual AFP screening resulted in the early detection and surgical resection of a 2 cm hepatoma in an asymptomatic 19–year–old Eskimo male who has since done well (14). This screening program was expanded to include all HBsAg-positive Alaskan natives, and a few asymptomatic hepatomas have been detected and successfully resected.

Similar programs are underway in high risk geographic areas. Unfortunately, not all hepatomas give rise to an abnormal AFP level. Moreover, serum AFP concentrations do not correlate with the size of the tumor, and the relationship between the changes in serum AFP levels and tumor growth is not clear (22). A further complicating factor is that smaller hepatocellular carcinomas slow down their growth rate with time for unknown reasons (17).

Secondary Liver Tumors

As mentioned earlier, metastases to the liver constitute the majority of hepatic neoplasms. Both surgical and medical approaches have in this category been directed, for the most part, at hepatic metastases from adenocarcinoma of the large bowel. The latter tumors, unlike other sites in the gastrointestinal tract, manifest a distinct pathologic pattern when they metastasize to the liver. The disease may remain confined to the liver with little or no extrahepatic disease, and is invariably fatal except for the occasional lesions that can be resected for cure.

Carcinoembryonic antigen (CEA) is a tumor marker discovered by Gold and Freedman in 1965 (12). It has been extensively studied in a variety of clinical situations with various solid tumors, particularly colorectal cancer. Determining the plasma

CEA level at periodic intervals is a simple and reliable test in detecting recurrent carcinoma of the large bowel, particularly, hepatic metastases (6, 8, 13, 21, 23, 28, 32, 34). Recently it has been noted that a rise in CEA levels may also be seen in the rare fibrolamellar hepatoma, which is usually seen in young adults (31).

Wanebo, *et al.* (32), found that 92% of patients with liver metastases had elevated plasma CEA levels, and among various patterns of recurrent disease, liver metastases had the highest CEA elevations. It is also well known that plasma CEA levels can be elevated several months prior to clinical, or even radiologic detection of liver metastasis (15, 19, 20, 30). This paved the way for an aggressive surgical approach of second–look laparotomy in asymptomatic patients who demonstrated persistently elevated plasma CEA levels; the expected result being the early detection of metastatic lesions at a stage when they can be resected with the potential for cure (3, 21, 23, 32).

Attiyeh and Stearns reported in 1981 on a prospective series of patients subjected to second–look laparotomy based on CEA elevations in colorectal cancer (3). Seventeen patients out of a total of 32 had hepatic metastasis, and seven had a curative hepatic resection; a resectability rate of 41% [7 of 17]. This compares quite favorably with a historically much lower resectability rate in patients explored after clinical and/or radiologic detection of their hepatic lesions.

A more recent update of this series, with a total of 48 patients, revealed hepatic metastases in 26 patients and a curative resection was possible in 13; a resectability rate of 50%. These patients continue to be followed by this author: Four patients are alive without evidence of disease from 36 to 66 months, two are alive with disease at 41 and 46 months, and 7 are dead of disease. Of the other 13 patients with unresectable disease, one is alive with disease and 12 are dead of disease.

LIVER FUNCTION TESTS

Liver function tests are rarely helpful in the early detection of hepatic neoplasms unless there is substantial involvement of the liver with tumor. Moreover, a high percentage of patients with hepatoma have varying degrees of liver damage due to underlying chronic active hepatitis and cirrhosis, which cause derangements in many of the parameters. Hepatic neoplasms in otherwise normal livers may occasionally give rise to an elevation in the serum alkaline phosphatase and/or lactic dehydrogenase. Jaundice, hypoalbuminemia, elevated serum transaminases, and coagulation defects usually denote an advanced stage of hepatic involvement with disease, which is diffuse and rarely, if ever, resectable. There may be rare instances of localized tumors causing obstructive jaundice by virtue of direct compression of major hepatic ducts and still be resectable, but on the whole, jaundice implies extensive bilobar disease. In brief, liver function tests are not generally useful in the early detection of liver tumors that can be resected for cure. However, these tests are of prime importance in the assessment of the patient's liver reserve which must be normal for a major hepatic resection to be successful.

RADIOACTIVE LIVER SCAN

Nuclear liver scans often show abnormal findings but may not be helpful in some patients because of the abnormal patterns seen in underlying cirrhosis. The liver scan can demonstrate focal defects, which would require further evaluation to elucidate their nature. A major deficiency, however, is the limitation of the scan in detecting small lesions in the liver less than 2.5 cm in diameter.

Liver scans are not always helpful when it comes to the extent of tumor involvement in the liver and its resectability. A study by Kim *et al.* (18). showed that liver scans detected tumors in 103 out of 110 patients (87%) documented by laparotomy. The scan diagnosed tumor location correctly in 62% for the right lobe, 27% for the left lobe, and 56% for bilobar disease, with an overall accuracy rate of 62%. As for the 39 patients who had resectable lesions, the scan detected tumors in only 30, and were correctly localized in 19.

In brief, the liver scan may be helpful in detecting tumors in the liver but falls short of expectations when it comes to extent and resectability of these tumors. Besides, it may miss small solitary tumors that are most amenable to curative resection.

ULTRASONOGRAPHY

In comparison with nuclear liver scan, ultrasonography of the liver has proved to be a more sensitive modality to detect early metastatic disease (27), the overall accuracy being 94%. It also permits differentiation of nonspecific filling defects on nuclear scans into those due to tumors and conditions such as cysts and abscesses.

Ultrasonography is, therefore, an easy, noninvasive, modality with a high sensitivity and specificity for the detection of hepatic neoplasms. It certainly can be utilized for detection in patients suspected of having disease based on abnormal CEA, alpha-fetoprotien, etc. . . . , or a high index of suspicion.

COMPUTERIZED TRANSAXIAL TOMOGRAPHY

Computerized transaxial tomography (CTT) is a very valuable diagnostic tool in verifying abnormalities detected on nuclear scan and/or ultrasound. It may shed further light as to the pathological process, and in most situations, accurately delineates anatomic relationships thereby giving a reasonable assessment of resectability. CTT is more sensitive than either nuclear scan or ultrasound in detecting smaller lesions in the liver, but it cannot be justified on a routine basis because of the hazards of excessive radiation exposure and cost effectiveness.

ANGIOGRAPHY

Selective angiography provides us with another method to evaluate the liver for space occupying lesions, and also delineates the vascular anatomy for the safe conduct of a major hepatic resection. This diagnostic modality is obviously invasive and not without risks, and, therefore, is not utilized in the initial steps of detecting liver tumors.

Angiography, CTT ultrasound and nuclear scanning are covered in greater detail in other chapters of this book.

SUMMARY

Surgical extirpation, when feasible, remains the hallmark of treatment for liver tumors, both primary and secondary, with a reasonable chance for long term survival. Unfortunately, the majority of these patients are not candidates for surgical resection when first seen. It is hoped that early detection would play a major role in increasing the resectability rate and, most importantly, long-term survival.

For a program of early detection to be successful, simple diagnostic screening tests will have to be applied to populations at risk. In the case of primary hepatocellular carcinoma, screening of high risk populations, mainly those with HBV infection, is in the form of yearly or twice yearly serum AFP determinations. As for secondary liver tumors, patients with a history of a GI malignancy, notably large bowel, are screened periodically with plasma CEA determinations. Other diagnostic tests for liver tumors, such as liver function tests, nuclear scan, etc. have a limited role in the early detection as well. Several investigations have shown that early detection did indeed increase resectability, but it remains to be seen whether this materializes into substantial gains in long-term survival.

REFERENCES

1. Abelev, GI, Perova, SD, Kramkova, NI, Postnikova, ZA, Irlin, IS: Production of embryonal α-globulin by transplantable mouse hepatomas. *Transplantation, 1:*174, 1963.

2. Adson, MA, Van Heerden, JA: Major hepatic resections for metastatic colorectal cancer. *Ann Surg, 191:*576, 1980.

3. Attiyeh, FF, Stearns, MW, Jr.: Second-look laparotomy based on CEA elevations in colorectal cancer. *Cancer, 47:*2119, 1981.

4. Attiyeh, FF, Wanebo, HJ, Stearns, MW: Hepatic resection for metastasis from colorectal cancer. *Dis Colon Rectum, 21:*160, 1978.

5. Beasley, RP, Lin, CC, Hwang, LY, Chien, CS: Hepatocellular carcinoma and hepatitis B virus: A prospective study of 22,707 men in Taiwan. *Lancet, 2:*1129, 1981.

6. Beatty, JD, Romero, C, Brown, PW, Lawrence, W, Jr., Terz, JJ: Clinical value of carcinoembryonic antigen. *Arch Surg, 114:*563, 1979.

7. Blumberg, BS, London WT: Hepatitis B virus: Pathogenesis and prevention of primary cancer of the liver. *Cancer, 50:*2657, 1982.

8. Booth, SN, Jamieson, GC, King, JPC, Leonard, J, Oates, GD, Dykes, PW: Carcinoembryonic antigen in management of colorectal carcinoma. *Br Med J, 4:*183, 1974.

9. Fortner, JG, Maclean, BJ, Kim, DK, *et al.*: The seventies evolution in liver surgery for cancer. *Cancer, 47:*2162, 1981.

10. Foster, JH: Survival after liver resection for cancer. *Cancer, 26:*493, 1970.

11. Furukawa, R, Tajima, H, Nakata, K, *et al.*: Clinical significance of serum alpha--fetoprotein in patients with liver cirrhosis. *Tumor Biol, 5:*327, 1985.

12. Gold, P, Freedman, SO: Demonstration of tumor — specific antigens in human colonic carcinomata by immunological tolerance and absorption techniques. *J Exp Med, 121:*439, 1965.

13. Herrera, MA, Chu, TM, Holyoke, ED: Cardinoembryonic antigen (CEA) as a prognostic and monitoring test in clinically complete resection of colorectal carcinoma. *Ann Surg, 183:*5, 1976.

14. Heyward, WL, Lanier, AP, Bender, TR, *et al.*: Early detection of primary hepatocellular carcinoma by screening for alpha–fetoprotein in high risk families: a case report. *Lancet, 2:*1161, 1983.

15. Holyoke, ED, Chu, TM, Murphy, GP: CEA as a monitor of gastrointestinal malignancy. *Cancer, 35:*830, 1975.

16. Hsu, HC, Lin WSJ, Tsai, MJ: Hepatitis-B surface antigen and hepatocellular carcinoma in Taiwan. *Cancer, 52:*1825, 1983.

17. Hsu, HC, Sheu, JC, Lin, YH, *et al.*: Prognostic histiologic features of resected small hepatocellular carcinoma (HCC) in Taiwan. A comparison with resected large HCC. *Cancer, 56:*672, 1985.

18. Kim, DK, McSweeney, J, Yeh, SDJ, Fortner, JG: Tumors of the liver as demonstrated by angiography, scan and laparotomy. *Surg Gynecol Obstet, 141:*409, 1975.

19. Mach, JP, Vienny, H, Jaeger, P, Haldemann, B, Egely, R, Pettavel, J: Long-term follow-up of colorectal carcinoma patients by repeated CEA radioimmunoassay. *Cancer, 42:*1439, 1978.

20. Mackay, AM, Patel, S, Carter, S, *et al.*: Role of serial plasma CEA assays in detection of recurrent and metastatic colorectal carcinomas. *Br Med J, 4:*382, 1974.

21. Martin, EW, Jr., James, KK, Hurtubise, PE, Catalano, P, Minton, JP: The use of CEA as an early indicator for gastrointestinal tumor recurrence and second look procedures. *Cancer, 39:*440, 1977.

22. Matsumoto, Y, Suzuki, T, Asada, I, Ozawa, K, Tobe, K, Honjo, I: Clinical classification of hepatoma in Japan according to serial changes in serum alpha–fetoprotein levels. *Cancer, 49:*354, 1982.

23. Minton, JP, James, KK, Hurtubise, PE, Rinker, L, Joyce, S, Martin, EW, Jr.: The use of serial carcinoembryonic antigen determinations to predict recurrence of carcinoma of the colon and the time for a second-look operation. *Surg Gynecol Obstet, 147:*208, 1978.

24. Oberfield, RA, Templeton, AC, Williams, L: Cancer of the liver. Cancer Manual American Cancer Society Massachusetts Division, 1982.

25. Sheu, JC, Sung, JL, Chen, DS, *et al.*: Growth rate of asymptomatic hepatocellular carcinoma and its clinical implications. *Gastroenterology, 89:*259, 1985.

26. Silverberg, E: Cancer statistics, 1986. *Ca, 36:*9, 1986.

27. Smith, IE, Taylor, KHW, McCready, VR, *et al.: Clin Oncol, 2:*47, 1976.

28. Staab, HJ, Anderer, FA, Struzef, E, Fischer, R: Slope analysis of the postoperative time course and its possible application as an aid in disease progression in gastrointestinal cancer. *Am J Surg, 136:*322, 1978.

29. Starzl, TE, Koep, LJ, Weil, R, III, Lilly, JR, Putman, CW, Aldrete, JA: Right trisegmentectomy for hepatic neoplasms. *Surg Gynecol Obstet, 140:* 208, 1980.

30. Sugarbaker, PH, Zamchek, N, Moore, FD: Assessment of serial carcinoembryonic antigen (CEA) assays in postoperative detection of recurrent colorectal cancer. *Cancer, 38:*2310, 1976.

31. Teitelbaum, DH, Tuttle, S, Carey, LC, Clausen, KS: Fibrolamella carcinoma of the liver. Review of three cases and the presentation of a characteristic set of tumor markers defining this tumor. *Ann Surg, 202:*36, 1985.

32. Wanebo, HJ, Stearns, MW, Jr., Schwartz, MK: Use of CEA as an indicator of early recurrence and as a guide to a selected second-look procedure in patients with colorectal cancer. *Ann Surg, 188:*481, 1978.

33. Wilson, SM, Adson, MA: Surgical treatment of hepatic metastases from colorectal cancers. *Arch Surg, 111:*330, 1976.

34. Wood, CB, Ratcliffe, JG, Burt, RW, Malcolm, JH, Blumgart, LH: The clinical significance of the pattern of elevated serum carcinoembryonic antigen (CEA) levels in recurrent colorectal cancer. *Br J Surg, 67:*46, 1980.

JOSEPH McCARTHY, M.D.

CHAPTER 3
Scintiscanning

When suspicion of recurrent, metastatic or primary tumor is aroused, it is important to go quickly to a simple investigation to set up the pattern for management. Scintiscanning, or radionuclide hepatic imaging, is a satisfactory first step.

There are two types of scans which are done. They depend on the mechanism of uptake of each of the two dominant cells within the liver.

Kupffer cells phagocytose injected radioactive technetium colloid and hence the common liver/spleen scan is obtained. 99m technetium sulphur colloid is utilized, and remains static in the liver, held by the Kupffer cells. It is used to demonstrate hepatic anatomy, and most of this chapter will be concerned with the colloid liver scan (Figure 3.1).

The second radionuclide hepatic imaging process depends on hepatocyte function. In this case, a radioactive technetium labelled organic molecule, such as 99m technetium disofenin, which is secreted by hepatocytes into the biliary system, is used. This is the basis of the hepato–biliary scan which evaluates cystic duct patency and provides a gross examination of the remainder of the ductal system.

COLLOID LIVER/SPLEEN SCAN

The use of colloid liver scanning to search for tumor in the liver depends upon the fact that the normal uniform distribution of Kupffer cells is disrupted by the presence and/or growth of lesions which are not typical normal liver structures. Because the tumor does not contain cells that have a phagocytic capability, as seen in the Kupffer cells, its expansion displaces normal liver tissue, and then the tumor shows up on the liver/spleen scan as a non–radioactive volume within the radioactive liver.

The liver scan is actually a reticuloendothelial scan, and the liver and spleen are well seen, but the bone marrow is barely seen with this examination. A short time after injection of technetium

colloid multiple views of the liver and spleen are taken from different angles. The images obtained are essentially two dimensional
projections of the three dimensional volume as seen from different
angles. The nature of the examination ensures that all aspects of
liver anatomy are included in the examination. It may be divided
into dynamic and static portions.

The dynamic examination is obtained in the left anterior
oblique position, immediately after intravenous injection of three
to four mCi/125MBq of 99m technetium sulphur colloid. Arterial
perfusion of the liver normally constitutes 20–25% of hepatic
flow. Dense hepatic images form after portal venous flow delivers
radiocolloid to the liver (Figure 3.1) and the colloid particles are
rapidly phagocytized by Kupffer cells.

Static images are obtained after a delay of 5–15 minutes.
Liver and spleen are well seen. Bone marrow may be barely seen,
depending upon the quality of the equipment utilized. Multiple
images are obtained in multiple projections, including anterior
views to show costal margin and hepatic size and position with a
lead strip (Figures 3.1 and 3.2).

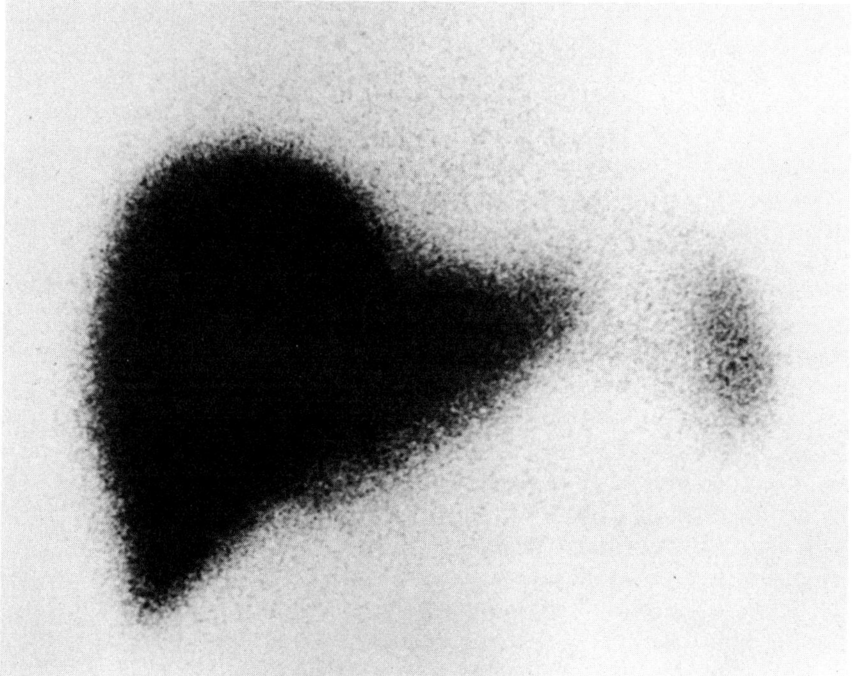

Figure 3.1. Normal dynamic liver/spleen scan.

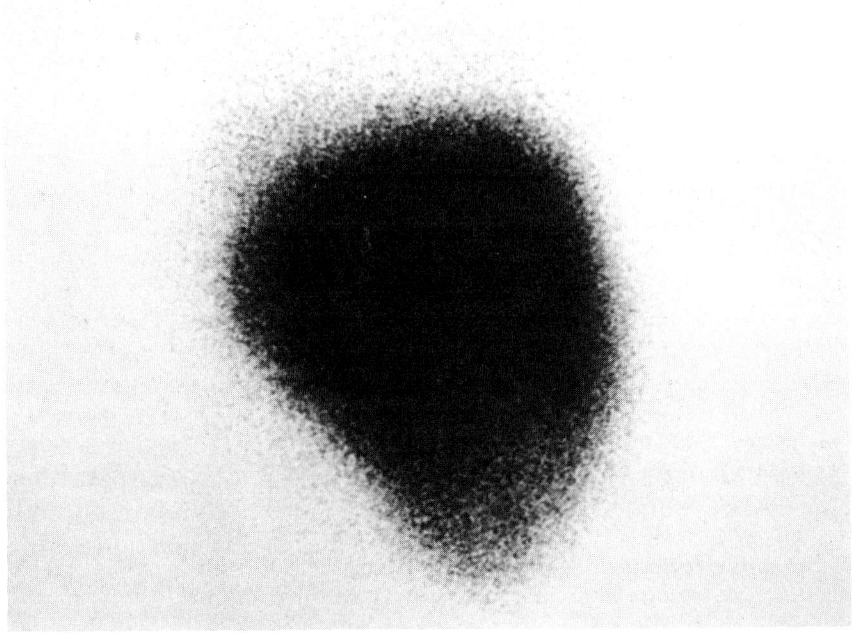

Figure 3.2. Normal static image.

Hepatic size may be evaluated on anterior view by measuring maximum vertical height by the lead measure (Figure 3.3). Maximum size of 18–19 cms has been proposed and used widely for the whole population. However, body weight should also be considered (Figure 3.4). A 40 kilogram woman may have a liver which measures 17 cms in vertical height and then the liver should be considered to be enlarged. A tall 115 kilogram man with a liver height of 23 cms is not likely to have an enlarged liver. Accurate evaluation of liver size may be made by "eyeballing" the images (1) and keeping the weight of the patients in mind.

Consideration should be given to hepatic shape, hepatic volume, pattern of activity in the liver and amount of activity in the liver. Livers come in many shapes and the ability to identify specific lobar boundaries is limited. Right lobes may be elongated (Riedeloid – Figure 3.5), elevated (diaphragmatic or superdiaphragmatic abnormality), or displaced. Left lobes may be prominent but gracile, and in the lateral view may be angulated very sharply, up to a right angle, by the costal margin in very obese patients.

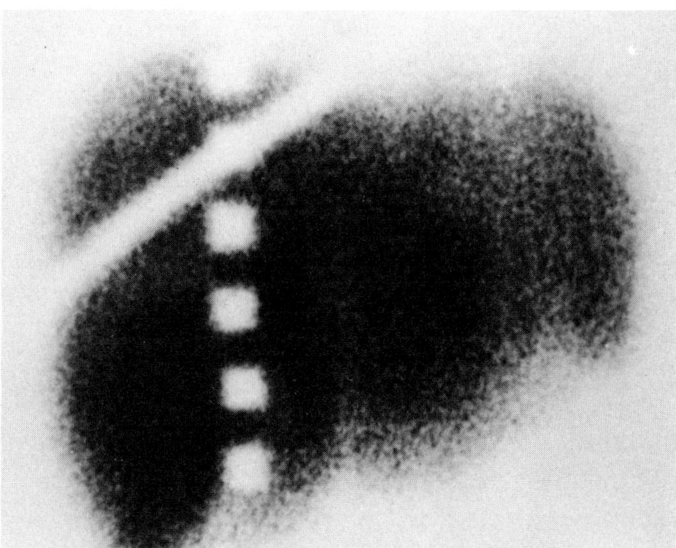

Figure 3.3. Measurement of maximum vertical height of the liver in a patient with chronic ethanol abuse who was also a heavy smoker. The liver is grossly enlarged, but is also pushed into the abdomen by hyper-aerated lungs. No space-occupying lesions are seen.

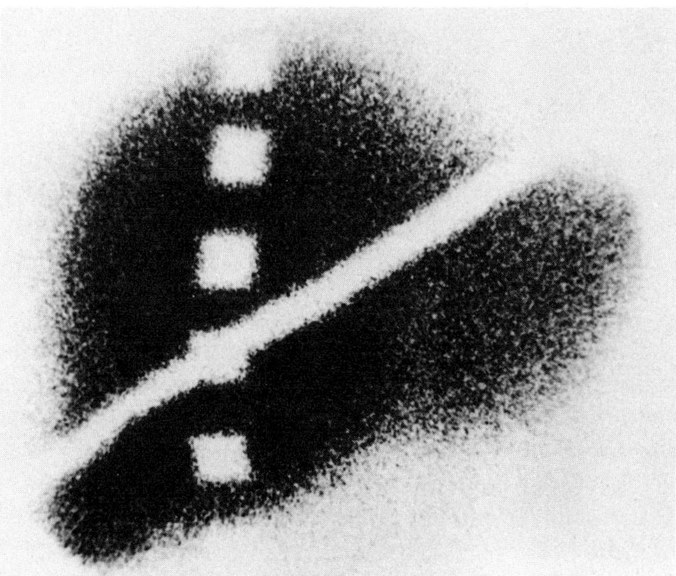

Figure 3.4. Hepatomegaly which may be due to the patient's obesity.

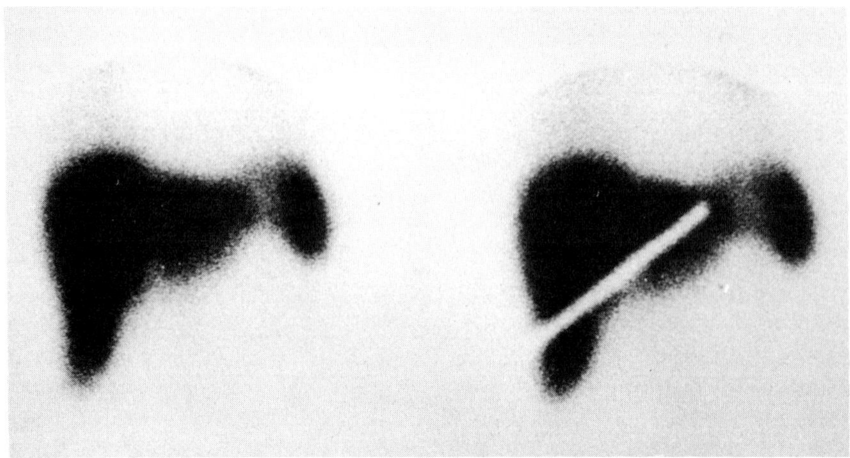

Figure 3.5. Normal liver with Riedeloid elongation of the right lobe.

The distribution of radiocolloid in the normal liver is called homogeneous. It is, in fact, homogeneous per unit of volume, but the volume of liver varies abruptly due ot its very irregular shape.

The net effect is a non-uniform final film density. The appreciation of the normal is mandatory for the detection of the abnormal. Focal defects in the homogeneous activity in the liver secondary to metastatic deposits are relatively easy to describe and by enumeration of size and site may be very helpful to the clinician. Heterogeneous activity (also called inhomogeneous in the United States of America) requires more interpretive skill and experience. Hepatocellular disease and diffuse small metastatic deposits are very difficult to differentiate: both may be present as heterogeneous activity (diffuse liver process).

Results

In the dynamic study increased hepatic arterial flow (arterialization) can be caused by severe hepatocellular disease, cirrhosis, hepatoma, metastatic deposits, arterio-venous malformation, hemangiomas and hyperplasia and adenomas.

Visualization of the cardiac blood pool in the late films indicates diffuse hepatic disease; the actual delivery of radioactive colloid by the blood stream is diminished and the rate of phagocytosis within the liver is also decreased in this condition so that the colloid shows up elsewhere.

Hepatocellular disease is the more likely diagnosis if a hetero-geneous pattern is accompanied by shrinkage of the right lobe, enlargement of the left lobe, splenomegaly, increased splenic colloid localization, increased bone marrow localization and pul-monary colloid activity (Figures 3.6 and 3.7). Further, Lee, *et al.* recently suggested that the multiple radiotracer approach may allow a more specific diagnosis of hepatocellular carcinoma to be made (2).

A patient clinically suspected of having metastases whose radionuclide liver scan is focally abnormal should be considered to have metastases until proven otherwise. On the other hand, a nega-tive radionuclide liver scan and a low index of suspicion are suffi-cient to terminate the investigation for liver metastases. If metas-

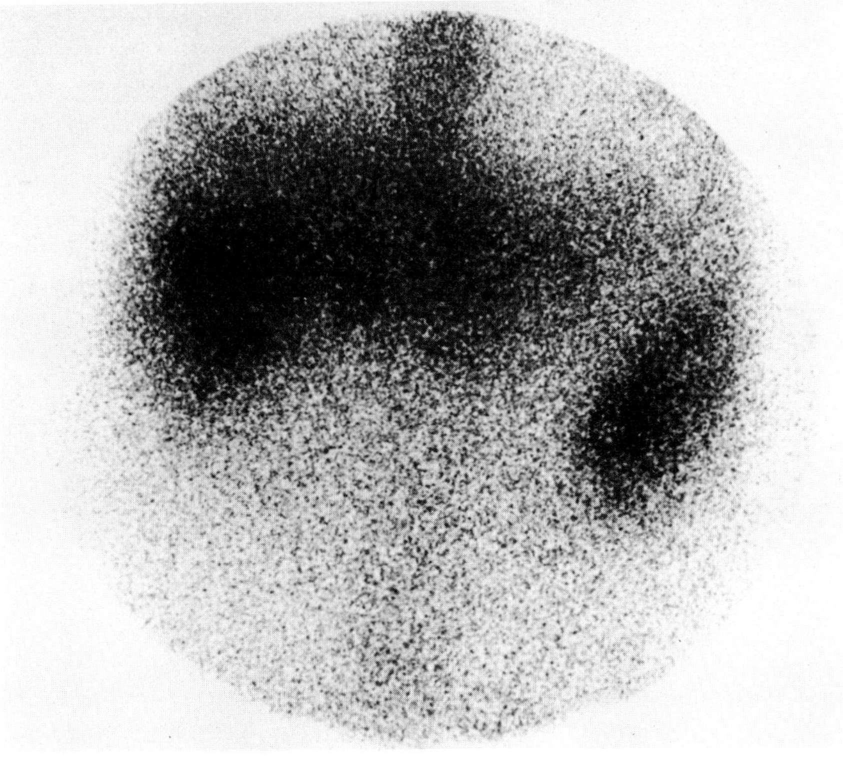

Figure 3.6. Space-occupying lesion in the right lobe of the liver; the pattern of colloid localization is suggestive of cirrhosis and hepatoma was clinically suspected.

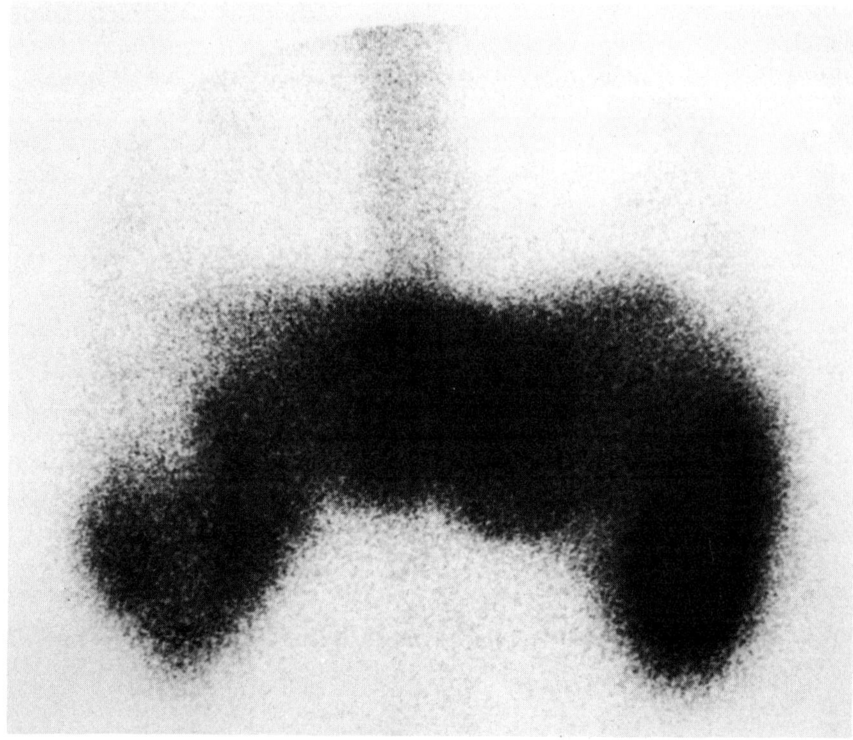

Figure 3.7. Space-occupying lesion of the right lobe of the liver; the pattern of colloid localization which is particularly marked with uptake in the spleen is highly suggestive of cirrhosis and therefore hepatoma would be suspected.

tases are still suspected, other modalities should be used to try and satisfy the question. For example, it has been suggested that it might be possible for these metastases, if colonic in origin, to directly take up 99m technecium labelled diphosphonate (DPD) (3).

Discussion

Nuclear imaging must be within or available to a hospital for that hospital to have JCAH approval. Therefore, by mandate, radionuclide imaging performed by a technologist is readily available. Nuclear imaging is not expensive.

Radioactive colloid liver scanning has a number of characteristics which make it an attractive means of evaluating the liver.

One is the non-invasive nature of the study. Other non-invasive means of evaluating the liver such as physical examination and blood tests of hepatic function are not as accurate in assessing the presence or absence of tumor in the liver. The liver may be of normal size and riddled with metastases (Figure 3.8). In addition, a grossly enlarged liver may have metastases which cannot be identified by palpation. Liver function tests are abnormal only when the metastatic involvement of the liver is advanced. In addition, abnormal liver function tests are not specific for tumor in the liver.

Non-invasive imaging examinations are preferred to invasive ones because they are safer, less traumatic, cheaper, easier to perform, easier to reproduce and retain accuracy. The radionuclide examination is the screening test of choice for the detection and follow-up of secondary deposits (Figure 3.9, 3.10). This is because of many factors, including sensitivity, specificity, radiation

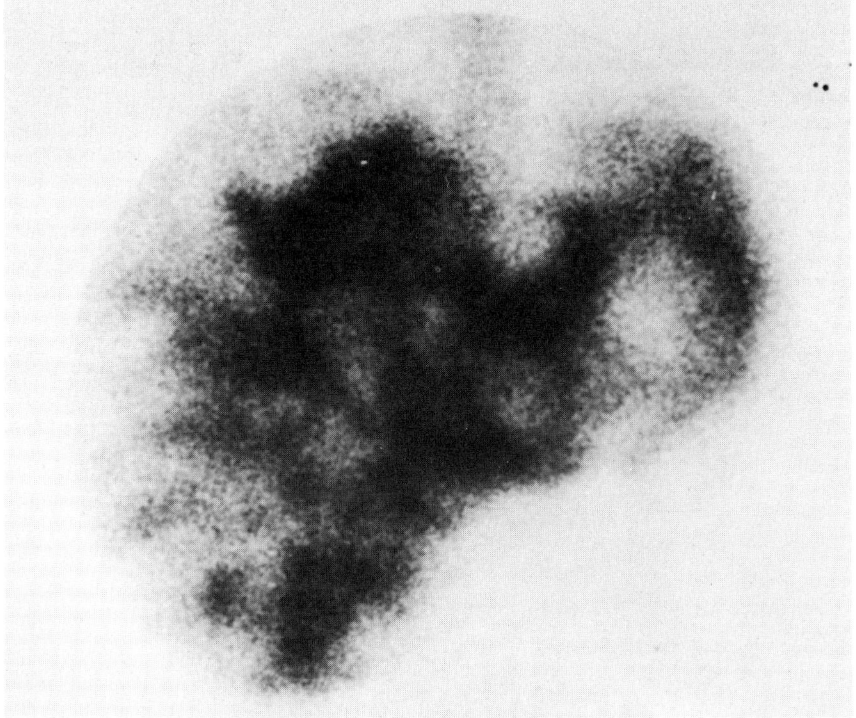

Figure 3.8. Minimal enlargement of the liver which is riddled with metastases from cancer of the colon.

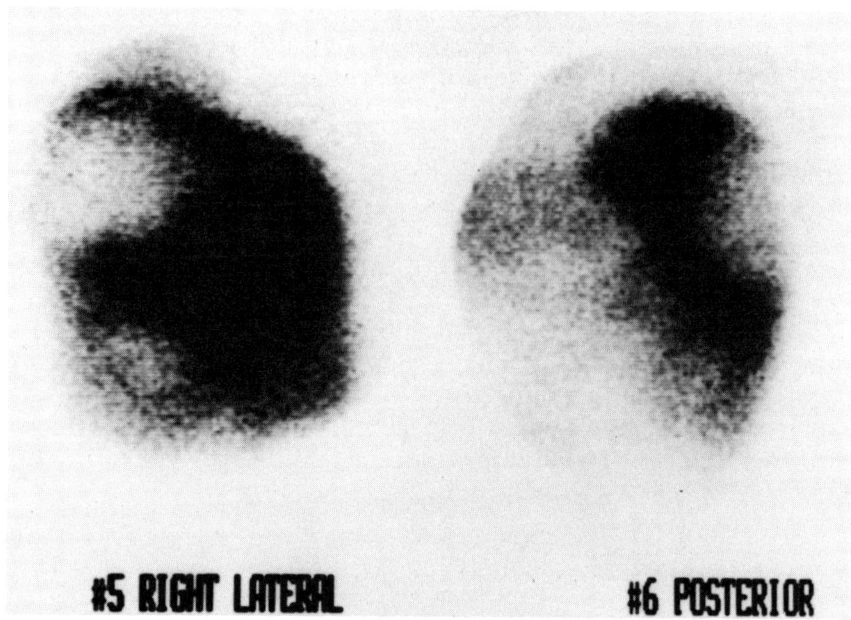

Figure 3.9. Detection of metastatic colon cancer. The largest lesion is postero-lateral in the right lobe.

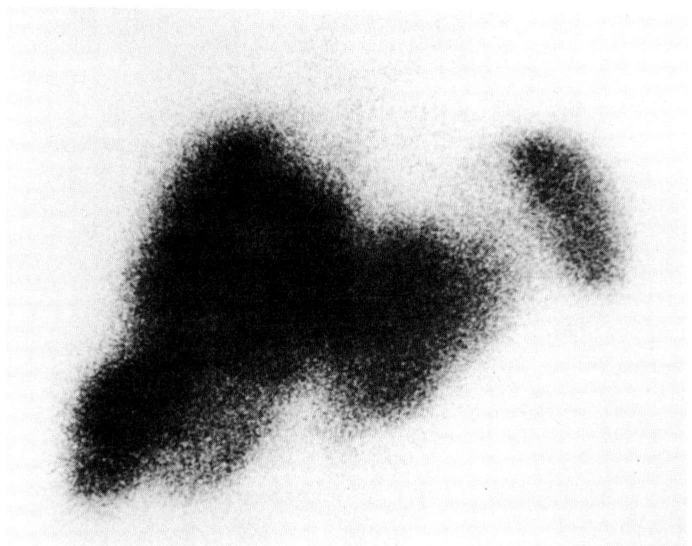

Figure 3.10. Multiple space–occupying lesions secondary to transitional cell metastases are seen in this patient's liver.

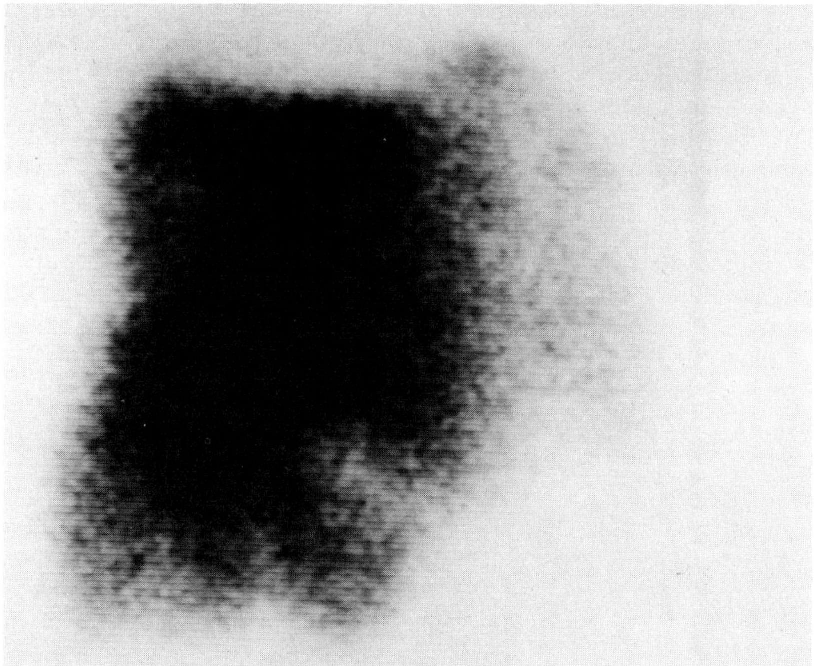

Figure 3.11. This patient has chronic myelogeneous leukemia with hepato-splenomegaly. The space-occupying lesions within the liver were demon-strated to be due to the patient's polycystosis.

burden, availability, reproducibility and the nature of the images used for analysis. It can not be assumed that the hepatic scinti-gram is not indicated in any particular clinical setting (4); the liver scan can be normal or abnormal due to non-malignant disease (Figure 3.11). Certainly one must have a baseline study to evaluate future abnormal patterns and their significance and the easiest way to follow the size of any detected abnormality or abnormalities within the liver is a nuclear scan (Figure 3.12, 3.13, 3.14, and 3.15). This remains the case even if other modalities first demon-strate an abnormality in the liver.

Where the clinical suspicion remains that tumor is within the liver and an equivocal nuclear study is obtained, then an ultra-sound examination should be carried out. This scheme only applies to initial evaluations. For the follow-up of previously described metastases, radionuclide imaging is well suited and can accurately demonstrate volume changes with more ease and less operator input than ultrasound (5). The proven lesions can be followed and new lesions detected. Splenic involvement can also be monitored or detected. Hepatomegaly may be demonstrated to be secondary to chemotherapy induced hepatocellular disease, rather than new metastatic deposits. The spleen is often influenced by hepatic disease or the same metastatic lesion which can afflict the liver. The spleen is easily and readily evaluated in a nuclear liver/spleen scan. As with the hepatic portion of the examination, the splenic distribution of radionuclide depends upon distribution of normal physiologic capabilities. Any disruption in the normal pattern of phagocytic cell distribution may result in an abnormality in the scintigram.

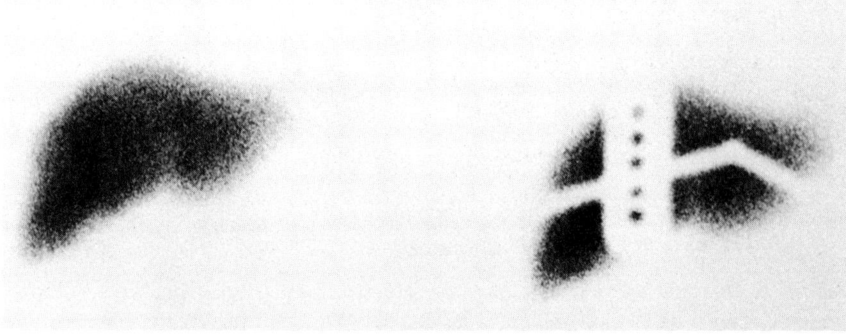

Figure 3.12. This patient's liver is displaced inferiorly by his hyperaerated lungs; there is no evidence of space-occupying lesions.

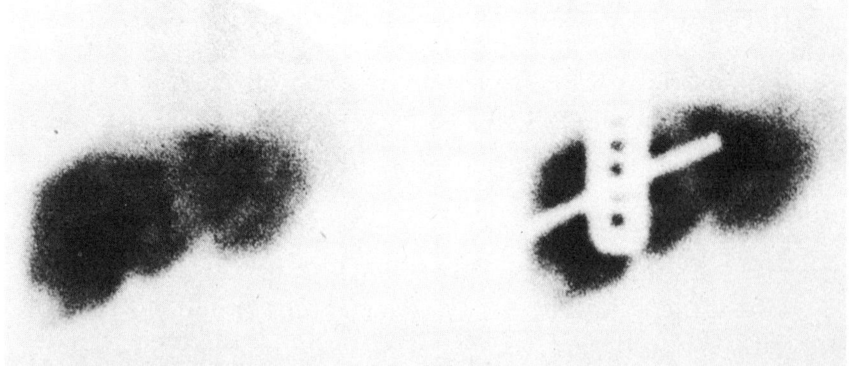

Figure 3.13. This is the same patient as in Figure 3.12 6 months later showing multiple space-occupying lesions in the liver and these are secondary to metastatic bronchogenic carcinoma.

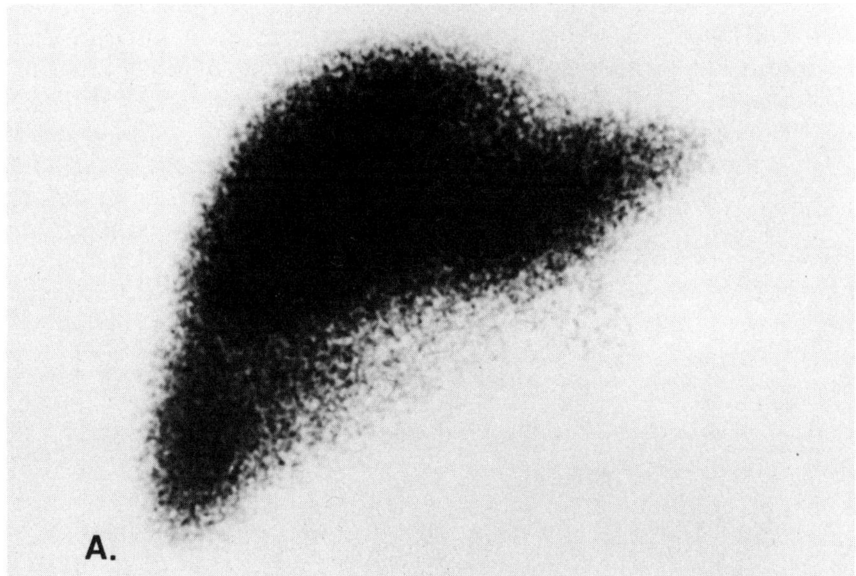

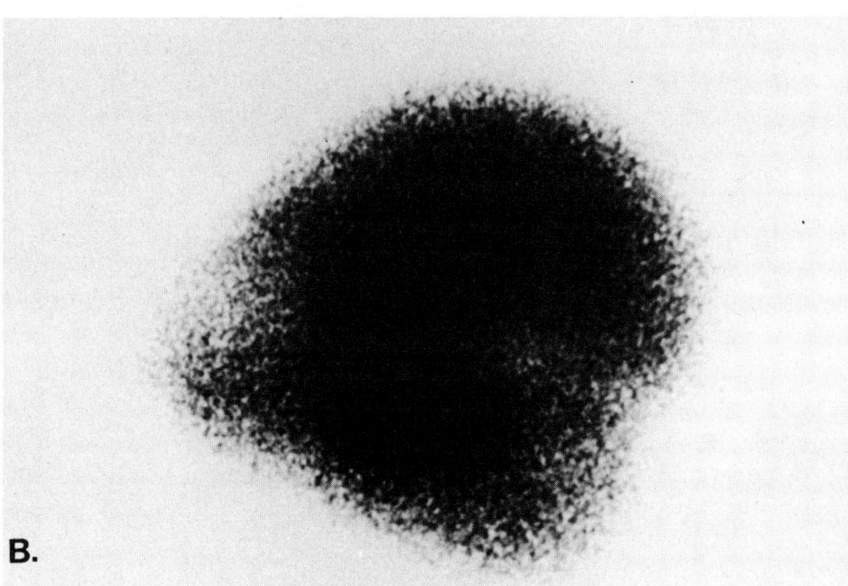

Figure 3.14. Large metastatic deposit in the posterior aspect of the right lobe of the liver.

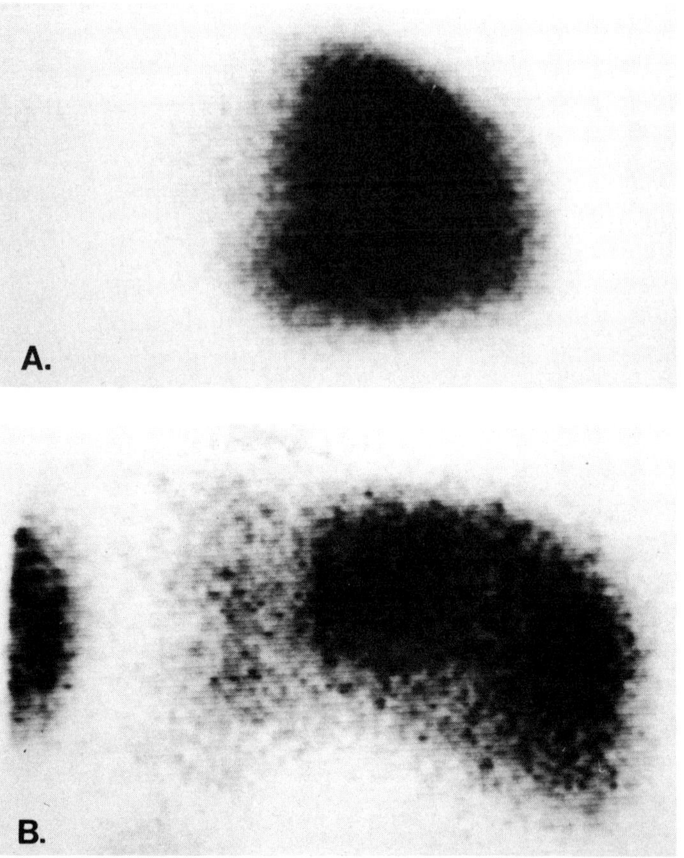

Figure 3.15. Same patient as in Figure 3.14 but following right hemihepatectomy. The remainder of the liver demonstrates poor liver function which is indicated because of bone marrow uptake and splenic uptake of radioactive colloid.

CT images and modern ultrasound images possess a greater capability for demonstrating anatomic detail than nuclear examinations. Spatial resolution of nuclear gamma cameras is worse than spatial resolution of ultrasound and CT machines; the resolution is further degraded by motion during the nuclear examination. All three modalities have improved their resolution in the past several years, but the nature of the nuclear hepatic imaging process dictates that resolution in modern nuclear examinations cannot approach the resolution of CT and ultrasound examination.

Resolution of an imaging method is an important determinant in the sensitivity of that method, and it must be remembered that comparison between imaging modalities is valid only for the equipment being evaluated. There are very few institutions which have state of the art equipment in arteriography, digital subtraction angiography, CT, ultrasound, and nuclear imaging. Hence, when evaluating the equipment in one's own institution or reading evaluations in the literature, one must be aware of the limitations of a particular imaging system, and its influence upon imaging accuracy.

Ultrasonography is quite widespread due to the low cost and affordability of machines. However, cost is a prime problem with CT imaging and will be more of a factor in NMR imaging. Angiography is also expensive.

The real world does not necessarily reflect research data. A particular imaging system may not be available for examining patients due to tight schedules, equipment breakdown or shortage, personnel sickness or shortage. In such a situation, which is all too common, the physician may be forced to move to other modalities before a radionuclide scan. It must also be borne in mind that the equipment available for imaging may be of the finest quality for one modality and markedly inferior for another. Quality control is another factor which is very important in nuclear medicine and can produce inferior images of low accuracy.

Usually, however, the accuracy of radionuclide scans is high. Yet, even when this is the case there are many times when a nuclear physician must say "I am not sure" since portions of the liver volume which are further away from the camera face, and deeper in the patient, present a problem of resolution and detection of abnormalities. Then, an ultrasound examination directed at the volume in question should be suggested. This directed examination becomes a definitive study; metastatic deposits are diagnosed or excluded by the impression of this examination. Also, in good hands, hepatocellular carcinoma can be detected early when ultrasonography is used as a screening technique (6).

Of course, ultrasonography, although it is quite widespread, requires highly trained personnel who are essential; physician participation is desirable. The knowledge, training and interest of the physician interpreting the image may reflect negatively on the accuracy of various modalities; This is particularly common with both nuclear and sonographic interpretive skills. However, both nuclear and CT scans are more highly reproducible than the ultrasound scan as there is a limited opportunity for operator influence. Ultrasound examination of the liver depends upon many factors including intestinal gas, obesity, scars, wounds, post-traumatic pain, individual echo factors, burns, and operator experience or inexperience. The ultrasound examination depends a great deal upon the capability of the person scanning (Figure 3.16) and also which scans (tomograms) are produced, seen and photographed; there is much art to ultrasound. Such limitations do not pertain to the nuclear examination of the liver.

Like the nuclear medical examination, anaphylactic reactions are not seen in the ultrasound examination. However, a CT examination is invasive in that IV contrast material may be administered and the potential for an anaphylaxis, therefore, exists.

Although the radionuclide examination provides the liver with a burden of two to four rads of ionizing radiation, this is insignificant. The CT examination also has a low radiation burn which is deposited in the skin and although this is more radio-

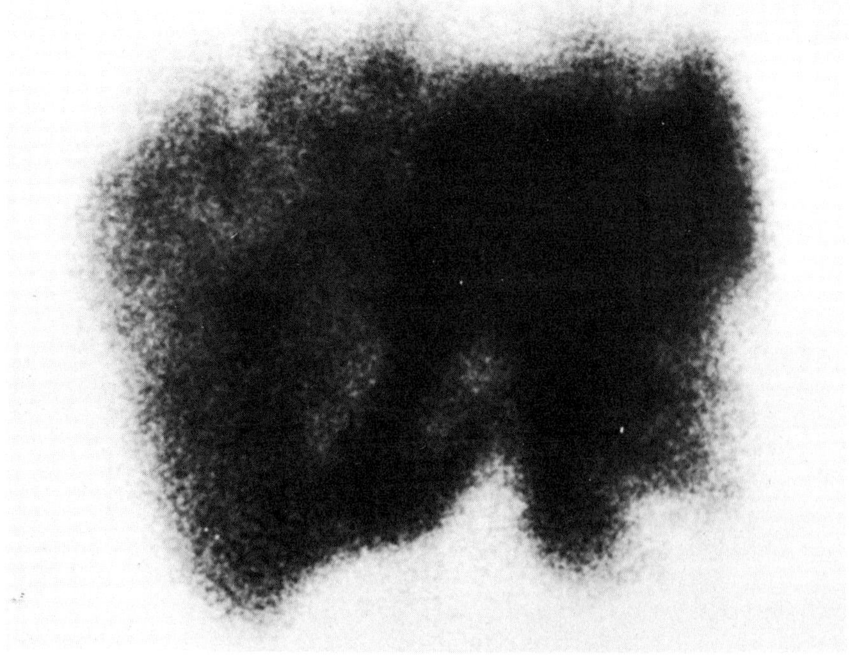

Figure 3.16. Hepatomegaly with enumerable space-occupying lesions secondary to metastatic breast carcinoma. Ultrasound examination did not demonstrate intrahepatic space-occupying lesions in this patient.

sensitive than the hepatocytes, again it is insignificant. Ultrasound, of course, is free of ionizing radiation.

Although CT scanning is fairly widespread throughout America it may not be readily available due to cost and constraints on portability.

Perfusion of the liver cannot be assessed by ultrasound and can be evaluated only to a limited extent by CT. Both arterial and portal venous phases of hepatic perfusion can be assessed via the radionuclide examination (7). Metastatic disease is one of the several causes of increased arterial perfusion.

Etiologic specificity varies with each type of procedure, depending upon the skills of the interpretor and pre-existing disease. The radionuclide examination of the liver which demonstrates a severely diseased liver, with a large irregular space-occupying lesion, enlarged spleen and increased bone marrow activity may be highly suggestive of hepatoma. Another pattern can be very suggestive of carcinoma of the colon. The number of hepatic lesions may be so great that one assumes that they represent metastatic deposits. Usually, however, the etiology of photon deficient volumes is obscured (Figure 3.17). CT imaging has similar

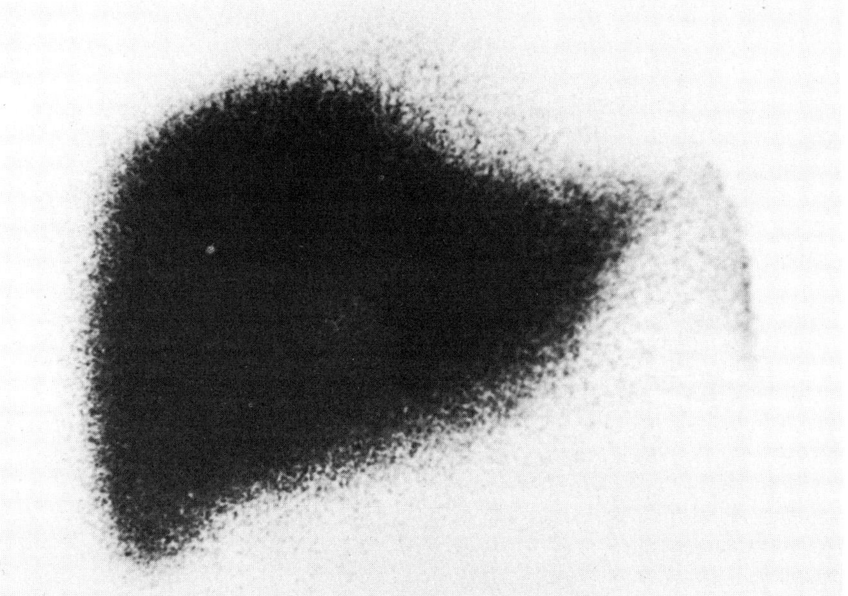

Figure 3.17. Central space-occupying lesion which was demonstrated subsequently to be secondary to inoperable cholangio-carcinoma.

drawbacks, unless hypervascularity can be seen as in hepatoma, or low density is detected as in cysts. Ultrasound can also differentiate between cysts and solid lesions; in addition the photo–deficient volumes in a radionuclide examination can be shown most likely to be regenerated nodules by the pattern of ultrasound scan, and it may be able to give the first clue in the diagnosis of hemangiomas (8).

In general, the "non–invasive" means of hepatic imaging include radionuclide examinations, ultrasound scans, computerized tomography; magnetic resonance imaging is still developing and is not widespread.

Far more invasive but still radiological is arteriography and this has all the potential untoward effects of arterial puncture and contrast injection, but with lower sensitivity and specificity than non–invasive liver imaging examinations; the radiation burden, the professional time, and cost are additional factors mitigating against the arteriogram in the search for metastases.

EMISSION COMPUTERIZED TOMOGRAPHY (ECT)

This method of hepatic imaging is another modality for radionuclide investigation. The general term includes Positron Emission Tomography (PET) and Single Photon Emission Computerized Tomography (SPECT). PET scanning is not widespread, for several reasons, not the least of which is capital equipment cost (several times CT costs). Other factors mitigating against widespread use of PET are the necessity of a nearby cyclotron and significant personnel increases. SPECT scanning utilizes the same radio–pharmaceutical as is used for the conventional liver/spleen scan; conventional gamma camera heads are attached to rotating devices and the data are computer acquired and processed. Additional capital cost is incurred in the rotating machinery, computer hardware and software.

Computer enhanced reconstruction provides images similar to CT images. Increased accuracy is obtained due to the slicing of hepatic volumes (9). Indeed, SPECT imaging has been demonstrated to be 10% more sensitive in detecting hepatic metastases than CT scanning (10). SPECT imaging has also been shown to be more sensitive than ultrasound (9) and has been demonstrated to have a sensitivity as high as 96% and ability to detect lesions as small as 8 mms (11). This technique will probably become much more widespread and its reliability will possibly result in more dependence on radionuclide imaging for detecting and following the course of hepatic metastases. Much of the increased accuracy is due to a markedly increased sensitivity for lesions deep within the liver.

The sensitivity of planar nuclear imaging is approximately the same as ultrasound imaging for detection of liver tumors (9). CT sensitivity is basically similar, but is improved by injection of intravenous contrast, and special dynamic techniques. The increase in sensitivity using this SPECT technology has already been discussed but serves to emphasize the point that the technology of gamma camera imaging and the cross–sectional anatomical knowledge utilized for CT imaging blend easily and to reinforce the point that SPECT imaging will likely become more widespread in the future for hepatic tumor screening.

Of course, estimations of hepatic size can be performed utilizing any imaging technique. For planar imaging, it has been demonstrated that the "eyeball" technique is just as accurate as geometric measuring techniques (1). However, SPECT imaging offers a superior method of evaluating liver volume, because the whole of the liver is included in the examination, while each individual slice is being obtained (12). In vitro measurements of hepatic volume using SPECT techniques show an incredibly high accuracy with almost a perfect correlation (r = 0.997) (5).

HEPATO–BILIARY IMAGING

Hepatocyte function is assessed by an intravenous injection of 99m technetium disofenin which provides hepato–biliary images and these may be utilized to evaluate the possibility of obstruction of the biliary tree, or part thereof. The relationship of ducts to tumor mass may be deducted from distortion of the ducts. Similarly, improvement of obstruction or displacement of biliary ducts by tumor mass may easily be assessed by hepato–biliary scan. Also, cystic duct obstruction is detected with great sensitivity using this technique.

However, it must be remembered that the cause of obstruction is not indicated by an abnormal hepato–biliary scan. Also, it must be emphasized that this modality has not been used frequently in the evaluation of liver tumors. Ultrasound and CT usually provide more accurate anatomic information and again the use of the colloid liver scan is a very simple method of quickly producing the same information.

GALLIUM IMAGING

Radionuclide gallium liver scanning may be useful in the diagnosis of hepatoma. Typically the colloid liver scan is abnormal with a photopenic lesion or lesions, typically involving at least the right lobe. Gallium scans are abnormal in the great majority of hepatomas. The increased gallium activity of the tumor will correspond to the decreased activity due to displacement of Kupffer cells by tumor.

The combination of gallium and colloid scan abnormalities described may also, but not commonly, be seen with metastases to the liver from malignancies of the lung, breast, hypernephroma, Hodgkin's disease, et al. the remainder of the clinical picture usually serves to limit the differential diagnosis.

CONCLUSIONS

In clinical practice, a simple repeatable investigation for early diagnosis of liver tumors and for following these tumors to ascertain response to therapy, is scintiscanning or radionuclide hepatic imaging. This investigation, being simple, is recommended as a first step. Sometimes, it needs to be supported by further investigations but exciting changes are becoming more widespread with the use of computer enhancement of these scintiscanning techniques. Indeed, the SPECT imaging method may become the preferred method for following hepatic tumors.

It is also advocated that as detailed a report as possible is always provided for the clinician. These details should include, whenever possible, exact anatomic details of the positions of the liver tumors, whether in right or left lobes and whether anterior or posterior and should also include the number of individual tumors seen. Clinicians find it relatively simple to visualize the tumor in the patient when observing the hepato–biliary scan but have more difficulty in comprehending ultrasound scans and sometimes also CT scans. Consequently, the aim of the nuclear medical physician should be to provide the clinician with information that is otherwise unobtainable.

REFERENCES

1. Rollo, FD, DeLand, FH: The determination of liver mass from radionuclide images. *Radiology, 91:*1191–1194, 1968.

2. Lee, VW, O'Brien, MJ, Morris, PM, *et al.*: The specific diagnosis of hepatocellular carcinoma by scintigraphy. Multiple radiotracer approach. *Cancer, 56:*25–36, 1985.

3. Wasylewski, AH, Fürst, G, Schmitt, G: Liver uptake of a 99mm Tc labelled diphosphonate (DPD) by metastatic lesions from large bowel carcinoma. *Eur J Nucl Med, 10:*467–468, 1985.

4. Evans, RA, Blank, KI, McMurtrey, MJ, Ballantyne, AJ: Radionuclide scans not indicated for clinical stage I melanoma. *Surg Gynecol Obstet, 150:* 532–534, 1980.

5. Strauss, LG, Clorius, JH, Frank, T, van Kaick, G: Single photon emission computerized tomography (SPECT) for estimates of liver and spleen volume. *J Nucl Med, 25:*81–85, 1984.

6. Sheu, JC, Sung, JL, Chen, DS, *et al.*: Early detection of hepatocellular carcinoma by real time ultrasonography. A prospective study, *Cancer, 56:* 660–666, 1985.

7. Fleming, JS, Humphries, NLM, Karran, SJ, *et al.*: In vivo assessment of hepatic arterial and portal venous components of liver perfusion; concise communication. *J Nucl Med, 22:*18–21, 1981.

8. Ricci, OE, Fanfani, S, Calabrò, A, *et al.*: Diagnostic approach to hepatic hemangiomas detected by ultrasound. *Hepato-gastroenterology, 32:* 53–56, 1985.

9. Berche, C, Aubry, F, Langlais, C, *et al.*: Diagnostic value of transverse axis tomoscintigraphy for the detection of hepatic metastases: Results of 53 examinations in comparison with other diagnostic techniques. *Eur J Nucl Med, 6:*435–452, 1981.

10. Britton, KD, Shapiro, B, Elliott, AT: Clinical results in quantitative single photon emission tomography. In: *Arch. Int. Symp. on Medical Radionuclide Imaging* SM-247/2 IAEA, Heidelberg, 1980.

11. Khan, O, Ell, PJ, Jarritt, PH, *et al.*: Comparison between emission and transmission computed tomography of the liver. *Brit Med J, 283:*1212–1214, 1981.

12. Kan, MK, Jopkins, GB: Measurement of liver volume by emission computed tomography. *J Nucl Med, 20:*514–520, 1979.

MARVIN WEINGARTEN, M.D.

CHAPTER 4
Computed Tomography

Since it was first introduced in 1974, Computed Tomography (CT) has been utilized in the evaluation of hepatic pathology (3, 4, 73, 75). The many advances in technology that have taken place since then now allow us to routinely obtain high resolution motionless images of the liver. CT, ultrasonography and radionuclide scintigraphy are all utilized in the evaluation of focal hepatic masses. CT is the most sensitive of these modalities. The accuracy of CT varies with the nature of the equipment and the technique used. Generally, it has an accuracy of greater than 90% and has been shown to have a lesion detection rate as high as 98% (19, 21, 43).

CT of the liver has two significant roles, the detection of lesions and differential diagnosis among them. Although certain entities have been shown to have fairly characteristic features, the diagnostic specificity of CT is still quite limited. The major role of hepatic CT is thus the detection of lesions and an accurate evaluation of their extent.

ANATOMY

Accurate CT evaluation of the liver is based on a detailed knowledge of its normal anatomy. Superiorly the liver is convex occupying the entire right upper quadrant. The caudal surface is concave with indentations formed by the kidney and gall bladder. The hepatic volume gradually diminishes caudally and the liver takes a more anterior and lateral position. There is considerable variation in the size and shape of the liver. The right lobe is generally larger than the left lobe. Reidel's lobe is an uncommon bulbous extension of the right lobe caudally which generally occurs in women. The left lobe is more inconsistent in shape. It may be very thin from front to back and may extend well across the midline into the left upper quandrant even as far as the left lateral abdominal wall. In others the left lobe, particularly its lateral segment, may be quite bulbous.

The normal liver parenchyma is homogeneous with a density greater than the kidneys and pancreas and equal to or slightly greater than the spleen. The intrahepatic vasculature is less dense than liver parenchyma (Figure 4.1). This relationship is reversed with intravenous contrast administration (Figure 4.2) as well as in cases of fatty infiltration of the liver (Figure 4.3). The gall bladder is an oval cystic water density structure seen on the caudal surface of the liver (Figure 4.4e). Occasionally invaginations of the diaphragm may cause pseudotumors or accessory fissures of the liver; this is particularly common along the superior and lateral surface of the right lobe (9).

The lobar and segmental anatomy of the liver is determined on the basis of blood supply. The liver is divided into right, left and caudate lobes. The right lobe is further divided into anterior and posterior segments while the left lobe is divided into medial and lateral segments. These divisions can be demonstrated by CT (68, 72) (Figure 4.4). The intersegmental fissures are identified on CT by the hepatic veins as well as certain other anatomic landmarks. On cephalad sections all three hepatic veins can be seen joining the inferior vena cava (IVC) (Figure 4.4a). The right hepatic vein (RHV) defines the right intersegmental fissure, a coronal

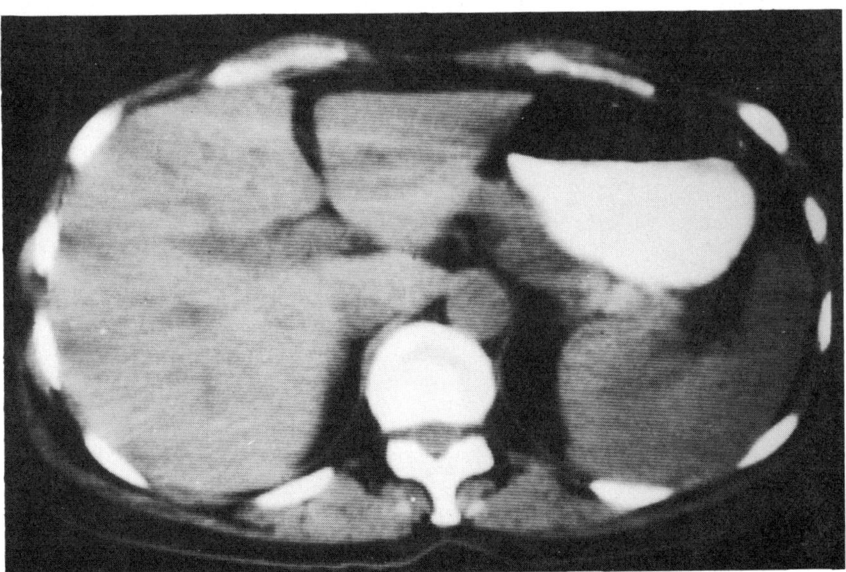

Figure 4.1. Normal liver without intravenous contrast. The intrahepatic vessels are lucent relative to liver parenchyma.

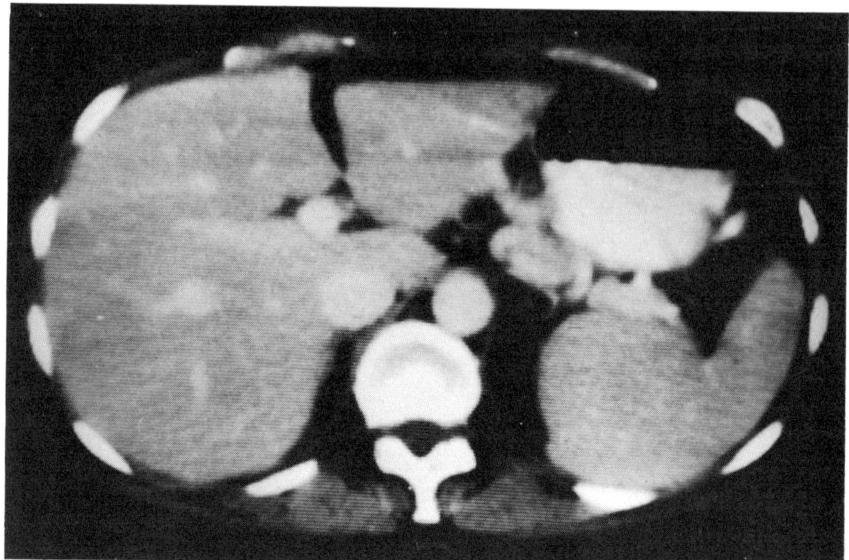

Figure 4.2. Normal liver after intravenous contrast. The intrahepatic vessels are denser than the liver parenchyma.

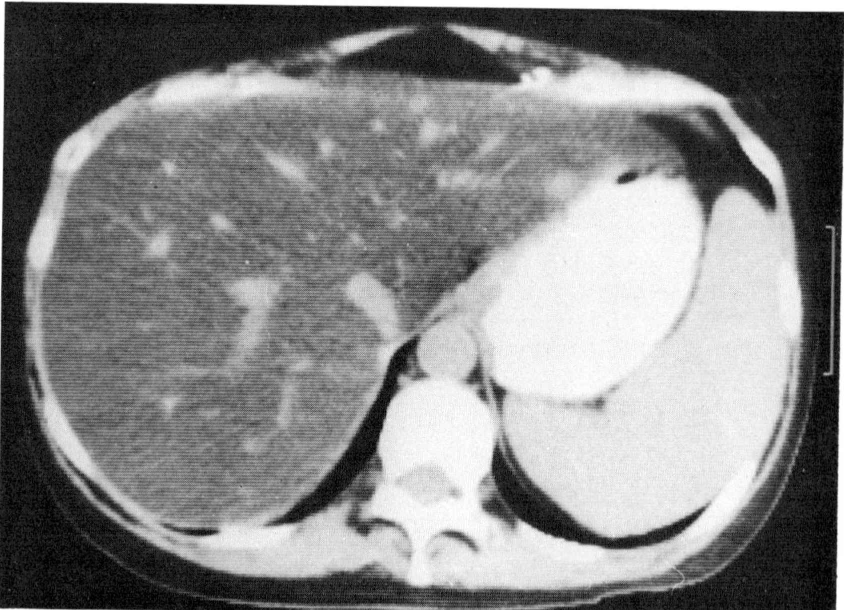

Figure 4.3. Fatty infiltration of the liver. The intrahepatic vessels are hyperdense to liver parenchyma without intravenous contrast.

plane separating the anterior and posterior segments of the right lobe. Superiorly the RHV runs obliquely medially and cephalad as it enters the IVC laterally on the right (Figure 4.4a). Inferiorly it has a nearly vertical course appearing as a round structure on CT as it is cut in cross-section (Figure 4.4b, c, d). The main interlobar fissure separating the right and left lobes is defined on cephalad sections by drawing a line from the IVC to the middle hepatic vein (MHV) (Figure 4.4a, b, c). The MHV has an oblique caudal-cephalic course entering the IVC antero-laterally on the right. On more caudal sections the main interlobar fissure is identified by a line extending from the IVC through a cleft at the neck of the gall bladder (Figure 4.4d) and even more inferiorly through the gall bladder fossa (Figure 4.4e). The left intersegmental fissure is a sagittal plane which separates the medial and lateral segments of the left lobe. On cephalad sections it is identified by the left

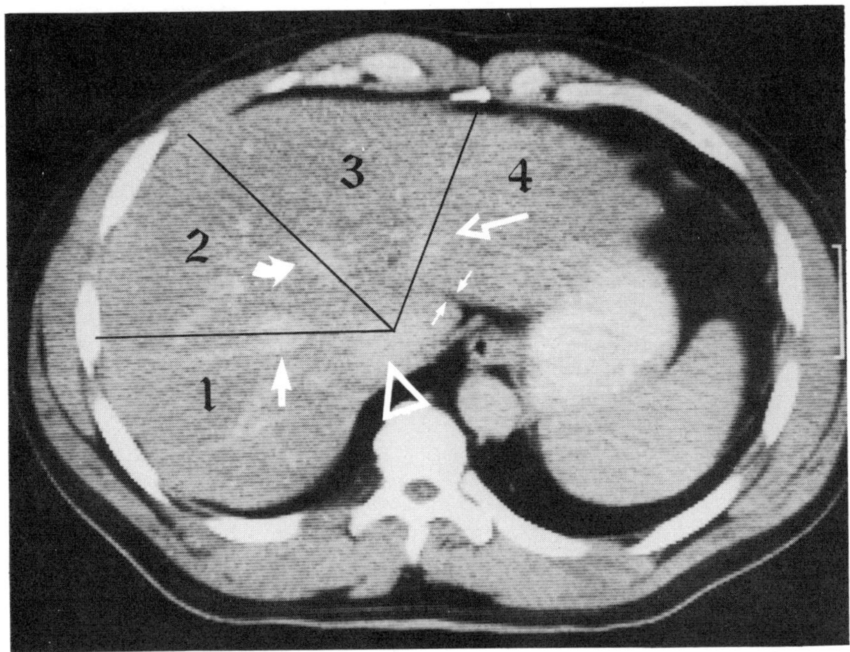

Figure 4.4 (A-E). Segmental hepatic anatomy.
(A) RHV (straight arrow), MHV (curved arrow), LHV (open arrow) divide the hepatic segments. 1-Posterior segment, right lobe, 2-Anterior segment, right lobe, 3-Medial segment, left lobe, 4-Lateral segment, left lobe. The caudate lobe lies anterior to IVC (arrowhead) and posterior to FLV (small arrows) which separates it from the lateral segment of the left lobe.

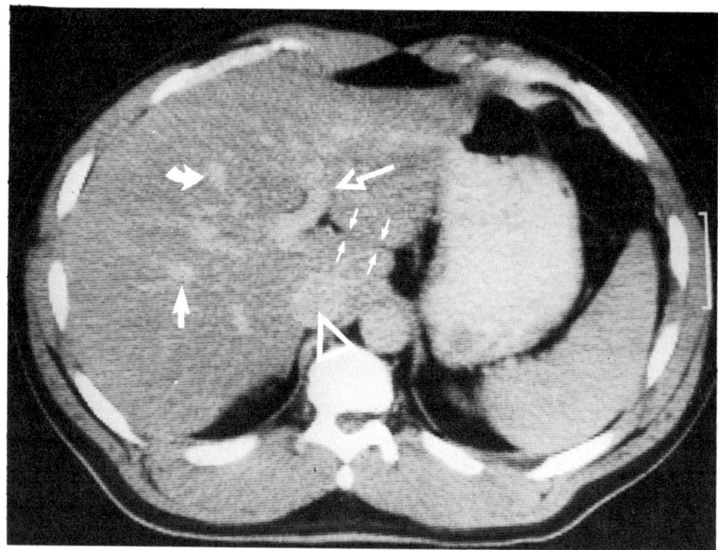

Figure 4.4(B). RHV (straight arrow) MHV (curved arrow), LPV (open arrow) divide the hepatic segments. FLV (small arrows) and IVC (arrowhead) border the caudate lobe.

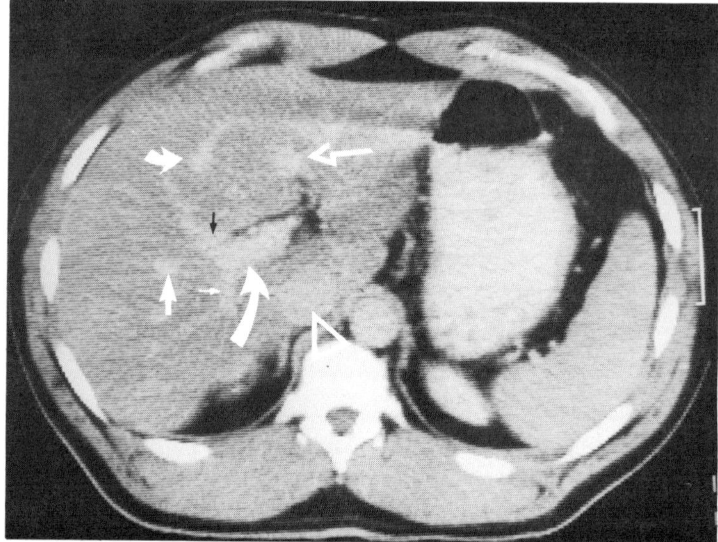

Figure 4.4(C). RHV (straight arrow), MHV (curved arrow), LPV (open arrow) divide hepatic segments. RPV (large curved arrow) divides into anterior segmental branch (small black arrow) and posterior segment branch (small white arrow) indicating the lateral extent of the caudate lobe. IVC (arrowhead).

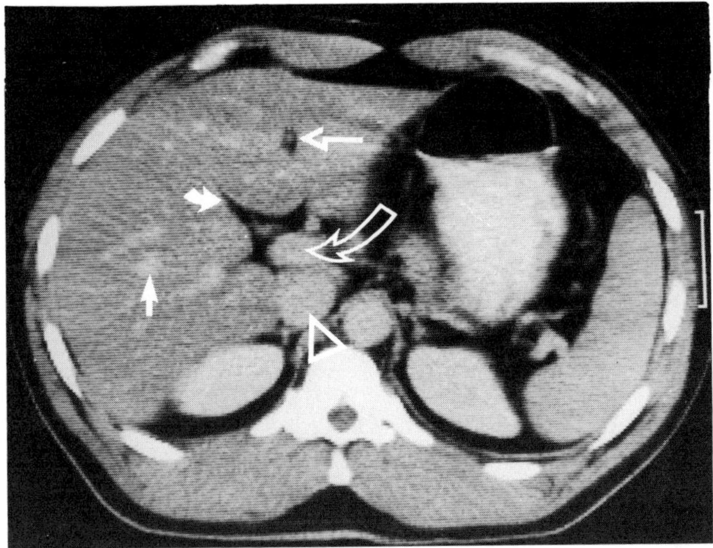

Figure 4.4(D). RHV (straight arrow), cleft at gall bladder neck (white curved arrow), FLT (open arrow) divide the hepatic segments. Main portal vein (open curved arrow), IVC (open arrowhead).

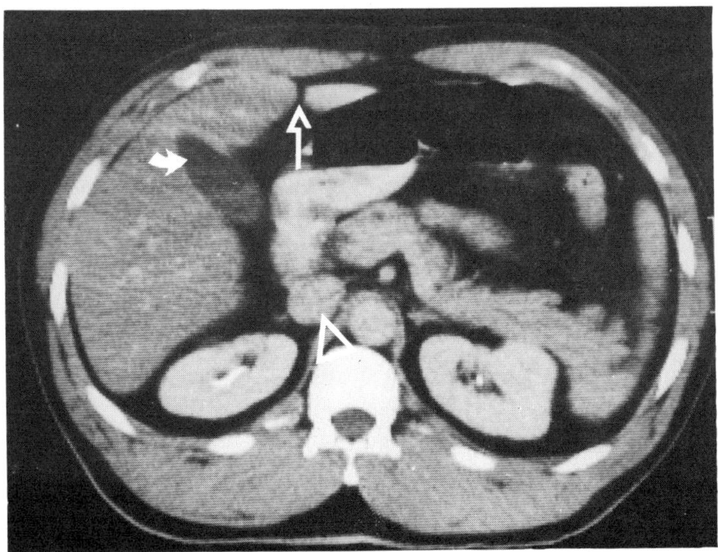

Figure 4.4(E). Gall bladder (curved arrow), FLT (open arrow), IVC, (open arrowhead).

hepatic vein (LHV) (Figure 4.4a). More caudally the left portal vein (LPV) marks the fissure (Figure 4.4b, c). Even further caudally the left lobe is divided by the fissure for the ligamentum teres (FLT), an intrahepatic extension of the falciform ligament containing the obliterated umbilical vein (Figure 4.4c, d). The caudate lobe is posterior lying between the IVC posteriorly and portal vein anteriorly. The majority of its volume is cephalic to the main portal vein and is separated anteriorly from the left lobe by the fissure for the ligamentum venosum (FLV) (Figure 4.4a, b). The lateral extent of the caudate lobe is marked by the margin of the FLV and more inferiorly by the lateral extent of the right portal vein where it divides into anterior and posterior segmental branches (Figure 4.4c). Occasionally a thin inferior extension, the papillary process, may appear as a structure separate from the liver between the IVC and portal vein (8).

The portal vein is formed posterior to the head of the pancreas by the union of the splenic vein and superior mesenteric

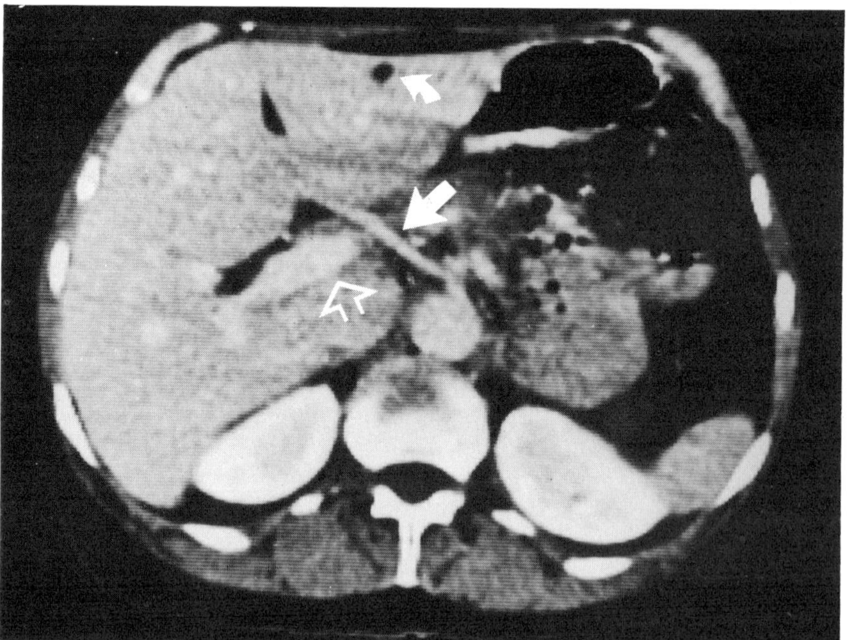

Figure 4.5. Hepatic artery (white arrow) anterior to main portal vein (open arrow) in the porta hepatis. Incidental simple cyst in the lateral segment of the left lobe (curved arrow).

vein. It then takes an oblique cephalad course within the hepato-duodenal ligament to enter the porta hepatis where is bifurcates into left and right branches. The main portal vein is posterior to the main hepatic artery (Figure 4.5) Occasionally the right hepatic artery arises from the superior mesenteric artery in which case it enters the liver by passing posterior to the portal vein and anterior to the IVC (Figure 4.6). The right portal vein runs horizontally to the right where it divides into anterior and posterior segmental branches (Figure 4.4c). The left portal vein turns anteriorly to the left to enter the left intersegmental fissure and then turns cephalad giving off branches to the medial and lateral segments (Figure 4.4b). Both left and right portal veins give off multiple small branches to the caudate lobe. Unlike the hepatic veins, the portal veins are within and not between the hepatic parenchymal segments, the exception being the intersegmental portion of the left portal vein. The hepatic arteries parallel the portal veins within the liver but are generally not identifiable by CT. The biliary tree also travels with the portal veins completing the portal triad. Normal sized intrahepatic biliary ducts are generally not visualized using CT.

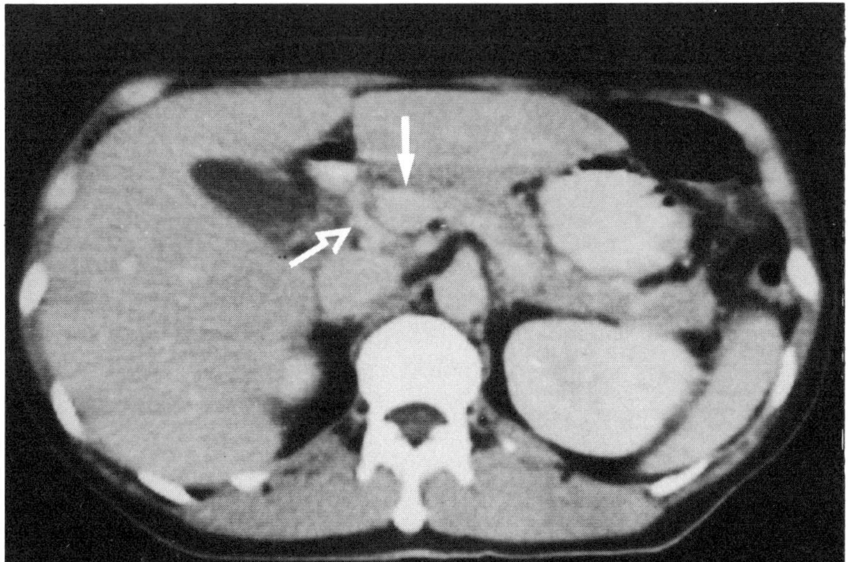

Figure 4.6. Right hepatic artery (open arrow) arising from superior mesenteric artery coursing posterior to the portal vein (white arrow).

TECHNIQUE

CT detection of a focal intrahepatic mass depends primarily on a difference in attenuation between the lesion and adjacent hepatic parenchyma. The smaller the size of the lesion the greater the attenuation difference must be. Plain or non-contrast CT relies on the inherent difference in density between normal and abnormal tissue. Nearly all masses, except those which are calcified, are hypodense relative to normal liver parenchyma (Figure 4.7). In cases of fatty infiltration of the liver masses may appear isodense or hyperdense (Figure 4.8). Several strategies to increase the tumor:organ attenuation difference have been devised most of which involve the administration of intravascular urographic contrast media. One may enhance the normal tissue so that tumors appear hypodense, or enhance the tumor tissue so it appears hyperdense. The differential enhancement of tumor vs. organ depends on the method of contrast administration as well as the timing of the scans obtained.

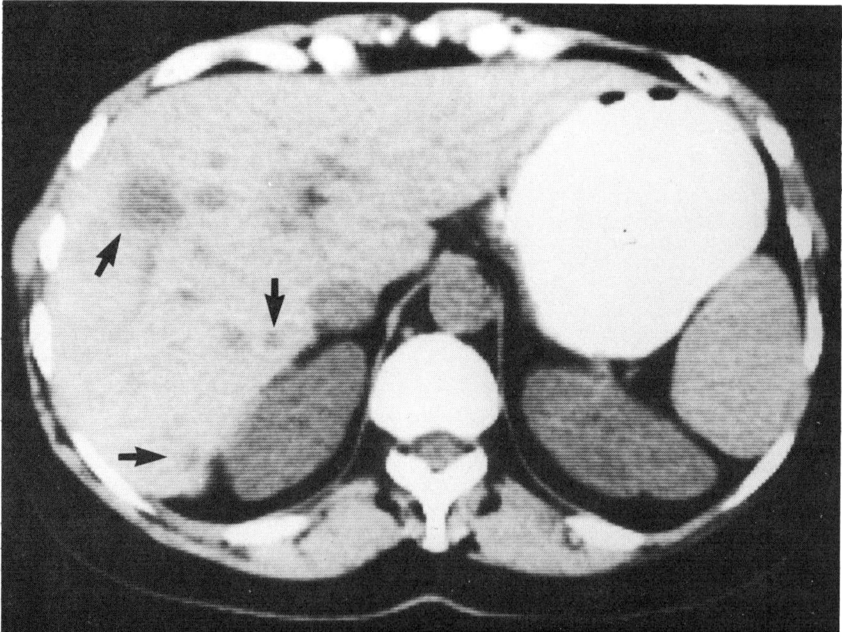

Figure 4.7. Scan without intravenous contrast: hypodense liver metastases (arrows) from breast carcinoma.

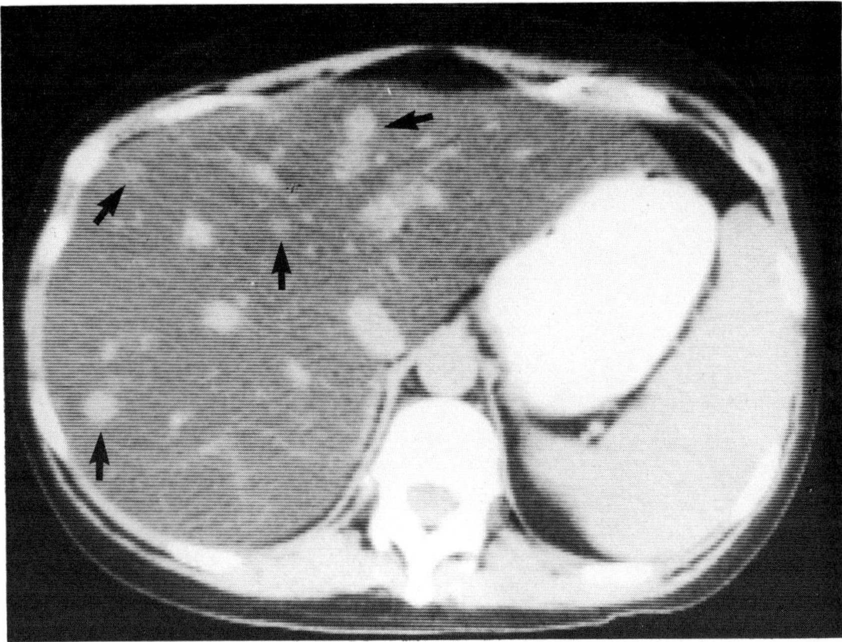

Figure 4.8. Scan without intravenous contrast: liver metastases from endo-metrial carcinoma (arrows) appearing hyperdense because of fatty infiltra-tion of the liver.

Intravenous Contrast

Urographic contrast may be given intravenously as a bolus or by drip infusion technique. Intravenous infusion is the least logical method of contrast administration (19). Both normal and abnormal tissue will be enhanced and the resultant effect on the relative tumor:organ attenuation difference is unpredictable. In a study comparing pre-contrast scans with scans obtained after intravenous contrast infusion Moss *et al.* found that 13% of lesions were seen only on the pre-contrast examination while only 3% were seen exclusively on the post-contrast scans and 58% were seen equally well both before and after contrast infusion (64). This is the least sensitive technique of contrast enhancement for lesion detection and is not recommended for evaluation of the liver. However, it is widely used because of its relative ease and simplicity.

It is now well established that bolus administration of intra-venous contrast is the method of choice for enhancement of the liver (14, 15, 27, 62). The maximum tumor:organ attenuation difference occurs in the two minutes immediately following an intravenous bolus of urographic contrast. The attenuation difference diminishes over the next few minutes as both tumor and normal tissue reach a similar plateau of density. Lesion detectability is, therefore, greatest during the immediate post–bolus period.

Software currently available allows a rapid sequence of scans to be obtained in a short period of time. Sequential Bolus Dynamic Incremental CT (SBDICT) utilizes this ability to maximize the sensitivity of CT in detecting focal lesions of the liver. Following an intravenous bolus of urographic contrast a rapid series of scans is obtained at contiguous anatomic levels during suspended respiration. The patient is then allowed to breathe, a repeat bolus is administered and another series of scans is obtained. The entire liver can usually be examined with three to four boluses. This is the most sensitive method for lesion detection in an overall screening survey of the liver (Figure 4.13). Unlike the infusion technique this takes full advantage of differential tumor:organ enhancement. In addition, the variability between patient respirations which may plague both non–contrast and infusion scan techniques is eliminated since each scan series is obtained during suspended respiration.

Rapid sequence scanning at a single anatomic level following a bolus of intravenous contrast is called Bolus Dynamic Non–Incremental CT (BDNCT). Although not a useful technique for an overall survey of the liver this can be utilized to evaluate the enhancement of a particular lesion during the different phases of circulation. Initially, this was thought to have great promise in increasing the diagnostic specificity of CT (7). However, tumors of varying histology may have similar enhancement patterns and separate tumor sites of like histology may behave differently (6, 16). Nevertheless, certain lesions such as cavernous hemangiomas have been shown to enhance in a characteristic fashion often allowing a specific diagnosis to be made. In addition, this technique may be applied prior to fine needle aspiration biopsy to avoid inadvertent biopsy of highly vascular lesions.

Intra–arterial Contrast

The liver receives approximately 75% of its blood supply

from the portal venous system. While some portal supply to hepatic neoplasms has been shown to exist, nearly all of the perfusion to tumors, both primary and metastatic, comes from the hepatic artery (1, 13, 49, 50). On rapid sequence scans obtained during injection of an angiographic catheter placed in the proper hepatic artery tumor tissue appears as intensely enhancing hyperdense masses relative to the normal parenchyma which receives mainly unopacified portal venous blood (20, 28, 62, 66, 69). This technique, which is extremely sensitive in lesion detection, is known as CT Arteriography (CTA). Freeny and Marks found that 55% of patients felt to have resectable disease on the basis of Sequential Bolus Dynamic Incremental CT had additional lesions which rendered their disease unresectable when examined using CTA (28) (Figure 4.14). However, this procedure is limited in application because of the frequent variations in hepatic arterial anatomy. The entire liver cannot be evaluated, for example, when the right hepatic artery arises from the superior mesenteric artery, a common variation. Furthermore, it can be confusing and difficult to interpret. Patients with cirrhosis exhibit a generalized patchy pattern of enhancement and small peripheral vessels may be difficult to distinguish from tumors (19).

The problems encountered with CTA are obviated by a technique called CT Arterial Portography (CTAP). Contrast is slowly infused through an angiographic catheter in the superior mesenteric artery. Following a 20–30 second delay after the start of the infusion, rapid sequence scans at contiguous anatomic levels are performed throughout the extent of the liver while the catheter infusion continues. The liver is thus examined during the portal venous phase. Normal parenchyma is maximally enhanced with only negligible enhancement of tumors and all tumors appear hypodense (19, 57) (Figures 4.15 and 4.16).

In a study of hepatocellular carcinoma, Nakao and coworkers found that detection of a lesion, particularly a small lesion, was more sensitive and easier with CTAP than with CTA (66). Matsui and colleagues were able to visualize lesions as small as 5 mm and found this to be the most sensitive technique of detecting hepatic lesions (57). Unlike CTA, with CTAP the entire liver can be examined in all patients regardless of their hepatic arterial anatomy by placing the catheter tip distal to any aberrant hepatic arterial supply. It also avoids the potential interpretive pitfalls of CTA.

Intravenous Iodolipids

Hepatosplenic specific iodolipid contrast media are presently being developed and evaluated (47, 58, 59, 80). Unlike the urographic contrast agents iodolipids localize exclusively in the hepatic and splenic reticuloendothelial systems and are retained there for an extended period. This eliminates the problem of the timing of the scans. Since only normal liver parenchyma is enhanced, the tumor:organ attenuation difference is maximized. However, there are drawbacks to the use of these agents. They must be administered slowly over a period of 20-60 minutes, are as entirely non-specific as radionuclide particulate agents, provide no information about lesion vascularity, are difficult to manufacture, and lastly are more toxic than the common urographic agents. Nevertheless, they do have great promise for increasing the sensitivity of CT in detecting focal hepatic masses. As of yet, they are not commercially available.

RADIOGRAPHIC FEATURES

CT of liver tumors is a highly sensitive but largely non-specific imaging modality. Most tumors appear as hypodense masses in the liver. Occasionally they may contain calcifications but in general the pattern of calcification is non-specific and does not aid in the differential diagnosis (71). Correlation with other imaging modalities may allow a specific diagnosis to be made. When necessary, CT guided percutaneous fine needle biopsy is a safe procedure yielding excellent diagnostic results (5, 55).

BENIGN TUMORS

Cavernous Hemangioma

Cavernous hemangioma is the most common benign tumor of the liver. It occurs more often in women than men, 4.5 to 1. Patients are typically asymptomatic and the mass is an incidental finding. It is usually solitary and is most commonly found in the posterior aspect of the right lobe. The majority are less than 5 cm in diameter. This is one of the few entities with specific characteristic features allowing the diagnosis to be made on CT in greater than 90% of cases (10, 29, 39, 41, 42, 60, 74). On non-contrast scans cavernous hemangioma is a well defined hypodense lesion indistinguishable from other solid benign and malignant masses. When evaluated using Bolus Dynamic Non–Incremental CT it will typically show early intense enhancement at its periphery which exceeds that of normal liver parenchyma. Delayed sequential scans show progressive centripetally advancing enhancement as the hypodense center becomes smaller (Figure 4.9). The margins of a cavernous hemangioma often become isodense to liver parenchyma on delayed scans making the entire lesion appear smaller. After contrast washout it returns to its original pre-contrast appearance. Hemangiomas typically remain hyperdense for prolonged periods of time indicating the slow transit of contrast that is seen on angiography. Smaller lesions may exhibit early diffuse or inhomogeneous enhancement rather than peripheral enhancement eventually becoming completely isodense to normal hepatic parenchyma on delayed scans, even after several

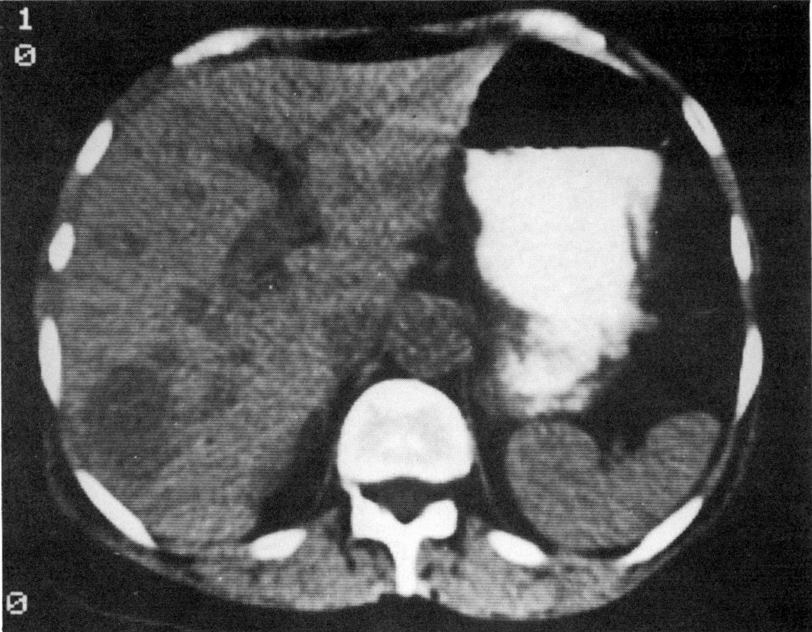

Figure 4.9 (A-D). Cavernous hemangioma with typical centripetally advancing enhancement (BDNCT).
(A) Prior to IV contrast there is a well-defined hypodense mass in the posterior segment of the right lobe.

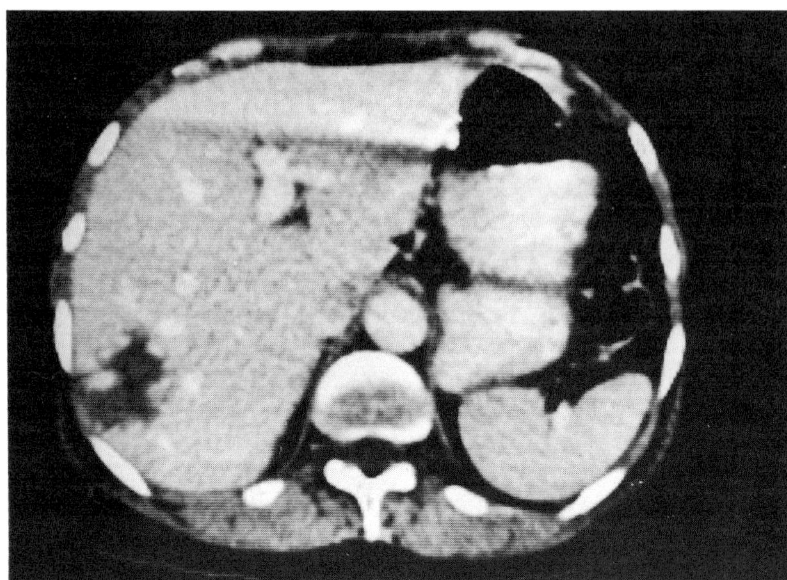

Figure 4.9 (B). 30 seconds after a bolus of intravenous contrast there is a discrete ring of peripheral enhancement at the margins of the lesion.

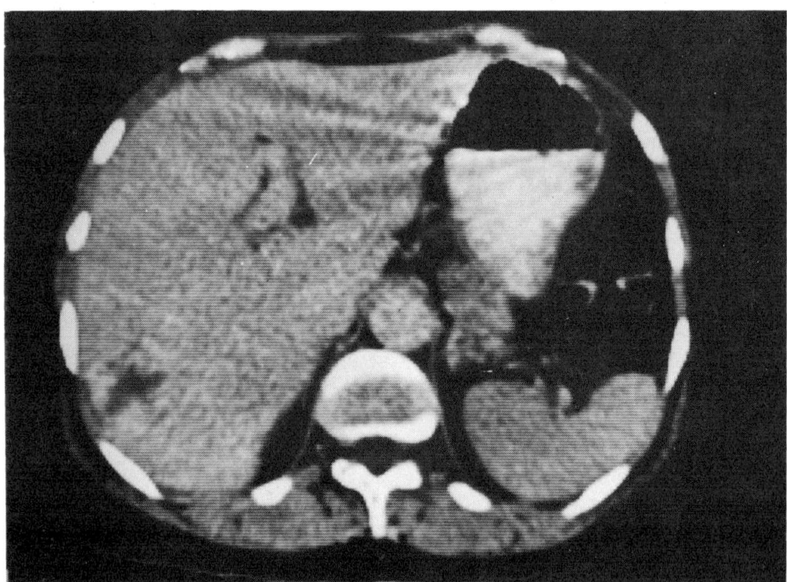

Figure 4.9 (C). 2 minutes following the bolus there is thickening of the rim of enhancement as the hypodense center appears smaller.

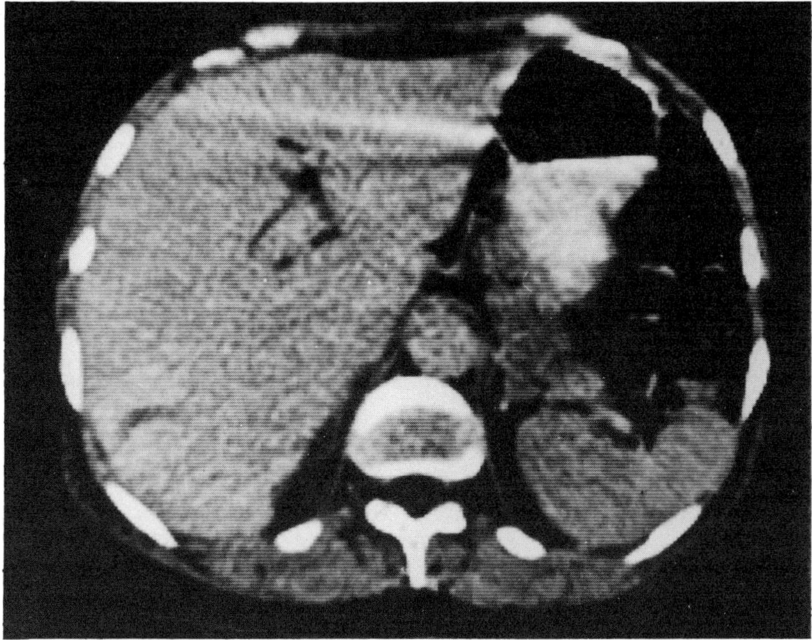

Figure 4.9 (D). 4 minutes after the bolus there is further progression of the enhancement.

minutes, allowing them to be distinguished from other masses which generally do not display such protracted enhancement (60).

Hepatic Adenoma

Hepatic adenoma is a benign well–encapsulated tumor composed exclusively of hepatocytes without Kupffer cells or bile ducts. It is usually a solitary lesion occurring in young women taking oral contraceptives. Clinically patients may present with severe abdominal pain as a result of spontaneous hemorrhage which can sometimes be fatal. The CT appearance is generally non–specific (19, 60, 74). On non–contrast scans hepatic adenoma is a solid hypodense mass. When seen immediately after an acute hemorrhage an hepatic adenoma may exhibit a hyperdense center on non–contrast scans secondary to freshly clotted blood, an appearance some authors consider diagnostic (26, 74). When the hemorrhagic episode is temporally remote the center appears hypodense and the lesion is no longer distinguishable from other masses. Evaluation with Bolus Dynamic Non–Incremental CT shows variable degrees of transient enhancement. It is important to differentiate hepatic adenoma from focal nodular hyperplasia because of the propensity of hepatic adenomas to spontaneously bleed.

Focal Nodular Hyperplasia

Focal Nodular Hyperplasia (FNH) is a rare non–encapsulated but well circumscribed benign mass composed of variable numbers of hepatocytes, Kupffer cells, and proliferating bile ducts. Grossly there is usually a central stellate scar with peripherally radiating septae. However, this is not a constant feature. FNH is more common in women than men 4 to 1. It is not related to oral contraceptive use and spontaneous hemorrhage is rare. Typically it is 4 to 7 cm in diameter and is solitary although it can be multiple in 20% of cases. Patients are usually asymptomatic and the mass is discovered incidentally. The CT appearance is often non–specific (19, 60, 70, 74). On non–contrast scans it is a solid hypodense mass. Using Bolus Dynamic Non–Incremental CT FNH exhibits transient intense diffuse enhancement. In some cases the central stellate scar can be seen as a hypodense area and the diagnosis can be made (26, 74). In most cases, FNH can be diagnosed by correlating the CT with radionuclide colloid scintigraphy (60, 70, 74). FNH usually accumulates colloid normally because it contains Kupffer cells. In 35% of cases, however, it may appear as a photopenic region. A focal mass greater than 2 to 3 cm in diameter which exhibits intense enhancement of BDNCT together with a normal radionuclide colloid scintiscan is diagnostic of FNH.

Biliary Cystadenoma

Biliary cystadenoma is a rare benign tumor arising from intrahepatic bile ducts. It is usually found in middle–aged women presenting with a painful epigastric mass often with intermittent jaundice. The findings on CT correlate well with the gross morphologic appearance (25, 30). It is seen as a large predominantly cystic mass with thick walls, internal septations and mural nodules. The mural nodules and septations enhance and are, therefore, more easily appreciated after intravenous contrast administration. The biliary tree may be dilated as a result of compression by the mass.

Occasionally a biliary cystadenoma may communicate with the biliary duct system which may then appear dilated because of excessive formation of mucinous material by the cystadenoma. Biliary cystadenoma cannot be reliably differentiated from other cystic masses including parasitic cysts, necrotic metastases, and biliary cystadenocarcinoma (25, 30). Fine needle aspiration may be necessary. However, it is usually easily distinguished from simple hepatic cysts using CT. Simple hepatic cysts appear as sharply defined, thin-walled, non-septated, homogeneous water density masses that exhibit no enhancement (Figures 4.5 and 4.10). Ultrasonography may be helpful in some cases since it is particularly good for defining septations, wall thickness, and mural nodules in cystic masses (25).

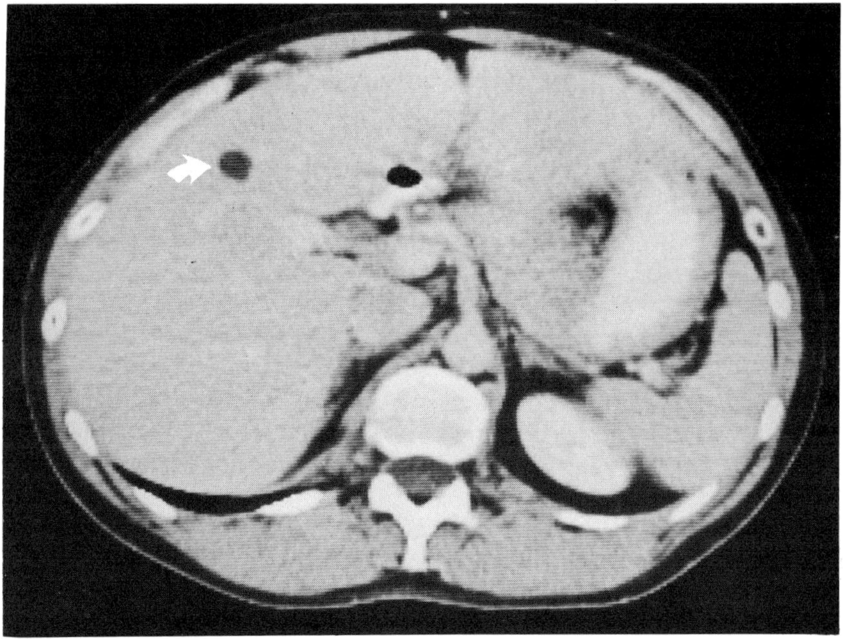

Figure 4.10. Simple hepatic cyst (arrow); the margins are sharp and well defined. The cyst contents have density characteristics of water.

Biliary cystadenocarcinoma is a rare malignant tumor thought to arise from malignant transformation of a biliary cystadenoma. The CT features are a large, multi-loculated, predominantly cystic mass with thick walls, internal septations and prominent internal papillary projections (19, 38, 60) (Figure 4.11). This is often indistinguishable from benign biliary cystadenoma as well as several other cystic masses, both neoplastic and non-neoplastic. Histological evaluation is required for diagnosis.

PRIMARY MALIGNANT TUMORS

Hepatocellular Carcinoma (Hepatoma)

Hepatocellular carcinoma is the most common primary malignant tumor of the liver. There is a high association of hepatocellular carcinoma with underlying liver disease, such as cirrhosis or hemochromatosis. There is also an increased incidence in Orientals and patients with positive HBsAG levels. Hepatoma is most com-

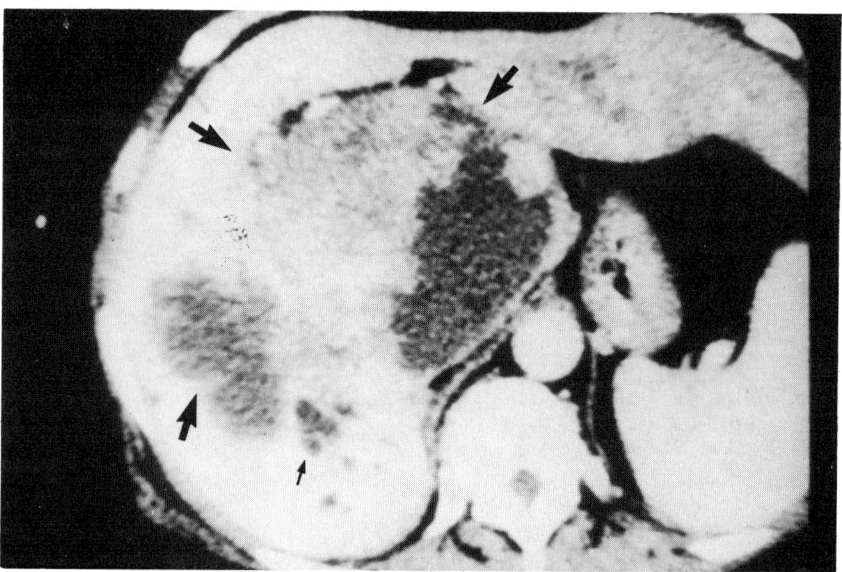

Figure 4.11. Biliary cystadenocarcinoma. Large cystic mass containing prominent internal projections of enhancing tissue (large arrows). Focally dilated bile ducts (small arrows) because of compression by the mass.

monly a solitary mass but it can also occur in a multinodular and a diffuse form. Pathologically it is characterized by a tendency toward vascular invasion of the hepatic veins and portal veins. Morphologic changes of cirrhosis are readily identified on CT (33) and the presence of a large mass in a cirrhotic liver is highly suspicious for hepatocellular carcinoma (60, 74) (Figure 4.12).

Hepatocellular carcinoma has a variable and generally non-specific appearance on CT (19, 24, 37, 40, 44, 60, 74). On non-contrast scans it most often presents as one or a small number of large hypodense inhomogeneous solid masses. Occasionally it may contain areas of calcification. In some cases hepatocellular carcinoma is isodense with normal liver parenchyma on non-contrast scans and its presence is indicated only by deformity of the liver contour. Examination with Sequential Bolus Dynamic Incremental CT usually shows hepatocellular carcinoma as a large hypodense mass. Hepatocellular carcinoma may sometimes become isodense after intravenous contrast. Usually this occurs when contrast is

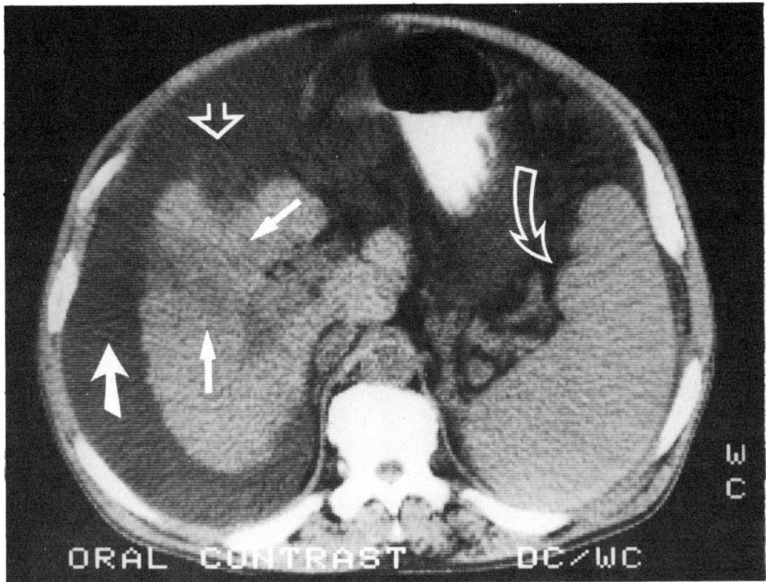

Figure 4.12 (A–C). Hepatocellular carcinoma in a cirrhotic liver.
(A) Before IV contrast: the liver is shrunken and nodular indicating cirrhosis and contains an ill-defined mass (small white arrows). Ascites (large white arrow), gall bladder (straight open arrow), large spleen (curved open arrow).

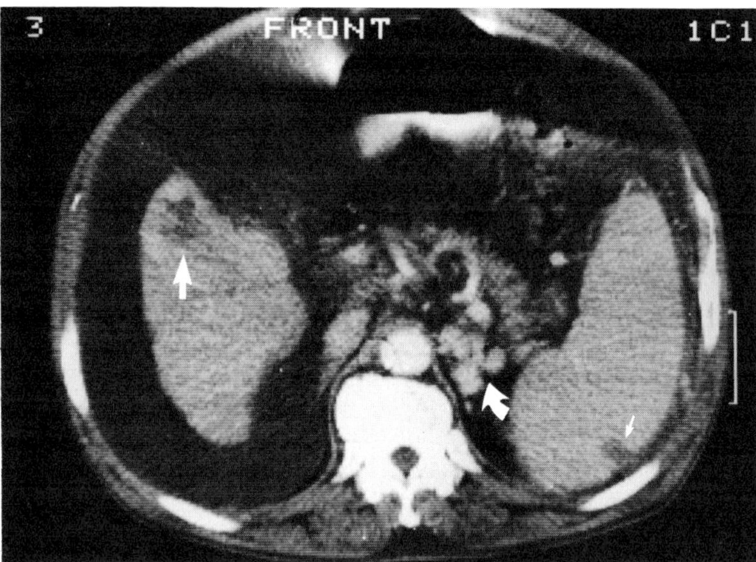

Figure 4.12 (B). After IV contrast: the mass is again seen (straight arrow). There is non-opacification of the right portal vein (curved arrow) as a result of tumor involvement.

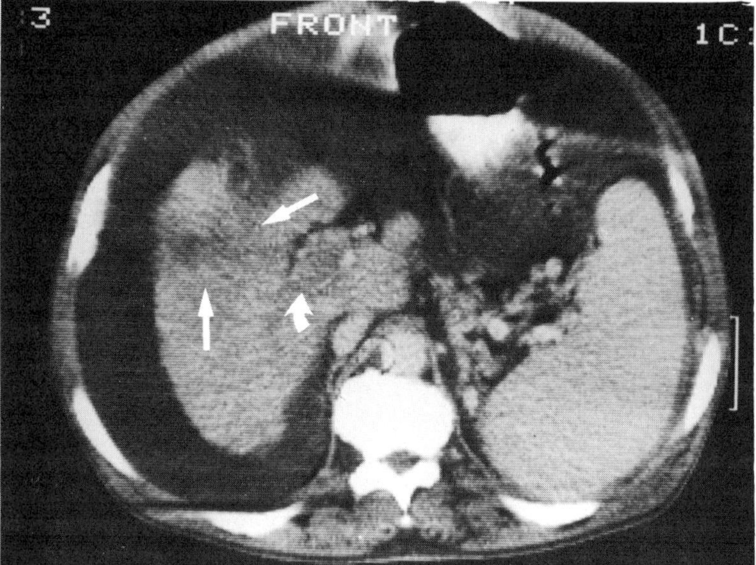

Figure 4.12 (C). More caudal section showing the mass (straight arrow). Note the retroperitoneal varices (curved arrow) and incidental splenic infarct (small arrow).

administered as an infusion. Even when contrast is given in bolus fashion hepatocellular carcinoma may infrequently become isodense; however, it will not be isodense both prior to and following an intravenous bolus of contrast. Therefore, both non–contrast scans and SBDICT are suggested when examining the liver for possible hepatocellular carcinoma. Bolus Dynamic Non–Incremental CT may be helpful in some cases as well. When examined using BDNCT hepatocellular carcinoma usually enhances intensely in the arterial phase and then becomes hypodense in the portal phase (6, 7, 34, 35, 36, 56, 60, 62, 67, 76). Both SBDICT and BDNCT have been shown to be useful in demonstrating arterial-portal shunting, vascular pooling and portal venous thrombosis, features characteristic of hepatocellular carcinoma and rare in other primary and secondary liver tumors.

Resectability of a hepatoma is determined by the extent of hepatic involvement and the presence or absence of venous invasion and extra–hepatic spread. This assessment is best accomplished with CT (45, 51). The combination of non–contrast scans and SBDICT provides the most detailed and accurate non-invasive evaluation of the intrahepatic extent of the tumor. BDNCT may also be utilized in selected cases when necessary. Portal vein or inferior vena cava occlusion may be detected by the presence of a lucent thrombus within the vascular lumen surrounded by enhancement of the vessel wall. Other signs of portal venous thrombosis are an enlarged portal vein diameter, failure to visualize a lobar or segmental branch of the portal vein, the presence of arterial–portal shunting and lobar or segmental regions of hypodensity in the distribution of an occluded intrahepatic portal vein (22, 34, 35, 56, 57, 67, 76) (Figure 4.11b and 4.17b). Ultrasonography may also be utilized in evaluating hepatocellular carcinoma and is particularly sensitive in detecting vascular involvement by the tumor (45). Distant metastases, such as to lymph nodes or other visceral organs, are most accurately detected by CT.

When the tumor appears to be resectable by these techniques the patient is sent for hepatic angiography followed by CT Arterial Portography. CTAP is the most sensitive technique for detecting intrahepatic lesions and is also the most sensitive means of detecting portal venous involvement (57, 66). All patients considered candidates for potential resection of hepatocellular carcinoma should undergo CTAP pre-operatively.

Cholangiocarcinoma

Cholangiocarcinoma usually develops in the extrahepatic biliary tree, most commonly at the distal common bile duct or at the junction of the right and left hepatic ducts in the porta hepatis. There is also a peripheral type arising from small intrahepatic bile ducts. Cholangiocarcinoma generally occurs in non-cirrhotic livers. It has a known association with chronic ulcerative colitis, Clonorchis sinensis infestation, gallstones and biliary papillomas. The usual clinical presentation is painless jaundice.

The CT features of hepatic cholangiocarcinoma are non-specific (19, 38, 60, 79). The most common finding is local or generalized dilatation of the biliary tree. In some cases dilated ducts may be the only finding on CT without any identifiable mass. However, widespread intraductal extension of tumor may be present microscopically (38). In others, multiple non-specific hypodense masses may be seen that are indistinguishable from metastases or hepatoma (38, 60, 79). Cholangiocarcinoma arising in the porta hepatis frequently invades the liver parenchyma locally presenting on CT as an ill-defined mass that enhances after intravenous contrast. The distinction from hepatoma can usually be made angiographically (60, 79).

SECONDARY MALIGNANT TUMORS
(METASTASES)

Metastases, as a group, are the most common malignant tumors of the liver. CT is the most sensitive technique for detecting liver metastases with an accuracy of greater than 90%. In a recent prospective study comparing CT, ultrasonography and radionuclide scintigraphy CT was found to be the most accurate means of detecting liver metastasis from colon and breast carcinoma with a detection rate of 93% (2). Others have found the rate of detection to be as high as 98% (43). CT with the use of intravenous iodolipids promises to increase the sensitivity even further.

The CT appearance of metastases is non-specific (19, 60, 74). Most metastases appear as solid hypodense masses on both non-contrast and post-contrast scans (Figures 4.7 and 4.13). Some metastases may appear to be cystic because of either tumor necrosis or the mucinous nature of the tumor. Occasionally speckled punctate calcifications may be found particularly in metastases

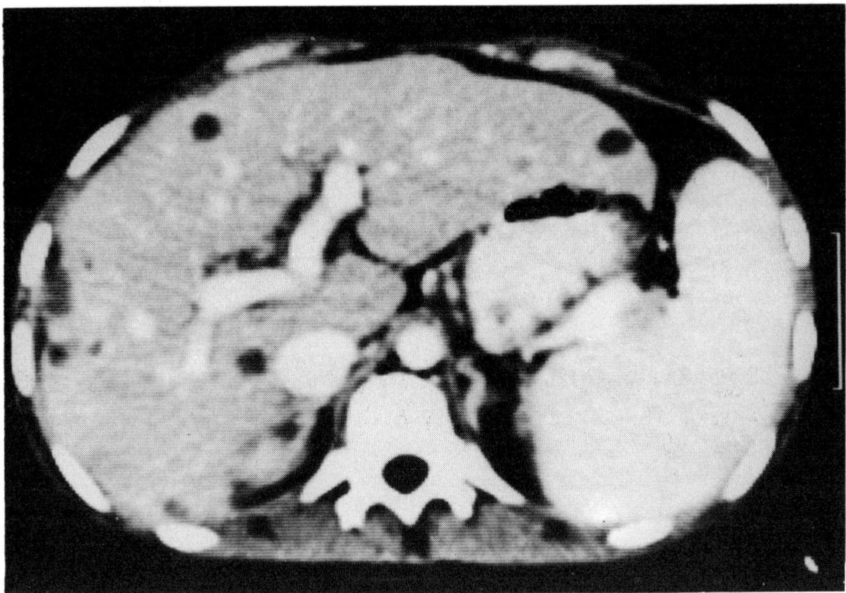

Figure 4.13. Multiple metastases from colon carcinoma involving all hepatic segments. Masses appear hypodense after IV contrast (SBDICT).

from mucin-producing adenocarcinoma of the colon. A few metastases may become isodense after intravenous contrast infusion but this is usually not a problem with Sequential Bolus Dynamic Incremental CT. On Bolus Dynamic Non-Incremental CT some metastases will have an enhancing rim or enhance diffusely. Unlike cavernous hemangioma, however, the enhancement is transient and does not generally persist.

The specific technique used in each case must be tailored to the individual patient. Our general approach is to begin with a non-contrast examination. This aids in detecting fatty infiltration of the liver, particularly focal fatty infiltration, which may confuse interpretation of the post-contrast examination. If the liver appears normal or there is only limited disease we proceed to SBDICT. In cases where only a solitary lesion is found, we evaluate the possibility of cavernous hemangioma with BDNCT. This is performed after allowing a delay for contrast washout.

In patients considered for potential resection of hepatic metastases a detailed evaluation of the extent of disease is essential. In order to be resectable, a tumor must be limited to a single segment or anatomically contiguous resectable segments. After the patient has been evaluated using SBDICT if the disease is considered resectable we proceed to hepatic angiography for a map of the hepatic arterial and venous anatomy followed by CT Arterial Portography. All patients being considered for potential hepatic resection should undergo either CT Arteriography or CT Arterial Portography pre-operatively (Figures 4.14, 4.15, and 4.16). These techniques provide the most sensitive and accurate assessment of the extent of disease and allow the surgeon to take the most appropriate course of action.

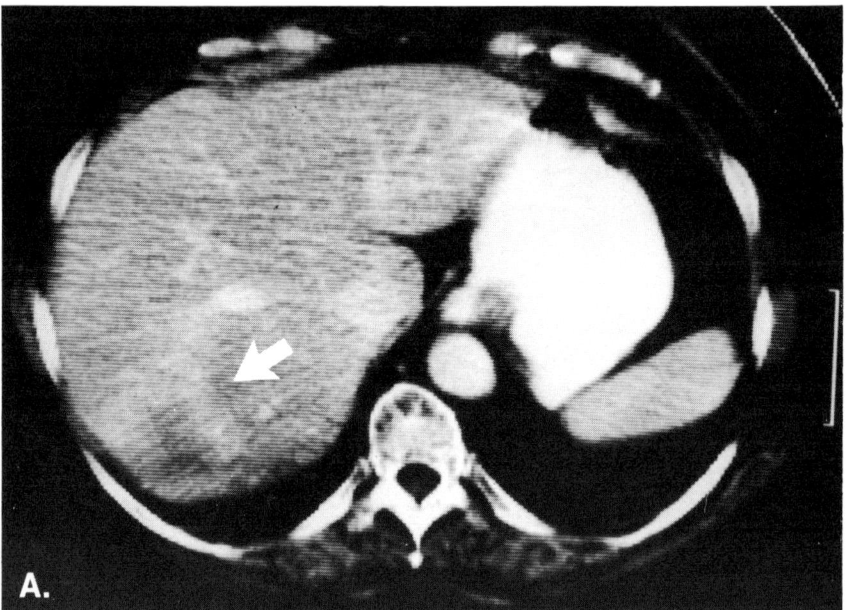

Figure 4.14 (A-D). Patient with colon CA.
(A & B). Using SBDICT a solitary metastasis in the posterior segment of the right lobe is seen (large arrow). The mass is hypodense with a slightly hyperdense rim. Incidental porcelain gall bladder (small arrow).

→

Figure 4.14 (C & D). Using CTA, the mass in the posterior segment of the right lobe appears as an intensely enhancing mass (large arrow). Additional masses are now seen in the anterior segment of the right lobe (open arrow) and the lateral segment of the left lobe (curved arrow) indicating that the disease is not resectable.

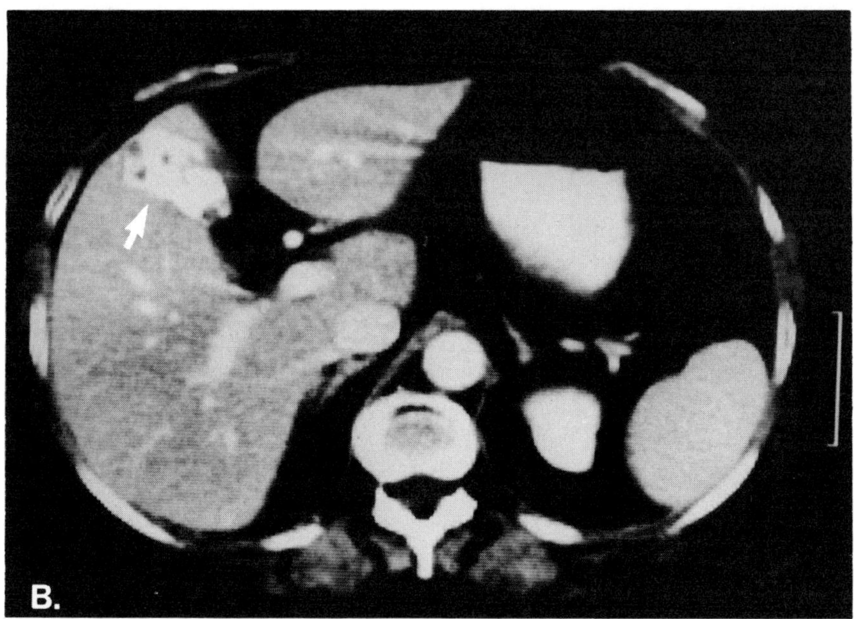

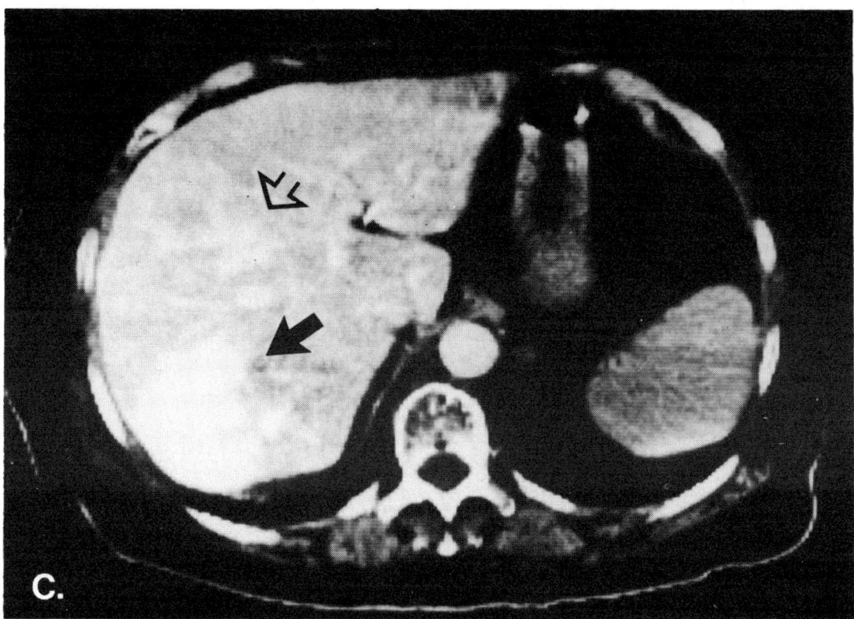

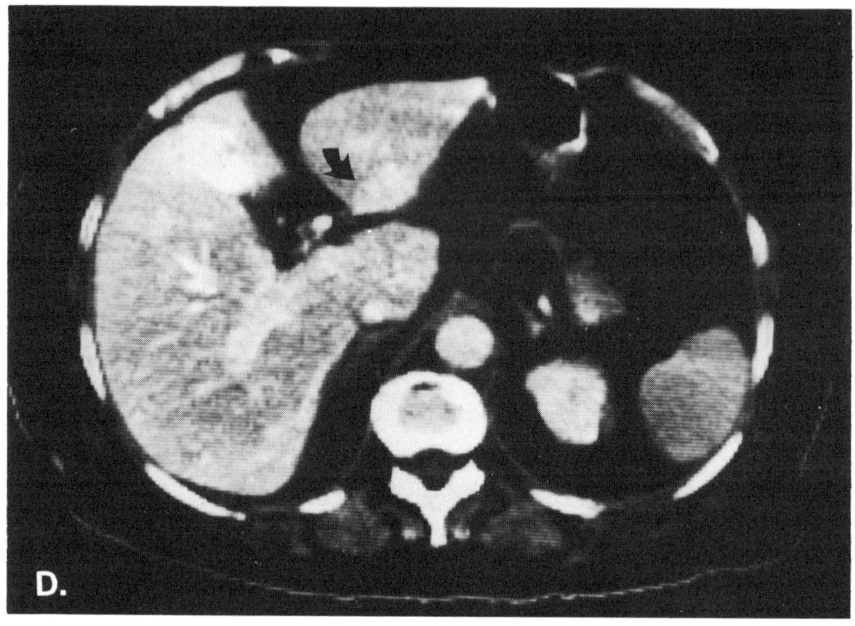

Figure 4.15 (A & B). CTAP in patient with colon CA showing three metastases in the right lobe but a normal left lobe indicating that the disease is resectable.

(A) Tumor masses in the anterior segment (open arrow) and posterior segment (closed arrow) of the right lobe.

Figure 4.15 (B). More caudal section showing third mass in the anterior segment of the right lobe (arrowhead). Gall bladder indicates main interlobar fissure (curved arrow).

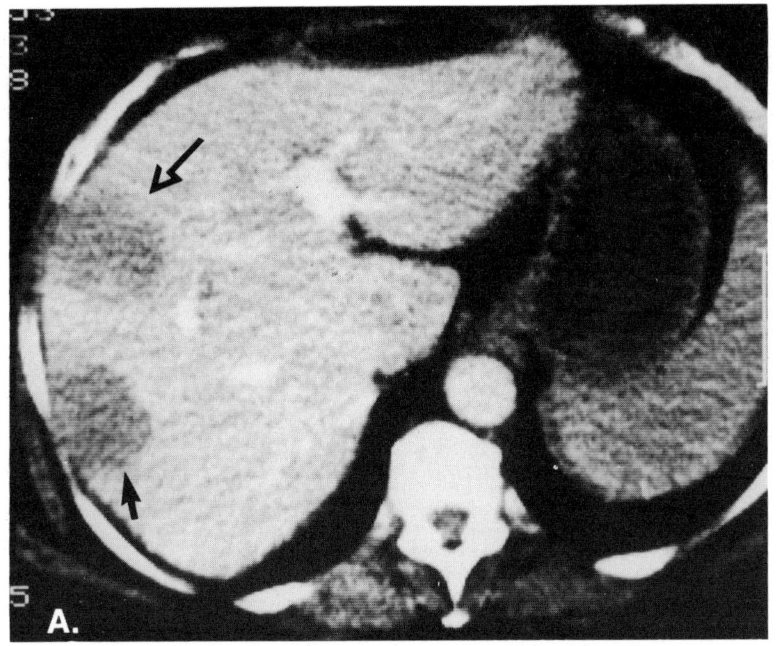
A.

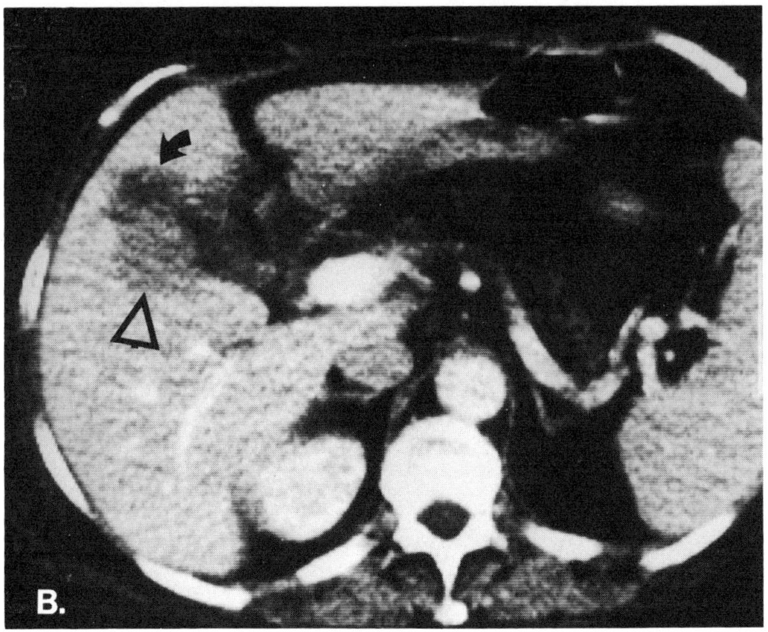
B.

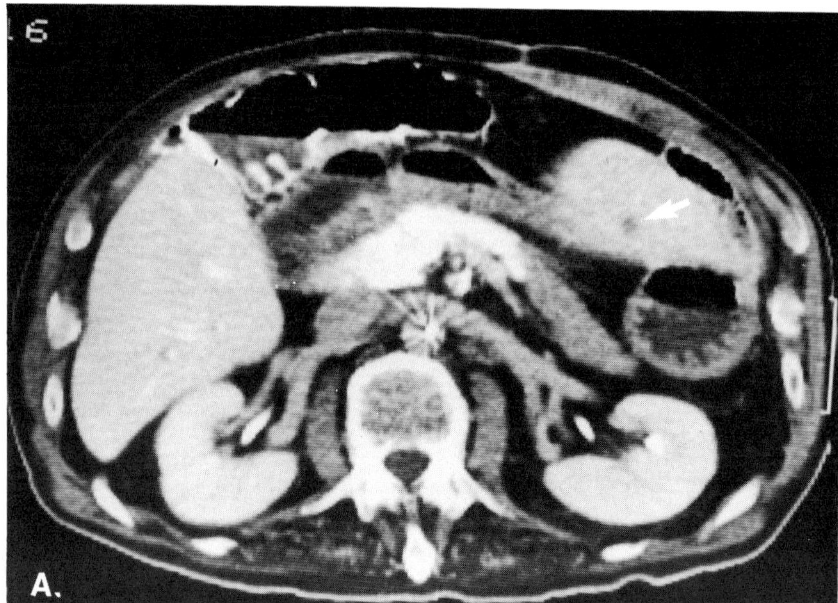

Figure 4.16 (A & B). Patient with colon carcinoma. The initial SBDICT showed a solitary mass in the posterior segment of the right lobe.
(A) CTAP shows an 8 mm mass in the lateral segment of the left lobe (arrow).

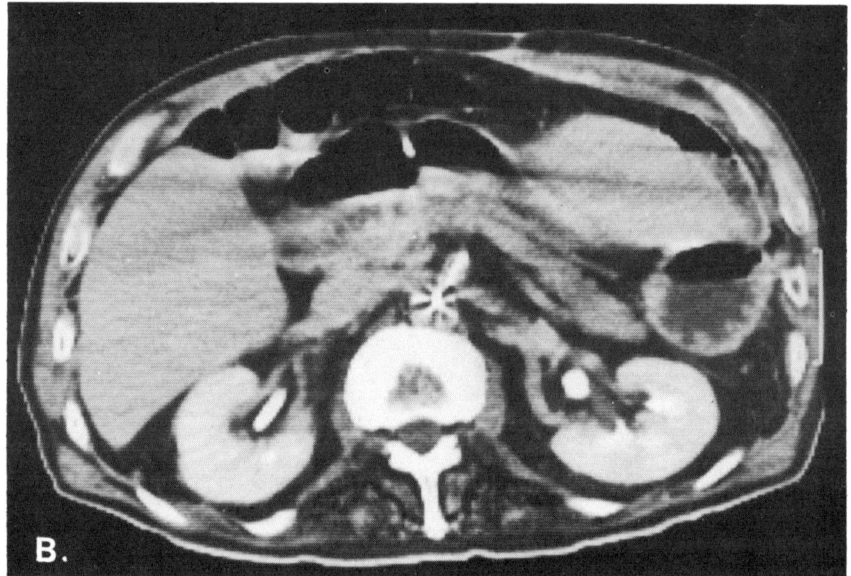

(B) Scan at the same level during equilibration phase shows no mass.

CT AFTER TUMOR EMBOLIZATION

Percutaneous transcatheter embolization of liver tumors is now accepted as a relatively non–invasive, safe and easy method of treating hepatic neoplasms. CT is the most efficacious means for follow–up in these patients (31, 52, 78). CT can measure the volume of a mass within approximately 5% accuracy (60, 61). This simply requires the appropriate software and the ability to trace a region of interest on a CT image. The computer can then calculate the volume on that single section or summate the volume on contiguous sequential sections to provide the volume of a mass. CT thus provides a simple means of assessing the success of the procedure by measuring a decrease in the volume of the embolized tumor.

It is important to recognize the normal appearance of the tumor following embolization (Figure 4.17). CT scans several days

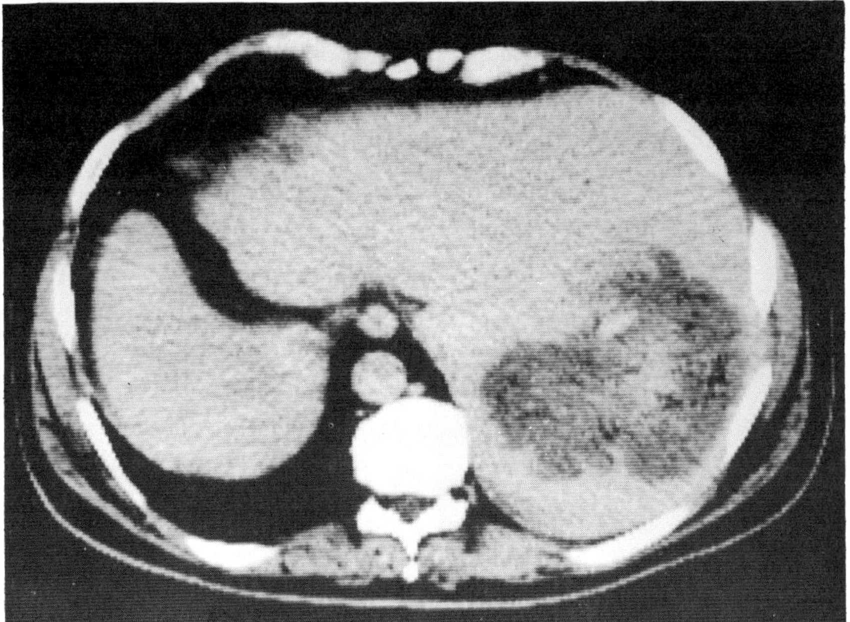

Figure 4.17 (A & B). Patient with hepatoma after undergoing transcatheter embolization of the tumor.
(A) Multiple small gas bubbles are seen throughout the tumor along with a hyperdense central portion probably secondary to hemorrhage in the infarcted tissue.

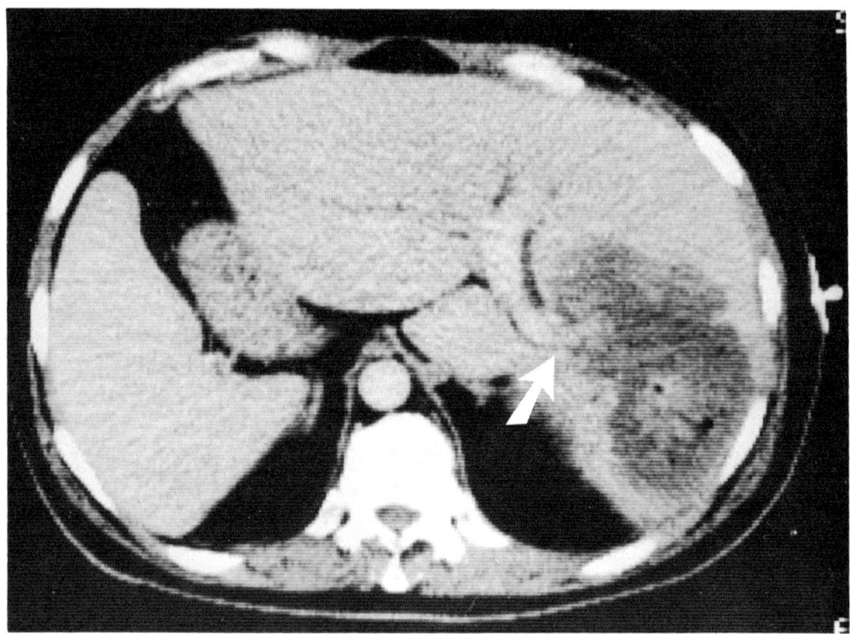

Figure 4.17 (B). Abrupt termination of the right portal vein (arrow) indicating thrombosis caused by the tumor.

after embolization often show small gas bubbles within the tumor. This generally reflects tumor necrosis and has been ascribed to oxygen released from oxyhemoglobin or carbon dioxide resulting from anaerobic metabolism (11, 31, 52, 60, 65, 78). Air introduced with the embolic material has also been offered as an explanation (17). This should not be confused with abscess formation, an infrequent complication. High density areas may also be seen within the tumor. This may be the result of hemorrhage into the infarcted tumor or may reflect contrast retained within the tumor because of the interrupted arterial perfusion (11, 31, 52, 78). Repeat CT scans weeks to months later show the necrotic tumor as a low density area that does not enhance. This finding correlates well with autopsy results (31, 65, 78).

CT facilitates early detection of tumor recurrence and is superior to angiography for follow–up of embolized tumors (31, 52, 78). The development of intrahepatic and extrahepatic collaterals may result in revascularization and tumor recurrence. In that case, enhancing regions are usually identified within the low density necrotic tumor on follow–up CT. This may signal the need for further or repeat intervention before it could otherwise be detected.

NEW TECHNOLOGY — MRI

Recent advances in technology have led to the development of Magnetic Resonance Imaging (MRI), a new imaging modality in the diagnostic armamentarium. MRI combines some of the advantages of CT and ultrasonography. It involves no ionizing radiation, can produce images in any desired plane and provides a high resolution tomographic image.

When nuclei containing an odd number of particles are placed in a strong magnetic field they align themselves in the direction of the field. This property is the basis for MRI. When a radiowave of a frequency equal to the resonant frequency of a particular nucleus, such as hydrogen, is applied to the magnetic field those nuclei become aligned in a direction different from the magnetic field. When the nuclei return to their original alignment they emit radiowaves of the same frequency as those they absorb. The resonant frequency of a nucleus varies with the magnetic field strength. By applying a non-uniform field of a known distribution, the spatial distribution of the nuclei can be determined and an image produced. In addition to the density of the nuclei, the rate at which the nuclei become aligned with the field (T_1) and the rate at which the nuclear energy emission decays (T_2) affect the MRI signal.

MRI of the liver seems to have great promise in the non-invasive evaluation of hepatic pathology. MRI is able to visualize the liver and its contents, particularly the hepatic vasculature, extremely well. Despite the fact that this is a modality in its infancy, MRI has been shown to be equal in sensitivity to CT in detecting focal hepatic lesions (12, 23, 54, 63). The ability to obtain images in any plane as well as the excellent demonstration of vascular structures produces a detailed anatomic display of the position of any masses that may be present. MRI is particularly good at demonstrating the internal architecture of masses, their relationship to vascular structures and any possible invasion of vessels by a mass (54, 63). Unlike CT no contrast media is necessary. In addition, MRI is not affected by artifacts from the ribs, stomach or surgical clips, all of which can be problems in hepatic CT.

The exact position MRI will hold in the diagnosis and evaluation of hepatic pathology has yet to be established.

REFERENCES

1. Ackerman, NB, Lien, WM, Kondi, ES, Silverman, NA: The blood supply of experimental liver metastases. I. The distribution of hepatic artery and portal vein blood to "small" and "large" tumors. *Surg, 66:*1067, 1969.

2. Alderson, PO, Adams, DF, McNeil, BJ, Sanders, R, Siegelman, SS, Finberg, HJ, Hessel, SJ, Abrams, HL: Computed tomography, ultrasound and scintigraphy of the liver in patients with colon or breast carcinoma: a perspective comparison. *Radiol, 149:*225, 1983.

3. Alfidi, RJ, Haagà, J, Meaney, TF, MacIntyre, WJ, Gonzales, L, Tarar, R, Zelch, MG, Boller, M, Cook, SA, Kelden, G: Computed tomography of the thorax and abdomen: a preliminary report. *Radiol, 117:*257, 1975.

4. Alfidi, RJ, Haagà, J, Havrilla, TR, Pepe, RG, Cook, SA: Computed tomography of the liver. *AJR, 127:*69, 1976.

5. Alspaugh, JP, Bernerdino, ME, Sewell, CW, Sones, PJ, Berkman, WA, Price, RB: CT directed hepatic biopsies: increased diagnostic accuracy with low patient risk. *J Comput Assist Tomogr, 7:*1012, 1983.

6. Araki, T: Diagnosis of liver tumors by dynamic computed tomography. *CRC Crit Rev Diagn Imaging, 19:*47, 1983.

7. Araki, T, Itai, Y, Furui, S, Tasaka, A: Dynamic CT densitometry of hepatic tumors, *AJR, 135:*1037, 1980.

8. Auh, YH, Rosen, A, Rubenstein, WA, Engel, IA, Whalen, JP, Kazam, E: CT of the papillary process of the caudate lobe of the liver. *AJR, 142:*535, 1984.

9. Auh, YH, Rubenstein, WA, Zirkinsky, K, Kneeland, BJ, Parges, JC, Engel, IA, Whalen, JP, Kazum, E: Accessory fissures of the liver: CT and sonographic appearance. *AJR, 143:*565, 1984.

10. Barnett, PH, Zerhouni, EA, White, RI, Siegelman, S: Computed tomography in the diagnosis of cavernous hemangioma of the liver. *AJR, 134:*439, 1980.

11. Bernardino, ME, Chuang, VP, Wallace, S, Thomas, JL, Soo, CS: Therapeutically infarcted tumors: CT findings. *AJR, 136:*527, 1981.

12. Borkowski, GP, Buonocore, E, George, CT, Go, RT, O'Donovan, PB, Meaney, TF: Nuclear magnetic resonance (NMR) imaging in the evaluation of the liver: a preliminary experience. *J Comput Assist Tomogr, 7:*768, 1983.

13. Breedis, C, Young, G: Blood supply of neoplasms in the liver. *Am J Pathol, 30:*969, 1954.

14. Burgener, FA, Hamlin, DJ: Contrast enhancement in abdominal CT: bolus vs. infusion. *AJR, 137:*351, 1981.

15. Burgener, FA, Hamlin, DJ: Contrast enhancement of hepatic tumors in CT: comparison between bolus and infusion techniques. *AJR, 140:*291, 1983.

16. Burgener, FA, Hamlin, DJ: Contrast enhancement of focal hepatic lesions in CT: effect of size and histology. *AJR, 140:*297, 1983.

17. Carroll, BA, Walter, JF: Gas in embolized tumors: an alternate hypothesis for its origin. *Radiol, 147:*441, 1983.

18. Casarella, WJ, Knowles, DM, Wolff, M, Johnson, PM: Focal nodular hyperplasia and liver cell adenoma: radiologic and pathologic differentiation. *AJR, 131:*393, 1978.

19. Clark, RA, Matsui, O: CT of liver tumors. *Semin Roentgenol, 18:*149, 1983.

20. Coin, CG, Chan YS: Computed tomographic arteriography. *J Comput Assist Tomogr, 1:*165, 1977.

21. Danielson, KS, Sheedy, PF, Stephens, DH, Hattery, RR, LaRusso, NF: Computed tomography and peritoneoscopy for detection of liver metastases: review of Mayo Clinic experience. *J Comput Assist Tomogr, 7:*230, 1983.

22. Doppman, JL, Dwyer, A, Vermess, M, Girton, M, Sugarbaker, P, Miller, D, Cornblatt, M: Segmental hyperlucent defects in the liver. *J Comput Assist Tomogr, 8:*50, 1984.

23. Doyle, FH, Pennock, JM, Banks, LM, McDonnell, MJ, Bydder, GM, Steiner, RE, Young, IR, Clarke, GJ, Pasmore, T, Gilderdale, DJ: Nuclear magnetic resonance imaging of the liver: initial experience. *AJR, 138:*193, 1982.

24. Dunnick, NR, Ihde, DC, Doppman, JL, Bates, HR: Computed tomography in hepatocellular carcinoma. *J Comput Assist Tomogr, 4:*59, 1980.

25. Federle, MP, Filly, RA, Moss AA: Cystic hepatic neoplasms: complementary roles of CT and sonography. *AJR, 136:*345, 1981.

26. Fishman, EK, Farmlett, E, Kadir, S, Siegelman, SS: Computed tomography of benign hepatic tumors. *J Comput Assist Tomogr, 6:*472, 1982.

27. Foley, WD, Berland, LL, Lawson, TL, Smith, DF, Thorsen, MK: Contrast enhancement technique for dynamic hepatic computed tomographic scanning. *Radiol, 147:*797, 1983.

28. Freeny, PC, Marks, WM: Computed tomographic arteriography of the liver. *Radiol, 148:*193, 1983.

29. Freeny, PC, Vimont, TR, Barnett, DC: Cavernous hemangioma of the liver: ultrasonography, arteriography and computed tomography. *Radiol, 132:*143, 1979.

30. Frick, MP, Feinberg, SB: Biliary cystadenoma. *AJR, 139:*393, 1982.

31. Furui, S, Ohtomo, K, Itai, Y, Iio, M: Hepatocellular carcinoma treated by transcatheter arterial embolization: progress evaluated by computed tomography. *Radiol, 150:*773, 1984.

32. Halvorsen, RA, Korobkin, M, Ram, PC, Thompson, WM: CT appearance of focal fatty infiltration of the liver. *AJR, 139:*277, 1982.

33. Harbin, WP, Robert, NJ, Ferrucci, JT: Diagnosis of cirrhosis based on regional changes in hepatic morphology. *Radiol, 135:*273, 1980.

34. Hosoki, T, Chatani, M, Mori, S: Dynamic computed tomography of hepatocellular carcinoma. *AJR, 139:*1099, 1982.

35. Hosoki, T, Toyonaga, Y, Araki, Y, Mori, S: Dynamic computed tomo-

graphy of isodense hepatocellular carcinoma. *J Comput Assist Tomogr, 8:* 263, 1984.

36. Inamoto, K, Sugiki, K, Yamasaki, H, Miura, T: CT of hepatoma: effects of portal vein obstruction. *AJR, 136:*349, 1981.

37. Inamoto, K, Sugiki, K, Yamasaki, H, Nakao, N, Miura T: Computed tomography and angiography of hepatocellular carcinoma. *J Comput Assist Tomogr, 4:*832, 1980.

38. Itai, Y, Araki, T, Furui, S, Yashiro, N, Ohtomo, K, Iio, M: Computed tomography of primary intrahepatic biliary malignancy. *Radiol, 147:*485, 1983.

39. Itai, Y, Furui, S, Araki, T, Yashiro, H, Tasaka, A: Computed tomography of cavernous hemangioma of the liver. *Radiol, 137:*149, 1980.

40. Itai, Y, Nishikawa, H, Tasaka, A: Computed tomography in the evaluation of hepatocellular carcinoma. *Radiol, 131:*165, 1979.

41. Itai, Y, Ohtomo, K, Araki, T, Furui, S, Iio, M, Atomi, Y: Computed tomography and sonography of cavernous hemangioma of the liver. *AJR, 141:*315, 1983.

42. Johnson, CM, Sheedy, PF, Stanson, AW, Stephens, DH, Hattery, RR, Adson, MA: Computed tomography and angiography of cavernous hemangiomas of the liver. *Radiol, 138:*115, 1981.

43. Knopf, DR, Torres, WE, Fajman, WJ, Sones, PJ: Liver lesions: comparative accuracy of scintigraphy and computed tomography. *AJR, 138:* 623, 1982.

44. Kunstlinger, F, Federle, MP, Moss, AA, Marks, W: Computed tomography of hepatocellular carcinoma. *AJR, 134:*431, 1980.

45. LaBerge, JM, Laing, FC, Federle, MP, Jeffrey, RB, Lim, RC: Hepatocellular carcinoma: assessment of resectability by computed tomography and ultrasound. *Radiol, 152:*485, 1984.

46. Lamki, N, Ravel, B: Computed tomographic diagnosis of hepatic metastases in fatty infiltration. *CT, 7:*227, 1983.

47. Lewis, E, AufderHeide, JF, Bernardino, ME, Barnes, PA, Thomas, JL: CT detection of hepatic metastases with Ethiodized Oil Emulsion 13. *J Comput Assist Tomogr, 6:*1103, 1982.

48. Lewis, E, Bernardino, ME, Barnes, PA, Parvey, HR, Soo, CS, Chuang, VP: The fatty liver: pitfalls in the CT and angiographic evaluation of metastatic disease. *J Comput Assist Tomogr, 7:*235, 1983.

49. Lien, WM, Ackerman, NB: The blood supply of experimental liver metastases. II. A microcirculatory study of the normal and tumor vessels of the liver with the use of perfusion silicone rubber. *Surg, 68:*334, 1970.

50. Lin, G, Hagerstrand, I, Lunderquist, A: Portal blood supply of liver metastases. *AJR, 143:*53, 1984.

51. Lunderquist, A, Owman, T: Preoperatove diagnosis and evaluation of hepatic tumor resectability. *Gastro-intest Radiol, 8:*227, 1983.

52. Magid, D, Fishman, EK, Kadir, S, Cameron, JL, Siegelman, SS: CT evaluation of therapeutic embolization of hepatic hemangiomas. *J Comput Assist Tomogr, 7:*1007, 1983.

53. Marchal, GJ, Baert, AL, Wilma, GE: CT of non-cystic liver lesions: bolus vs. infusion. *AJR, 137:*351, 1981.

54. Margulis, AR, Moss, AA, Crooks, LE, Kaufman, L: Nuclear magnetic resonance in the diagnosis of tumors of the liver. *Semin Roentgenol, 18:*123, 1983.

55. Martino, CR, Haagá, JR, Bryan, PJ, LiPuma, JP, ElYousef, SJ, Alfidi, RJ: CT guided liver biopsies: eight years experience. *Radiol, 152:*755, 1984.

56. Mathieu, D, Grenier, P, Larde, D, Vasile, N: Portal vein involvement in hepatocellular carcinoma: dynamic CT features. *Radiol, 152:*127, 1984.

57. Matsui, O, Kadoya, M, Suzuki, M, Inoue, K, Itoh, H, Ida, M, Takashima, T: Work in progress: dynamic sequential computed tomography during arterial portography in the detection of hepatic neoplasms. *Radiol, 146:*721, 1983.

58. Miller, DL, Rosenbaum, RC, Sugarbaker, PH, Vermess, M, Willis, M, Doppman, JL: Detection of hepatic metastases: comparison of EOE-13 computed tomography and scintigraphy. *AJR, 141:*931, 1983.

59. Miller, DL, Vermess, M, Doppman, JL, Simon, RM, Sugarbaker, PH, O'Leary, TJ, Grimes, G, Chatterji, DG, Willis, M: CT of the liver and spleen with EOE-13: review of 225 examinations. *AJR, 143:*235, 1984.

60. Moss, AA: Computed tomography of the hepatobiliary system. In: Moss, AA, Gamsu, G, Genant, HK (eds.), *Computed Tomography of the Body.* Philadelphia: W.B. Saunders Co., 1983, pp. 599-698.

61. Moss, AA, Cann, CE, Friedman, MA, Marcus, FS, Resser, KJ, Berninger, W: Volumetric CT analysis of hepatic tumors. *J Comput Assist Tomogr, 5:*714, 1981.

62. Moss, AA, Dean, PB, Axel, L, Goldberg, HI, Glazer, GM, Friedman, MA: Dynamic CT of hepatic masses with intravenous and intra-arterial contrast material. *AJR, 138:*847, 1982.

63. Moss, AA, Goldberg, HI, Stark, DB, Davis, PL, Margulis, AR, Kaufman, L, Crooks, LR: Hepatic tumors: magnetic resonance and CT appearance. *Radiol, 150:*141, 1984.

64. Moss, AA, Schrumpf, J, Schnyder, P, Korobkin, M, Shimshak, RR: Computed tomography of focal hepatic lesions: a blind clinical evaluation of the effect of contrast enhancement. *Radiol, 131:*427, 1979.

65. Nakamura, H, Tanaka, T, Hori, S, Yoshioka, H, Kuroda, C, Okamura, J, Sakurai, M: Transcatheter embolization of hepatocellular carcinoma: assessment of efficacy in cases of resection following embolization. *Radiol, 147:*401, 1983.

66. Nakao, N, Miura, K, Takayasu, Y, Wada, Y, Miura, T: CT angiography in hepatocellular carcinoma. *J Comput Assist Tomogr, 4:*59, 1980.

67. Nakayama, T, Hiyama, Y, Ohnishi, K, Tsuchiya, S, Kohno, K, Nakajima, Y, Okuda, K: Arterioportal shunts on dynamic computed tomography. *AJR, 140:*953, 1983.

68. Pagani, JJ: Intrahepatic vascular territories shown by computed tomography (CT): the value of CT in determining resectability of hepatic tumors. *Radiol, 147:*173, 1983.

69. Prando, A, Wallace, S, Bernardino, ME, Lindell, MM: Computed tomographic arteriography of the liver. *Radiol, 130:*697, 1979.

70. Rogers, JV, Mack, LA, Freeny, PC, Johnson, ML, Sones, PJ: Hepatic focal nodular hyperplasia: angiography, CT, sonography and scintigraphy. *AJR, 137:*983, 1981.

71. Scatarige, JC, Fishman, EK, Saksouk, FA, Siegelman, SS: Computed tomography of calcified liver masses. *J Comput Assist Tomogr, 7:*83, 1983.

72. Sexton, CC, Seman, RK: Correlation of computed tomography, sonography and gross anatomy of the liver. *AJR, 141:*711, 1983.

73. Stephens, DM, Sheedy, PF, Hattery, RR, MacCarty, RL: Computed tomography of the liver. *AJR, 128:*579, 1977.

74. Stanley, RJ: Liver and biliary tract. In: Lee, JKT, Sagel, SS, Stanley, RJ (eds.), *Computed Body Tomography.* New York: Raven Press, 1983, pp. 167–211.

75. Stanley, RJ, Sagel, SS, Levitt, RG: Computed tomography of the liver. *Radiol Clin N Am, 15:*331, 1977.

76. Suzuki, M, Itoh, H, Konishi, H, Ida, M, Matsui, O, Takashima, T: Hepatocellular carcinoma involving the portal vein. *J Comput Assist Tomogr, 6:*831, 1982.

77. Tada, S, Fukuda, K, Aoyagi, Y, Harada, J: CT of abdominal malignancies: dynamic approach. *AJR, 135:*455, 1980.

78. Takayasu, K, Moriyama, N, Muramatsu, Y, Suzuki, M, Yamada, T, Kishi, K, Hasagawa, H, Okazaki, N: Hepatic arterial embolization for hepatocellular carcinoma: comparison of CT scans and resected specimens. *Radiol, 150:*661, 1984.

79. Thorsen, MK, Quiroz, F, Lawson, T, Smith, DF, Foley, WD, Stewart, ET: Primary biliary carcinoma: CT evaluation. *Radiol, 152:*479, 1984.

80. Vermess, M, Doppman, JL: CT of the liver with intravenous lipoid contrast material: review of the current status. *Semin Roentgenol, 18:*102, 1983.

HOWARD L. BERMAN, M.D.
STUART G. KATZ, M.D.

CHAPTER 5
Angiography and Interventional Therapy

INTRODUCTION

Despite the development of newer imaging modalities including CT, ultrasound and NMR, angiography maintains a vital role in the diagnosis, evaluation and treatment of liver tumors.

For the surgeon, the arteriogram is critical for determining the type of tumor, extent of spread, resectability and variation of vascular anatomy. In addition, angiographic embolization and infusion of chemotherapeutic agents may serve as important adjuncts to therapy.

ANATOMY

The liver is composed of two main lobes which are subdivided into segments based upon arterial anatomy. Classically, the common hepatic artery arises from the celiac axis as the major arterial supply of the liver. After giving off the gastroduodenal artery, the hepatic artery ends in right and left branches, supplying the right and left hepatic lobes. These two main arteries continue to branch dividing the right hepatic lobe into four sub–segments and the left lobe into two. Only 50 to 60% of patients will have this classic vascular anatomy. In the remaining patients, there are variations of the origins of the hepatic arteries. The most common alternatives are: the entire right hepatic replaced to the superior mesenteris artery (SMA) in 14%, an accessory right hepatic from the SMA in 6%, the left hepatic artery entirely replaced to the left gastric in 10%, and an accessory left hepatic from the left gastric in 8%. In 3% of patients, the hepatic artery will be totally replaced to the SMA (1, 2, 3). Knowledge of these variations is especially important when considering chemical infusion or embolization.

93

ATLAS

Hepatic tumors include benign lesions, such as focal nodular hyperplasia, hepatic adenoma, cavernous hemangioma and regenerating nodules. Malignant liver tumors include hepato–cellular carcinoma (hepatoma), cholangiocarcinoma and metastatic lesions. The following will be a short description of the angiographic findings of each. These findings will be summarized in Table 1.

TABLE 1
SUMMARIZED ANGIOGRAPHIC FINDINGS OF HEPATIC TUMORS

FOCAL NODULAR HYPERPLASIA (FNH)

Size:	Usually 4 to 7 cm, 15 cm reported
Neovascularity:	Yes. Vessels arranged like spokes of a wheel but vessels are not encased or obstructed (no tumor vessels).
Nodular Appearance:	Round. Usually subcapsular but may be pedunculated (20%) or multiple (20%).
Size of Feeding Vessels:	Large feeding vessels at periphery surrounding lesions with small vessels penetrating to center of mass (no portal flow).
Arterial-Venous Shunting:	No shunting.
Blush or Stain and Persistence:	Fine diffuse granularity. Focal hemorrhage and necrosis do not occur.
Differential Points:	One–third will take up Sulfur Colloid on liver–spleen scan.
Comments:	Usually asymptomatic but occasionally may be difficult to tell from adenoma or hepatoma.

HEPATIC ADEMONA

Size:	8 to 15 cm
Neovascularity:	Yes. Rich, coarse neovascularity but not as densely packed as FNH or as bizarre as hepatoma.
Nodular Appearance:	Round or lobulated truly encapsulated usually solitary maybe multiple — 20%.
Size of Feeding Vessels:	Main hepatic artery may be dilated, multiple surrounding peripheral arteries which are not dilated with small penetrating arteries.
Arterial-Venous Shunting:	No shunting
Blush or Stain and Persistence:	Blush is homogenous except for lucent areas of central necrosis or hemorrhage which may rarely have associated contrast puddling.
Differential Points:	Cold on Sulfur Colloid Scan. May take up but not excrete on Tc99^{m} Hida Scan.
Comments:	Associated with females taking birth control pills. Marked propensity for life threatening spontaneous hemorrhage.

CAVERNOUS HEMANGIOMA

Size:	Usually small occasionally may involve entire liver.
Neovascularity:	No. Normal small hepatic arteries fill the hemangioma.
Nodular Appearance:	Yes. Usually small and single occasionally may be multiple and large.
Size of Feeding Vessels:	Small normal–sized hepatic arteries supply mass.
Arterial-Venous Shunting:	No shunting.
Blush or Stain and Persistence:	Well marginated pooling "C" or irregular ringed shaped spaces persisting up to 18 to 20 seconds.
Differential Points:	Irregular amorphous calcification may be seen on plain films (calcification in interstitial septae).
Comments:	May be painful or rupture when large.

REGENERATING NODULE

Size:	Varies
Neovascularity:	No. Vessels within tumor show stretching and displacement but distinct tumor vascularity is absent.
Nodular Appearance:	Yes. Often very large.
Size of Feeding Vessels:	Vascularity of regenerating nodule is similar to normal liver.

<table>
<tr><td>Arterial-Venous Shunting:</td><td>Hepatic vessels near periphery show stretching and displacement.
Uncommon.</td></tr>
</table>

Arterial-Venous Shunting: Uncommon.
Blush or Stain and Similar to surrounding liver but may be more or less pronounced.
Persistence:
Differential Points: Occurs in cirrhosis particularly post–necrotic may have normal to increased uptake of Sulfur Colloid on liver scan.
Comments: The presence of patent hepatic and portal venous branches within tumor is important to differentiate from hepatoma.

CHOLANGIO–SARCOMA

Size: Varies
Neovascularity: Yes. Predominantly a hypovascular lesion showing encasement and obstruction of surrounding vessels, but fine neovascular vessels may be present.
Nodular Appearance: No. Poorly defined infiltrative lesion.
Size of Feeding Vessels: Small–Infiltrating lesion which encases and obstructs surrounding arterial and portal vessels.
Arterial-Venous Shunting: No
Blush or Stain and Not pronounced and only occasional; poorly marginated.
Persistence:
Differential Points: Associated with obst. jaundice with narrowing of main biliary ducts on P.T.C.
Comments: May be difficult to differentiate from hypovascular mets or anaplastic hepatoma

HEPATOMA WELL–DIFFERENTIATED

Size: Varies
Neovascularity: Yes. Neovascularity with dilated vessels with variable size lumens arranged irregularly with diffuse vessel distribution.
Nodular Appearance: Solitary, may be multiple.
Size of Feeding Vessels: Large may steal from multiple vessels.
Arterial-Venous Shunting: Present in 70% with invasion of portal and hepatic veins.
Blush or Stain and Pronounced tumor stain with vascular lakes and channels.
Persistence: (Doesn't persist as long as cavernous hemangioma.)
Differential Points: Usually hypervascular with tumor stain, A–V shunting and portal vein invasion mass effect on surrounding vessels.
Comments: Predominate form of hepatoma.

ANAPLASTIC

Size: Varies
Neovascularity: Neovascularity and tumor vessels present small tumor vessels penetrate mass from surrounding vessels.
Nodular Appearance: Diffuse or poorly marginated.
Size of Feeding Vessels: Enlarged but smaller than well differentiated.
Arterial-Venous Shunting: Uncommon.
Blush or Stain and Much less pronounced tumor stain poorly defined and uneven.
Persistence:
Differential Points: More commonly hypovascular may be difficult to differentiate from cholangiosarcoma or hypovascular mets.
Comments: Uncommon.

METS

Size: Varies.
Neovascularity: Yes. Minimally enlarged vessels supplying mets with irregular tumor vessels.
Nodular Appearance: Yes. Usually multiple may be singular.
Size of Feeding Vessels: Supplied usually by small hepatic arteries although somewhat larger than normal.
Arterial-Venous Shunting: No
Blush or Stain and *Hypervascular.* Malignant carcinoid islet cell tumor (present with intense stain) leiomyosarcoma and renal cell Ca (large tumor vessels).
Persistence:
Differential Points: *Slight to moderate blush.* Adeno Ca of breast, endometrium colon, Ca of adrenal, seminoma, pancreas other than adeno Ca. *Avascular.* Malignant melanoma–adenocarcinoma of pancreas, gall bladder, bile ducts, squamous cell of lungs and esophagus.
Comments: All mets appear as filling defects on portal phase of hepatic angiogram.

FOCAL NODULAR HYPERPLASIA (FNH)

The angiographic findings are consistent with the histopathology of this benign lesion (4). Proliferating hepatocytes, Kupffer cells and biliary radicals develop along fine septae arranged like the spokes of a wheel, radiating from an area of central scarring. Although the lesion is well demarcated, it is not encapsulated. Large dilated arteries surround the tumor with smaller neovessels penetrating along the septae to the center of the lesion. The capillary phase shows a diffuse, homogeneous granular appearance. Areas of central necrosis or hemorrhage are uncommon (see Figure 5.1).

The lesion is usually solitary and subcapsular but may be pedunculated in 20% and multiple in 20%. One third of these lesions will accumulate ^{99m}Tc sulfur–colloid on nuclear imaging scans.

LIVER CELL ADENOMA

The diagnosis of hepatic adenomas is especially important because of the high incidence of life threatening spontaneous hemorrhages. The hepatic adenoma differs from FNH, as it is composed entirely of well differentiated hepatocytes. It also is truly encapsulated. Although usually solitary, it may be multiple in 20%. There is a high incidence in women using oral contraceptives and the lesion has only been reported in men who were treated with androgen or anabolic steroids.

Nuclear medicine studies show a cold defect on sulfur–colloid liver spleen scans consistent with the absence of reticuloendothelial cells. Uptake of biliary scanning agents such as ^{99m}Tc HIDA has been reported. This is as expected since the tumor is composed solely of sheets of hepatocytes without portal triads, central veins or biliary duct connections (5).

The tumor is usually larger than FNH measuring 8 to 15 cm. The main hepatic artery is routinely dilated and blood supply to the tumor usually runs peripherally with neovascular vessels penetrating the tumor. These penetrating vessels are not as densely packed as in FNH, or as bizarre and malignant appearing as in hepatoma. The capillary blush may be irregular with areas of central necrosis and focal hemorrhage present. Hemorrhagic areas

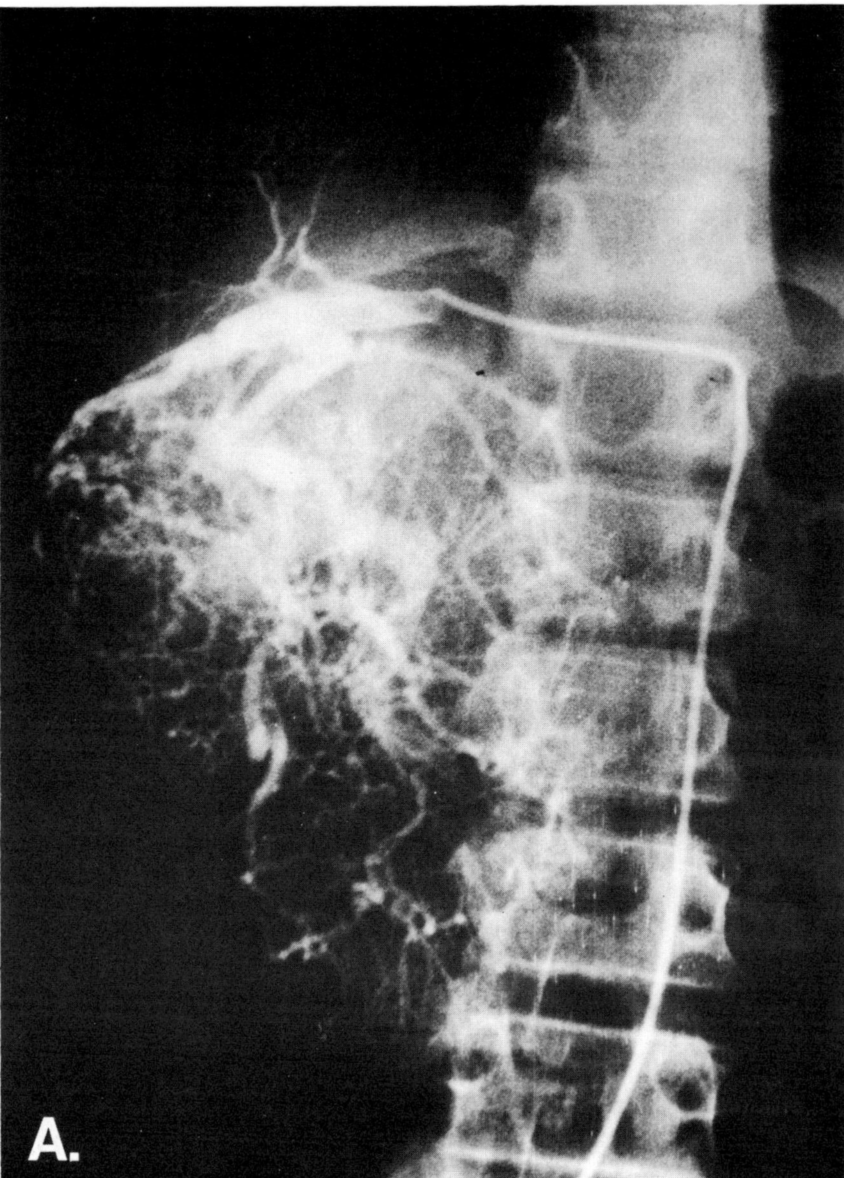

Figure 5.1 (A & B). Focal Nodular Hyperplasia. Arterial phase (A) demonstrating multiple spoke wheel radiating hepatic arteries supplying a large mass lesion of the right lobe of the liver. The parenchymal phase (B) demonstrates the homogeneous coarse granular enhancement.

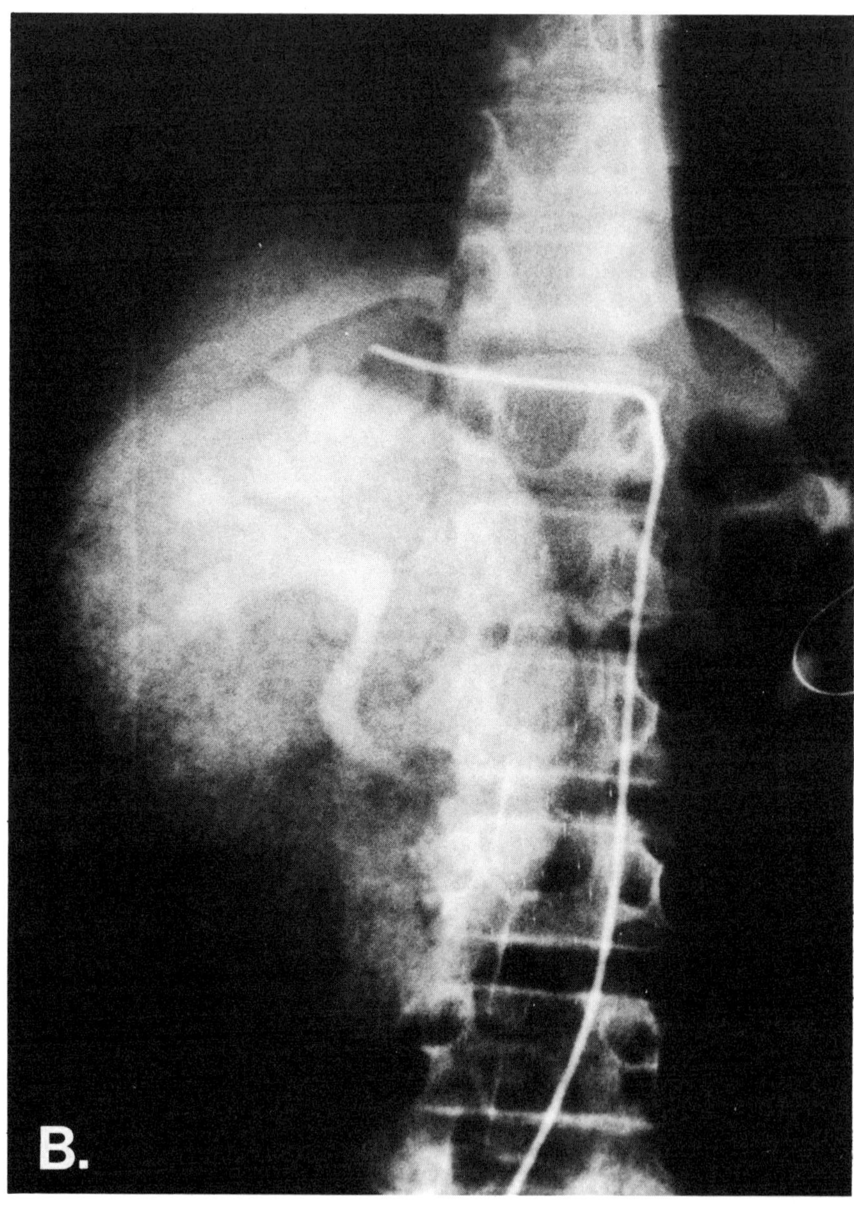

may infrequently present with areas of contrast puddling. Although usually hypervascular, as many as one third may be hypovascular (see Figure 5.2) (6, 7).

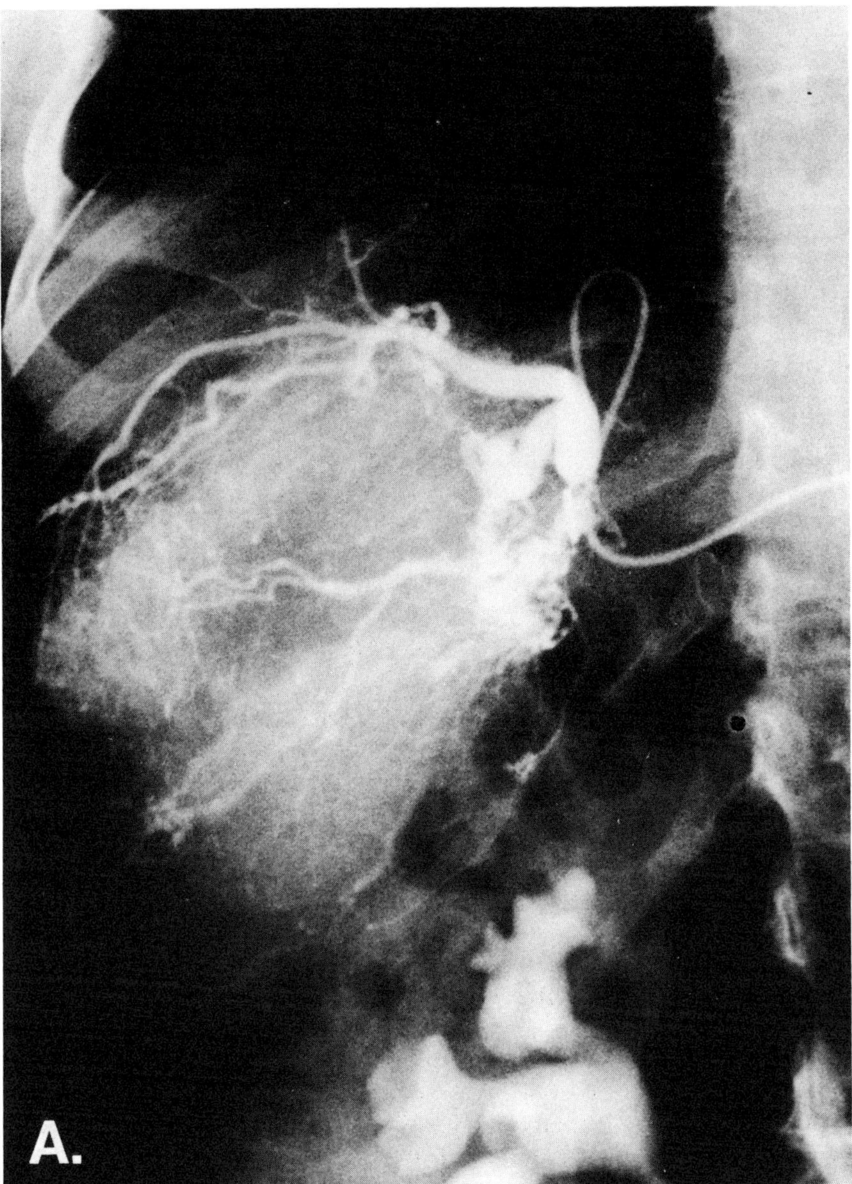

Figure 5.2 (A & B). Hepatic Adenoma. Arterial phase (A) demonstrates the rich neovascular blood supply to the hypervascular mass lesion. The parenchymal phase (B) demonstrates the irregular homogeneous enhancement of the lesion.

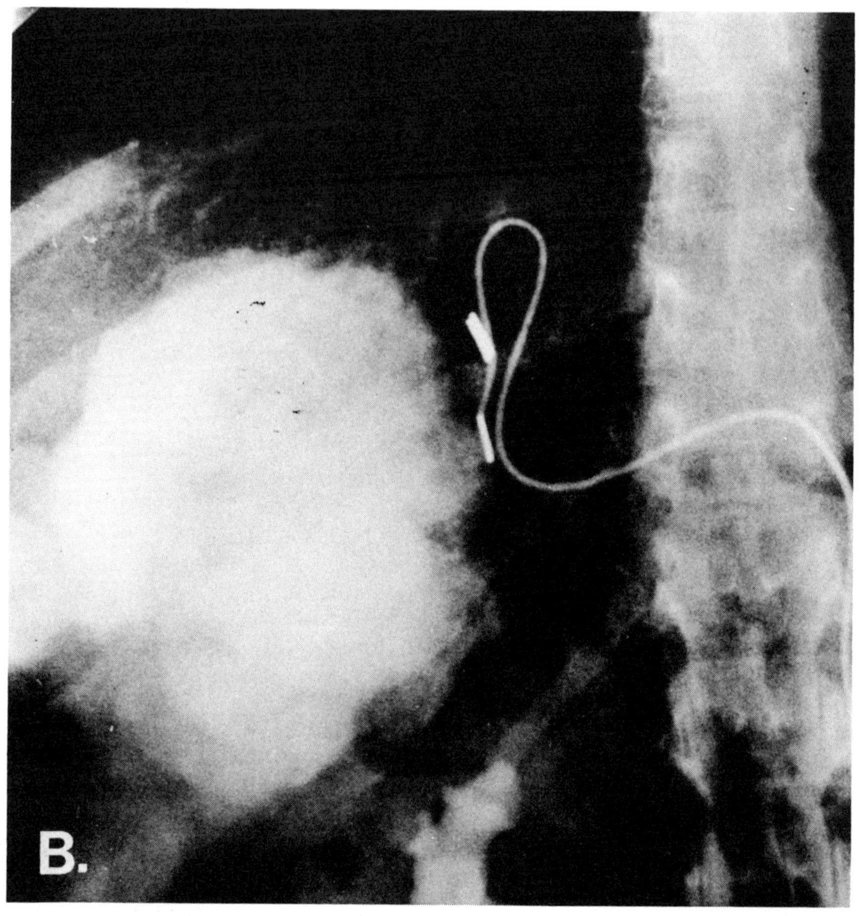

CAVERNOUS HEMANGIOMA

Cavernous hemangioma is the most common benign tumor of the liver. The tumor consists of blood filled spaces separated by fibrous septae and lined by flattened endothelium. These lesions are usually small and single, and discovered as an incidental finding. Occasionally they will cause pain and even rupture if the lesion grows large enough.

Angiographically, this lesion is very vascular, but the tumor is supplied by small unremarkable hepatic arteries which show normal tapering. Although small normal appearing hepatic arteries supply the nodular appearing lesion, the hemangioma itself, due to its size, may cause displacement and crowding of surrounding vessels. No neovascularity is present. The hallmark of these lesions is their prolonged blush or opacification which may last up to 20 seconds. This is far longer than the blush of a hepatoma or metastic deposit. The vascular spaces of the hemangioma opacify in irregular rings or "C" shapes due to the fibrous obliteration of the centers of the lesions. (This opacification appearance is almost pathognomonic.) Rarely fine calcification can be seen in the septae on plain films of the abdomen (see Figure 5.3) (8).

REGENERATING NODULES

Regenerating nodules occur when there has been significant damage to the liver parenchyma. There is a marked association between cirrhosis, especially post–necrotic, and regenerating nodules. The presence of these nodules is especially important because of the need to differentiate them from hepatomas which also have an increased incidence in cirrhosis.

Regenerating nodules appear similar in vascularity to surrounding liver. If they grow large enough, they may displace or stretch surrounding vessels. The feeding vessels are not enlarged and vascularity within the tumor may be tortuous, but actual tumor vascularity does not develop. No invasion of the portal system occurs. Continued patency of the portal and hepatic veins is an important factor ruling against hepatoma. Another useful difference is that regenerating nodules may show minimal to increased activity on nuclear medicine sulfur–colloid liver spleen scan. Unfortunately, uptake may also be totally absent as it is in a hepatoma (9).

HEPATOMA

Hepatocellular tumor or hepatoma shows a wide range of presentations ranging from a well differentiated, solitary lesion to multifocal, multinodular or diffuse anaplastic lesions (10) (see Figure 5.4).

The presentation of the hepatoma angiographically may be an indication of its histopathology. The well differentiated hepatoma forms a pattern of hepatocytes arranged in trabeculae, joined by endothelial cells with blood containing spaces between the trabe-

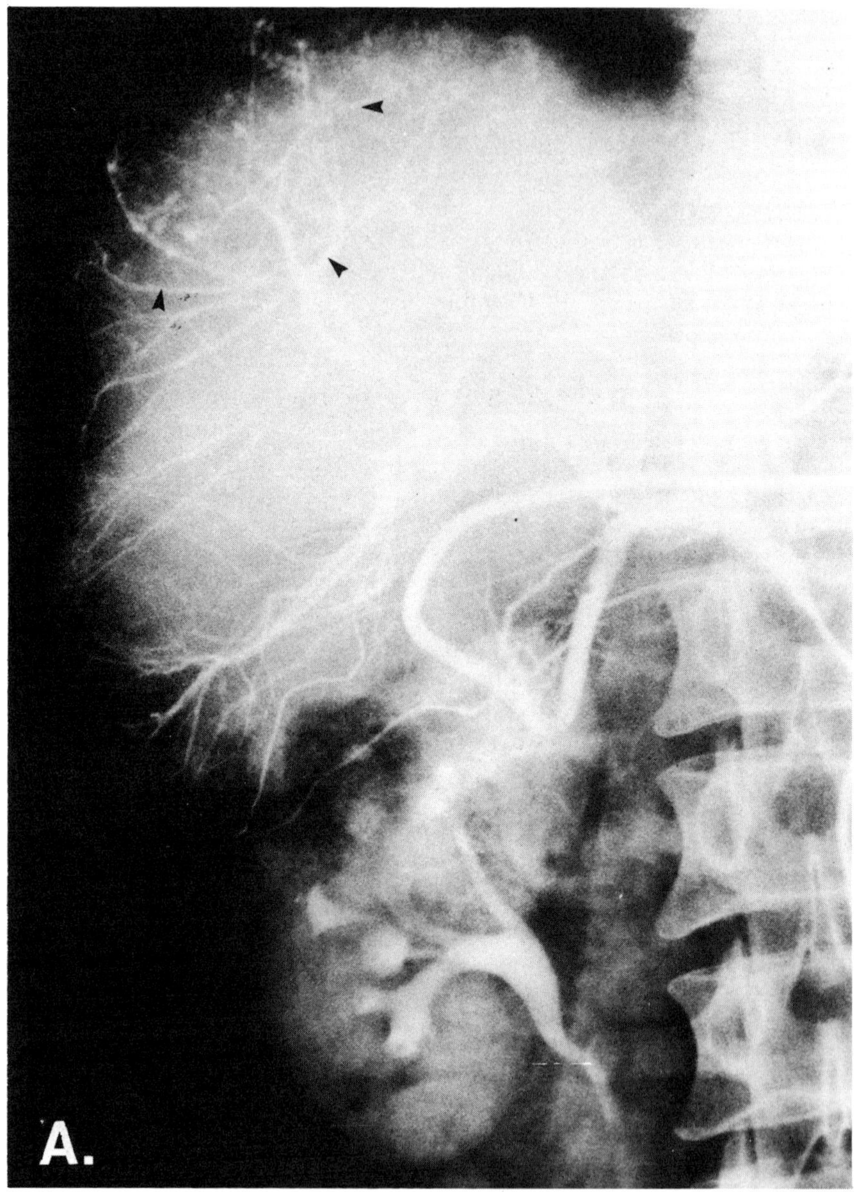

Figure 5.3 (A & B). Cavernous Hemangioma. The arterial phase (A) demonstrates the early visualization of the cavernous hemangioma with small focal areas of enhancement. B shows continued enhancement of the lesion well into and beyond the venous phase.

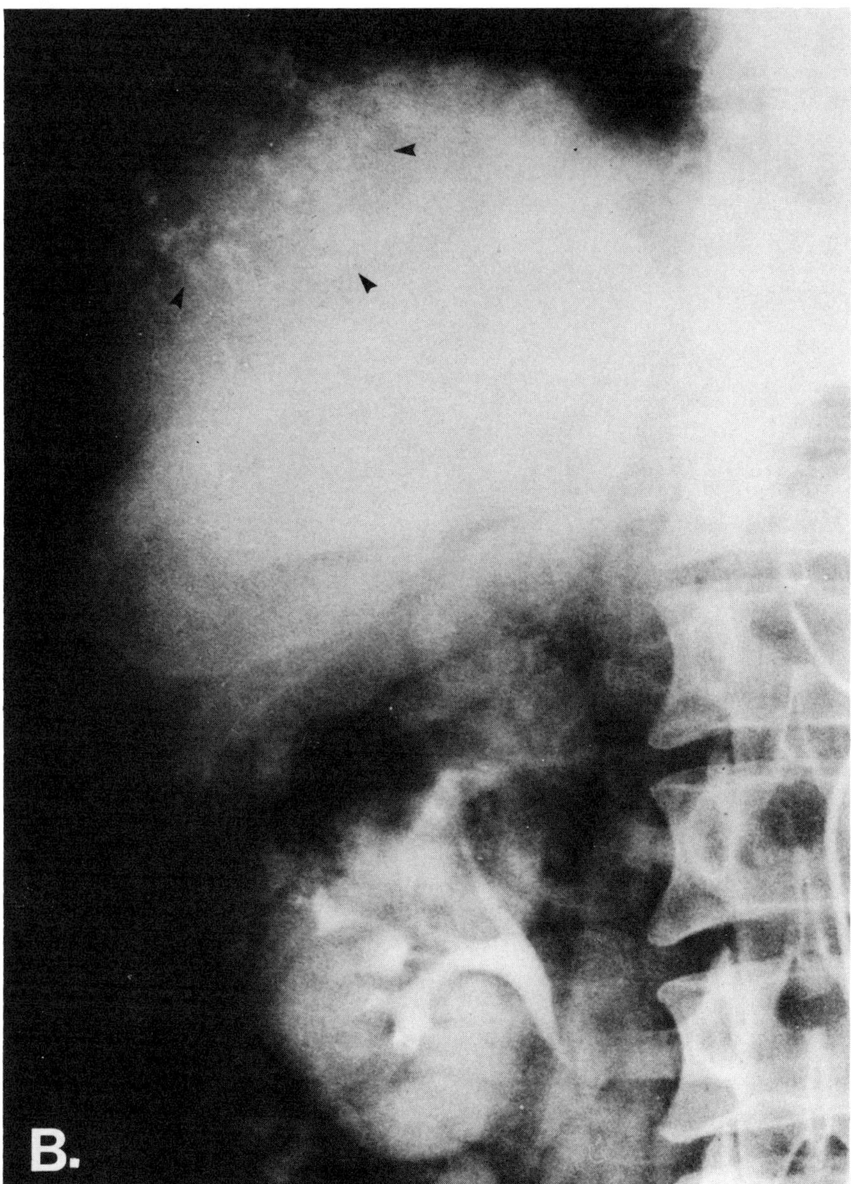

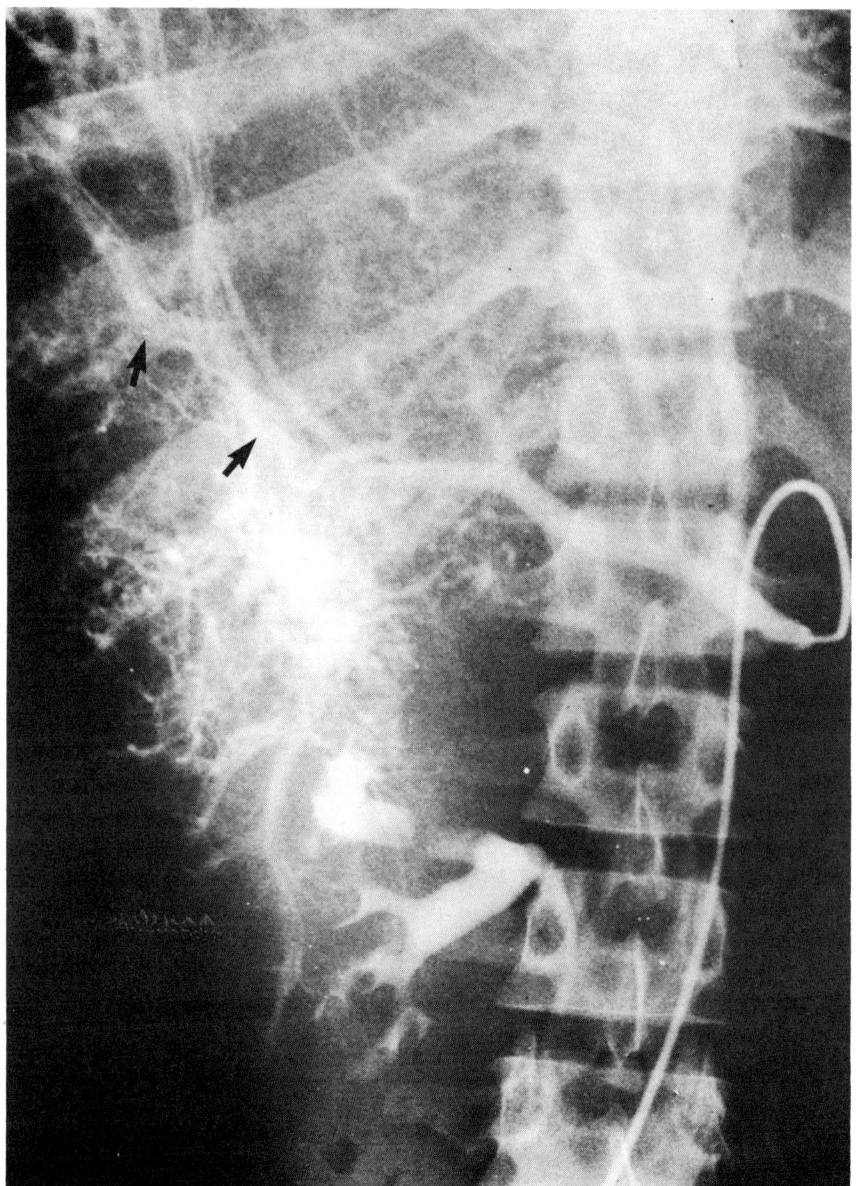

Figure 5.4. Hepatoma. The arterial phase shows the irregular malignant blood supply to a large hepatoma of the liver with rapid shunting to the portal vein (arrow). This case is courtesy of Dr. Sidney Glanz, Downstate Medical Center, New York.

culae. These blood filled spaces account for the pronounced tumor stain of the well differentiated hepatoma. In the normal liver, the sinusoids are bathed mostly by portal blood, with only 25% coming from the artery, but in hepatomas the blood filled spaces are filled solely with arterial blood. This explains the pronounced tumor stain.

Vascular blood supply enlarges to supply this tumor. Arteriovenous shunting occurs as does portal and hepatic vein invasion (11). Venous thrombosis can result in uneven opacification of the tumor. As the tumor enlarges, areas of necrosis may occur.

At the other end of the range of presentation is the anaplastic or "solid" form of hepatoma. In this cell–type, the tumor cells do not form the well organized trabecular pattern with surrounding blood-filled spaces. Instead, the tumor is solid with a poorly vascularized interstitium. The absence of the blood-filled spaces explains the minimal tumor stain with small neoplastic feeding vessels. Arteriovenous shunting is infrequent.

The blood supply to the hepatoma has been described by Kido *et al.* (12) as massive (diffusely enlarged penetrating arteries supply the tumor), arborization (tree like) and basket-type (fine neo–vessels proliferating from the displaced hepatic arteries that surround the surface of the tumor with poor vascularization within the tumor itself). In the well–differentiated hepatoma, the massive form of blood supply is most common. But as well–differentiated tumors undergo central necrosis, the basket-type develop.

In the anaplastic form, arborization and basket form predominate (13, 14, 15).

CHOLANGIOCARCINOMA

Cholangiocarcinoma is difficult to differentiate from hypovascular metastasis or anaplastic hepatoma. Cholangiocarcinoma is usually hypovascular and infiltrative, causing encasement of surrounding vessels. As the tumor spreads, especially about the liver hilum, fine neovascular vessels may develop. These may result in a tumor stain. More commonly the lesion is hypovascular and is only recognized because of obstructive jaundice with associated encasement and obstruction of surrounding vessels on angiogram (16, 17).

METASTASES

Metastases to the liver range from hyper to hypovascular. Their appearances are similar to the primary tumor. Hypervascular metastases producing a pronounced tumor stain include malignant carcinoid and islet cell pancreatic tumor. Leiomyosarcoma and renal cell carcinoma are also hypervascular, but present with large tumor vessels.

Slight to moderate neovascularity is seen in adenocarcinoma of the breast, endometrium and colon. Similar presentation is also noted of cancer of the adrenals, seminoma and pancreas except adenocarcinoma of the pancreas.

Avascular metastases include adenocarcinoma of the pancreas, gall bladder, bile ducts, squamous cell cancer of the lung and esophagus and malignant melanoma.

All metastases appear as filling defects on portal phase, since all are predominantly supplied by hepatic arterial branches and not portal vein.

Although hepatic metastases are supplied by small hepatic arteries, these vessels are somewhat larger than surrounding uninvolved arteries and they do not taper normally as they approach the lesion forming irregular tumor vessels (18, 19, 20, 21) (see Figure 5.5).

SURGICAL CRITERIA FOR RESECTABILITY

Surgery is the only curative therapy for malignant liver tumors. Survival is possible even after three segments of the liver are resected, as long as the remaining segment is normal. This aggressive approach includes a tri-segmentectomy which removes all the liver except the lateral segment of the left lobe (22).

Classic criteria for selection of patients for hepatectomy, therefore, require:
1. One or more segments must be free of tumor
2. Absence of tumor invasion of hepatic vein, portal vein and I.V.C.

Imaging of hepatic tumors by CT and ultrasound can confirm non-resectability due to multi-segment or diffuse involvement, but angiography is required to demonstrate precise segmental anatomy as well as anatomy of involvement based on arterial supply.

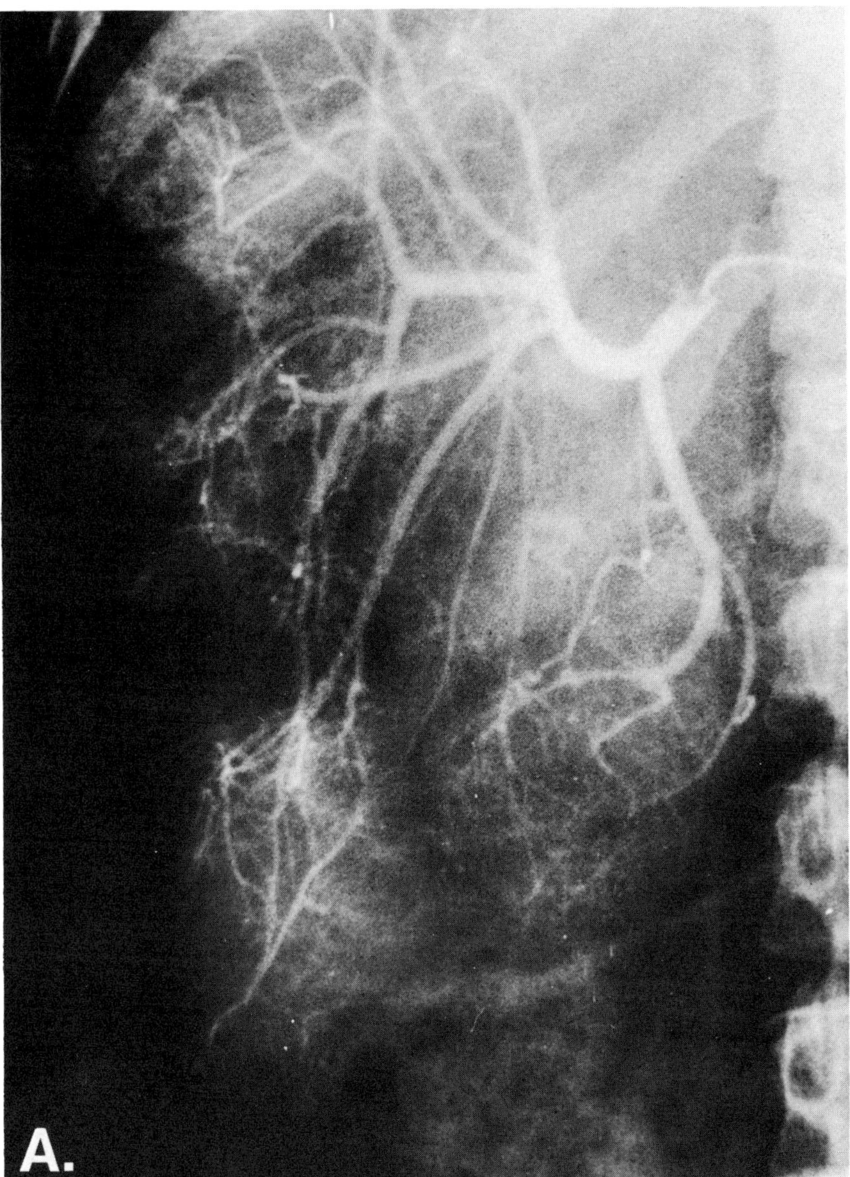

Figure 5.5 (A & B). Colonic Metastases. The arterial phase demonstrates the arterial blood supply to multiple colonic metases to the liver. Late arterial phase (B) shows the enhancement at each of these focal deposits.

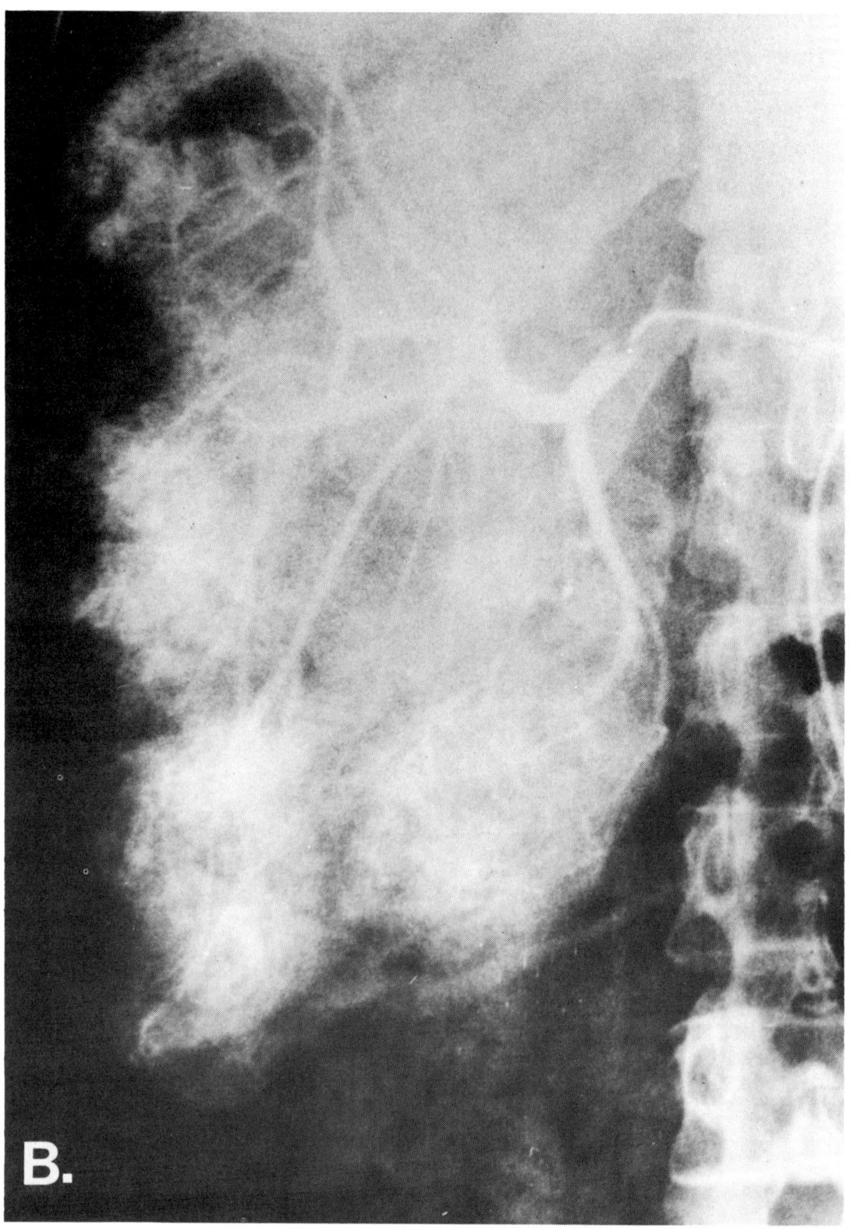
B.

Angiographic findings indicating involvement by tumor include: (23, 24, 25)
1. Hypervascularity
2. Neovascularity
3. Mass effect
4. Encasement of large arteries
5. Arteriovenous shunting
6. Intravascular tumor thrombus, especially portal vein (threads and streaks sign) (11).

Although arteriography can demonstrate extent of vascular involvement as well as arterial variation, hypovascular lesions as well as vascular invasion by small lesions may be missed. The left lobe in particular may be difficult to evaluate. Direct intra–arterial injection of the hepatic artery during CT may be of value in clearing questionable areas. Close correlation between all imaging modalities is recommended prior to resection.

INTERVENTIONAL ANGIOGRAPHY AS AN ADJUNCT TO TREATMENT OF LIVER TUMORS

A significant contemporary development is the utilization of angiographic techniques for adjunctive therapy of primary hepatic and metastatic neoplasms. Applications include the placement of hepatic arterial catheters for selective infusion of chemotherapeutic agents and transcatheter embolization.

Although surgery is the most definitive therapy for malignant tumors of the liver, angiography for selective intra–arterial infusion of cytotoxic agents as well as direct embolization of hepatic tumors may improve surgical results or offer an alternative treatment for unresectable tumors (26, 27).

Tumors of the liver, both primary and metastatic, derive their blood supply from the hepatic artery. The normal liver, though, receives only 25% of its blood supply from the artery and the remainder from the portal vein. This dual blood supply makes arterial infusion or selective arterial embolization especially inviting for the treatment of liver tumors.

Selective hepatic arterial chemotherapeutic infusion permits the delivery of higher drug concentrations to the target tumor than the same dose delivered intravenously. Intra–arterial infusion also yields fewer systemic side effects than peripheral injection, possibly because of augmented "first pass" drug extraction by the tumor.

Transcatheter therapy (for infusion and embolization) requires that super–selective catheterization be performed. Therapeutic effects are maximized and side effects minimized by placement of the catheter as close to the tumor as possible.

For hepatic infusion, catheter placement is crucial to prevent delivery of chemotherapeutic agents to stomach, gall bladder or pancreas by collateral vessels (28, 29, 30). This risk can be minimized by prophylactic embolization of the origin of the gastro-duodenal artery (31, 32). Nonetheless, cases are now being reported in which sclerosing cholangitis occurs even after correct placement of the catheters. This can be a fatal complication and seems dose and time related (33, 34).

Effective hepatic arterial perfusion can also be limited by multiple hepatic arteries (this occurs in 45% of patients). Since hepatic arteries serve as readily available collaterals for each other, angiographic embolization of the origins of all replaced or accessory vessels except one, will allow infusion through a single catheter to treat the entire liver (35). The distribution of infusate can be assessed by observing contrast injection through the catheter (fluoroscopically or on CT), or by scanning the transcatheter injection of ^{99m}Tc labeled macro–aggregated albumin (a nuclear medicine scanning agent used for lung scans). (36).

Infusion catheters have been placed by the traditional trans-femoral arterial approach using the Seldinger percutaneous puncture technique. Since most infusion protocols require prolonged cycles of treatment lasting several weeks, the transfemoral catheter position becomes inconvenient as the patient must be immobilized throughout this period. Alternative approaches include transaxillary and transbrachial arterial placement (37). Although catheter insertion in the arm is more convenient for the patient, there are increased local complications secondary to puncture of a smaller artery, and the actual selective catheterization may be more difficult. Recently there has been increased interest in long term infusion of cancercidal agents via transarterial catheters connected to surgically placed indwelling pumps.

When liver tumors fail to respond to systemic or direct intra-arterial chemotherapy, an alternative approach is arterial embolization (38). Embolization has also been used to control pain, hemorrhage, and to occlude arteriovenous shunts. Preoperative embolization also helps to demarcate tumor and decrease vascularity and, therefore, blood loss during surgery. Again, the dual blood supply or normal liver protects uninvolved parenchyma while arterial embolization causes devascularization of the tumor. Intrahepatic arteries can rapidly re-establish blood flow via collaterals following embolization. Therefore, the effectiveness of embolization becomes dependent on the size of embolizing agent and thus the level of vascular blockade.

If occlusion coils were used to occlude large arteries, collaterals would readily develop to supply the intact distal circulation of the embolized vessel. Thus, while proximal embolization employing coils is useful for occluding accessory hepatic arteries when a selective infusion catheter is to be placed or to protect the gastroduodenal artery during chemotherapeutic infusion, proximal embolization is inappropriate for infarction of tumors. Instead, occlusion of the pre-capillary or arteriolar level vessels must be performed (39). This can be done using small particulate matter such as Gelfoam or Ivalon (Figure 5.6A) or newer agents such as cyano-acrylate, a rapidly polymerizing glue, and absolute alcohol. Absolute alcohol is thought to infarct vessels by causing a capillary level vasculitis (40). Use of these liquid agents requires careful catheter placement and slow arterial flow. Although the balloon occlusion technique of embolization of the common hepatic artery has now been advocated (41) because of its immediate effect, the problem of collateral circulation remains and it does appear from our experience that very satisfactory results are obtained by pre-capillary or arteriolar embolization.

One complication of infarction is superimposed infection. It may be difficult to diagnose abscess formation as all the classic findings of infection, such as pain, fever, tenderness, WBC elevation, abnormal biochemical values of liver function and gas bubbles on abdominal x-ray may be produced by nonseptic infarction of the tumor. Of most value in differentiation, is the severity of symptoms with infarction resulting in only mild findings reaching a peak in the first few days following infarction and then improving. Nonseptic bubble formation (Figure 5.6B) is thought to be produced by gas liberation from the breakdown of highly vascular tumors (42). Another major concern with hepatic artery embolization is the development of gall bladder necrosis (29). This can be avoided by selective catheterization of hepatic artery branches and using an embolic material such as a mixture of absorbable cellulose and contrast which does not reflux (43). This might also help to avoid the far worse disaster of bile duct necrosis after hepatic artery embolization (44).

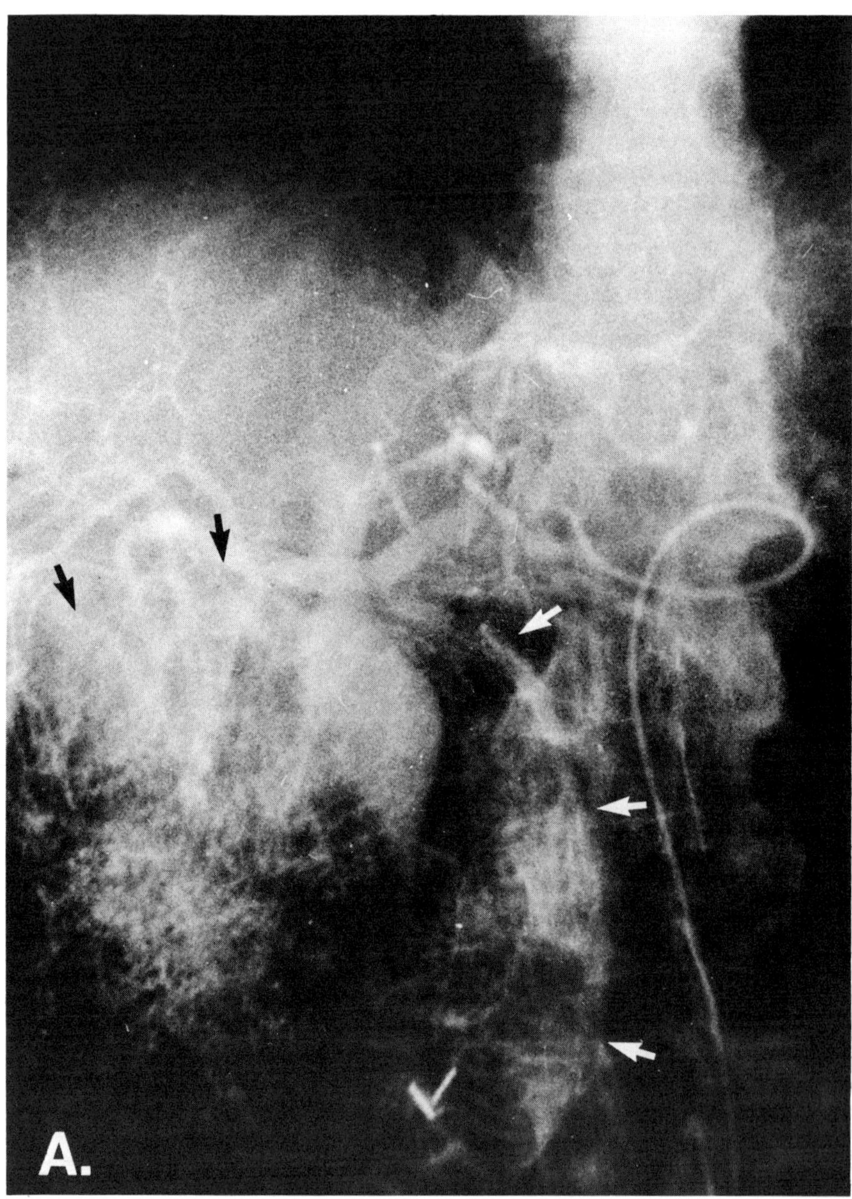

Figure 5.6 (A & B). Embolization of Colonic Metastases. A massive metastatic deposit to the right lobe of the liver is seen on the arterial phase demonstrating malignant vascularity, with areas of hypervascularity intermixed with

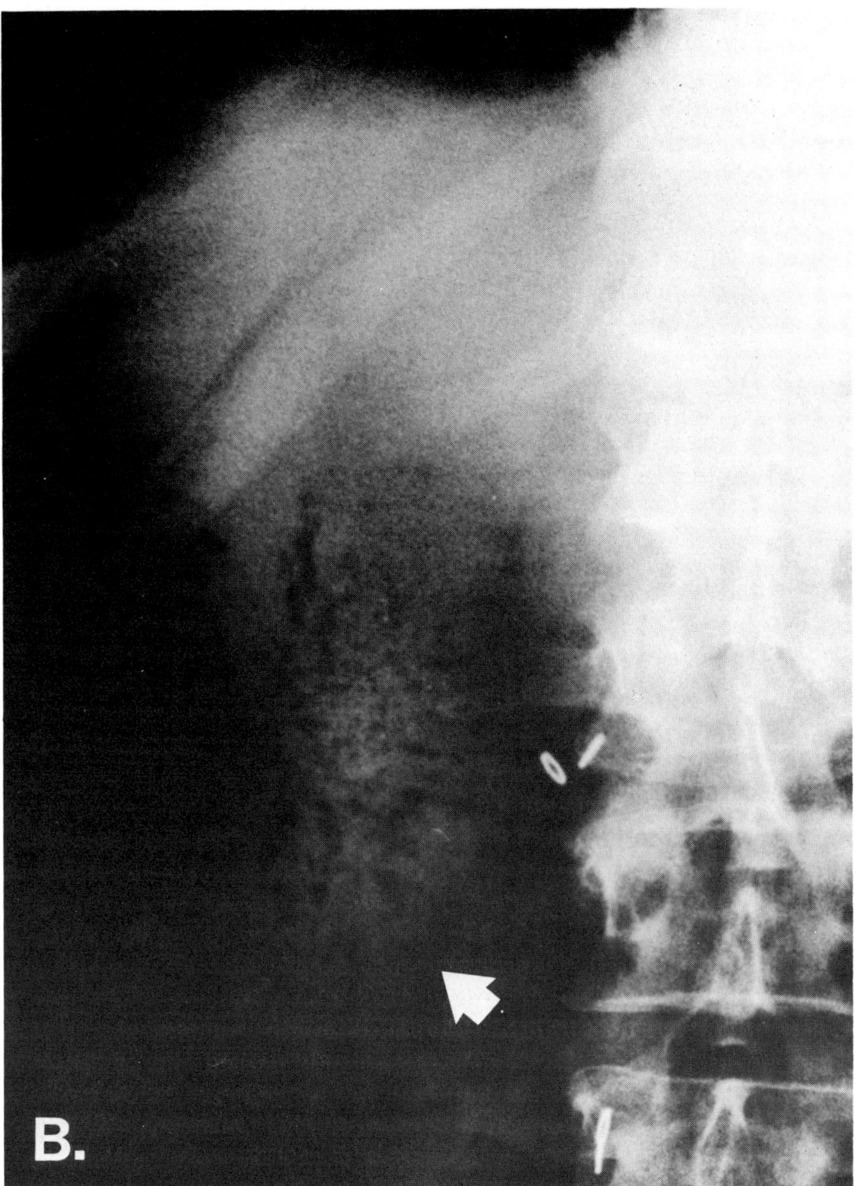

areas of necrosis (A). This lesion was embolized. A follow-up plain film study showed necrosis of the lesion with multiple gas bubbles easily seen (B). The gas bubbles represent sterile tumor necrosis.

Relative contraindications to hepatic arterial embolization include conditions which make the normal parenchyma more dependent upon arterial flow, such as underlying cirrhosis, portal vein occlusion and extensive replacement of normal tissue by tumor. Drs. Wallace and Chuang have successfully embolized such patients using a serial approach, treating one territory at a time (45).

With experience gained in hepatic arterial chemotherapeutic infusion and in embolization, the next step is chemo–embolization. This has been done successfully at Chiba University in Japan by selective intra–arterial infusion of Mitomycin C in micro-capsule form in patients with unresectable hepatocellular carcinoma, and a mean survival rate of 8.4 months (median 9 months) was achieved (46).

CONCLUSION

The emphasis upon angiography as a means for primary detection of hepatic neoplasms has decreased markedly with technical improvement in noninvasive or minimally invasive imaging modalities, such as, nuclear medicine liver spleen scan, ultrasound, computed tomography and nuclear magnetic resonance. The importance of angiography for differential diagnosis has simultaneously increased, however, as many incidental lesions are detected through the use of these newer imaging procedures in patients presenting with a variety of nonspecific abdominal complaints as well as in patients with known primary malignant disease elsewhere in the body. Angiographic techniques are increasingly being employed for therapeutic applications, such as focal infusion of chemotherapeutic agents and selective embolization, in addition to demonstration of vascular anatomy prior to surgery.

REFERENCES

1. Michels, NA: *Blood Supply and Anatomy of the Upper Abdominal Organs with a Descriptive Atlas.* Philadelphia: Lippincott Co, 1955.

2. Lunderquist, A: Arterial segmental supply of the liver, an angiographic study. *Acta Radiol Suppl, 272:*1–68, 1967.

3. Ruzicka, FF, Jr., Rankin, RS: Normal arterial anatomy of the abdominal viscera. *CRC Crit Diagn Imaging, 9:*337–385, 1977.

4. McMullen, CT, Montgomery, JL: Arteriographic findings of focal nodular hyperplasia of the liver and review of the literature. *Am J Roentgenol,* *117:*380-387, 1973.

5. Belfer, AJ, Grijm, R, VanderSchoot, JB: Hepatic adenoma, imaging with different radionuclides. *Clin Nucl Med, 4:*375-378, 1979.

6. Casarella, WJ, Knowles, DM, Wolff, M, Johnson, PM: Focal nodular hyperplasia and liver cell adenoma. Radiologic and Pathologic Differentiation. *Am J Roentgenol, 131:*393-402, 1978.

7. Goldstein, HM, Neiman, HL, Mena, E, *et al.*: Angiographic findings in benign liver cell tumors. *Radiol, 110:*339-343, 1974.

8. McLoughlin, MJ: Angiography in cavernous hemangioma of the liver. *Am J Roentgenol, 113:*50-55, 1971.

9. Rabinowitz, JG, Kinkabwala, M, Ulreich, S: Macro-regenerating nodule in cirrhotic liver. *Am J Roentgenol, 121:*401-411, 1974.

10. Reuter, SR, Redman, HC, Siders, DB: The spectrum of angiographic findings in hepatoma. *Radiol, 94:*89-94, 1970.

11. Okuda, K, Musha, H, Yoshida, T, *et al.*: Demonstration of growing casts of hepatocellular carcinoma in the portal vein by celiac angiography, the thread and streaks sign. *Radiol, 117:*303-309, 1975.

12. Kido, C, Sasaki, T, Kaneko, M: Angiography of primary liver cancer. *Am J Roentgenol, 113:*70-81, 1971.

13. Okuda, K, Obata, H, Jinnouchi, S, *et al.*: Angiographic assessment of gross anatomy of hepatocellular carcinoma: comparison of celiac angiograms and liver pathology in 100 cases. *Radiol, 123:*21-29, 1971.

14. Jewel, KL: Primary carcinoma of the liver, clinical and radiologic manifestations. *Am J Roentgenol, 113:*84-91, 1971.

15. Yu, C: Primary carcinoma of the liver (hepatoma) its diagnosis by selective celiac arteriography. *Am J Roentgenol, 99:*142-149, 1967.

16. Reuter, SR, Redman, HC, Bookstein, JJ: Angiography in carcinoma of the biliary tract. *Br J Radiol, 44:*636-641, 1971.

17. Kaude, J, Rian, R: Cholangiocarcinoma. *Radiol, 100:*573-580, 1971.

18. Reuter, SR, Redman, HC: *Gastrointestinal Angiography*, 2nd Edition. Philadelphia: W.B. Saunders Co, 1977.

19. Watson, RC, Baltaxe, HA: Angiographic appearance of primary and secondary tumors of the liver. *Radiol, 101:*539-548, 1971.

20. Nebesar, RA, Pollard, JJ, Stone, DL: Angiographic diagnosis of malignant disease of the liver. *Radiol, 86:*284-291, 1966.

21. Moss, AA, Clark, RE, Palubinskas, AJ, Delorimer, AA: Angiographic appearance of benign and malignant hepatic tumors in infants and children. *Am J Roentgenol, 113:*61-69, 1971.

22. Starzl, TE, Bell, RH, Beart, RW, Putnam, CW: Hepatic trisegmentectomy and other liver resections. *Surg Gynecol Obstet, 141:*429-437, 1975.

23. Gammill, SL, Takahashi, M, Kawanani, M, Fort, R, Sparks, R: Hepatic angiography in the selection of patients with hepatomas for hepatic lobectomy. *Radiol, 101:*549-554, 1971.

24. Gammill, SL, Takahashi, M, Jingu, K, Stumpe, W, Font, R: A com-

parison of scans and angiograms in selecting patients with hepatomas for hepatic lobectomy. *Am J Roentgenol, 123:*522-530, 1975.

25. Marks, WM, Jacobs, RP, Goodman, PC, Lim, RC: Hepatocellular carcinoma, clinical and angiographic findings and predictability for surgical resection. *Am J Roentgenol, 132:*7-11, 1979.

26. Chuang, VP, Wallace, S: Arterial infusion and occlusion in cancer patients. *Sem Reontgenol, 16:*13, 1981.

27. Chuang, VP, Wallace, S: Interventional approaches to hepatic tumor treatment. *Sem Roentgenol, 18:*127, 1983.

28. Hall, DA, Clause, ME, Gramm, HF: Gastroduodenal ulceration after hepatic arterial infusion chemotherapy. *Am J Roentgenol, 136:*1216, 1981.

29. Kuroda, C, Iwasaki, M, Tanaka, T, *et al.*: Gall bladder infarction following hepatic transcatheter arterial embolization. *Radiol, 149:*85, 1983.

30. Chuang, VP, Wallace, S, Stroehlein, JR, *et al.*: Hepatic artery infusion chemotherapy, gastroduodenal complications. *Am J Roentgenol, 137:* 347, 1981.

31. Granmayeh, M, Wallace, S, Schwarten, DE: Transcatheter occlusion of the gastroduodenal artery. *Radiol, 131:*59, 1979.

32. Kuribayashi, S, Phillips, DA, Harrington, DP, *et al.*: Therapeutic embolization of the gastroduodenal artery in hepatic artery infusion chemotherapy. *Am J Roentgenol, 137:*1169, 1981.

33. Pien, EH, Zeman, RK, Benjamin, SB, *et al.*: Iatrogenic sclerosing cholangitis following hepatic arterial chemotherapy infusion. *Radiol, 156:* 329-330, 1985.

34. Botet, JF, Watson, RC, Kemeny, N, *et al.*: Cholangitis complicating intra-arterial chemotherapy in liver metastases. *Radiol, 156:*335-337, 1985.

35. Chuang, VP, Wallace, S: Hepatic arterial redistribution for intra-arterial infusion of hepatic neoplasms. *Radiol, 135:*295, 1980.

36. Bledin, AG, Kantarjian, HM, Kim, EE, *et al.*: Tc 99^{m}-Labeled macroaggregated albumin in intrahepatic arterial chemotherapy. *Am J Roentgenol, 139:*711, 1982.

37. Cason, WP, Whaley, RA: Intra-arterial hepatic infusion via the axillary artery using the headhunter catheter. *Radiol, 134:*247, 1980.

38. Chuang, VP, Wallace, S: Hepatic artery embolization in the treatment of hepatic neoplasms. *Radiol, 140:*51, 1981.

39. Clause, ME, Lee, RGL, Duszlak, ES, *et al.*: Peripheral hepatic artery embolization for primary and secondary hepatic neoplasms. *Radiol, 147:*407, 1983.

40. Ellman, BA, Green, CE, Eigenbrodt, E, Garriott, JC, Curry, TS: Renal infarction with absolute ethanol. *Invest Radiol, 15:*318-322, Jul-Aug, 1980.

41. Nakamura, H, Tanaka, M, Oi, H: Hepatic embolization from the common hepatic artery using balloon occlusion techniques. *Am J Radiol, 145:*115-116, 1985.

42. Rankin, RN: Gas formation after renal tumor embolization without abscess. A benign occurrence. *Radiol, 130:*317-320, 1979.

43. Onodera, H, Oikawa, M, Abe, M, Goto, Y,: Gall bladder necrosis after transcatheter hepatic arterial embolization: A technique to avoid this complication. *Radiol, 152:*209-210, 1984.

44. Makuuchi, M, Sukigara, M, Mori, T, *et al.*: Bile duct necrosis: Complication of transcatheter hepatic arterial embolization. *Radiol, 156:*331-334, 1985.

45. Chuang, VP, Wallace, S, Soo, CS, *et al.*: Therapeutic ivalon embolization of hepatic tumors. *Am J Roentgenol, 138:*289, 1982.

46. Ohnishi, K, Tsuchiya, S, Nakayama, T, *et al.*: Arterial chemo-embolization of hepatocellular carcinoma with Mitomycin C microcapsules. *Radiol, 152:*51-55, 1984.

W. JOHN B. HODGSON, M.D.

CHAPTER 6
Incisions

Extirpation of liver tumors requires appropriate access. The left lateral hepatic segment, that is the portion of the liver to the left of the falciform ligament, is the easiest to resect and therefore its approach will be discussed first.

MIDLINE INCISIONS

Most surgeons encounter the left lateral segment of the liver in the course of performing vagotomies and then this segment simply gets in the way. Its attachments are usually divided and the liver retracted out of the way. The approach is usually through an upper midline incision (Figure 6.1) and this seems to be a good place to start for tumor resection. The incision, however, must be long enough. It should be carried up past the xiphoid process (which can always be resected if it is prominent or otherwise interferes with the resection), and the other end should be extended below the umbilicus. Retraction on the margins of this incision will provide quite adequate exposure of the left lateral segment of the liver.

Patients with narrow costal angles make particularly good subjects for such an incision, but it can be rather short in a patient with a wide costal margin. Closure is simple, the author preferring interrupted Jones-type sutures of #0 Vicryl. A good strong scar results.

Although the right paramedian incision is the preferred approach in many Centers to the gall bladder, it seems to be more difficult to perform and is no stronger than the midline incision. Therefore, I use the latter for hepatic artery ligation or cannulation, provided no other procedures are contemplated on the right side of the liver.

If the surgeon is considering formal left hemihepatectomy through the gall bladder fossa to the inferior vena cava, again, the upper midline is a perfectly satisfactory incision. Madding and

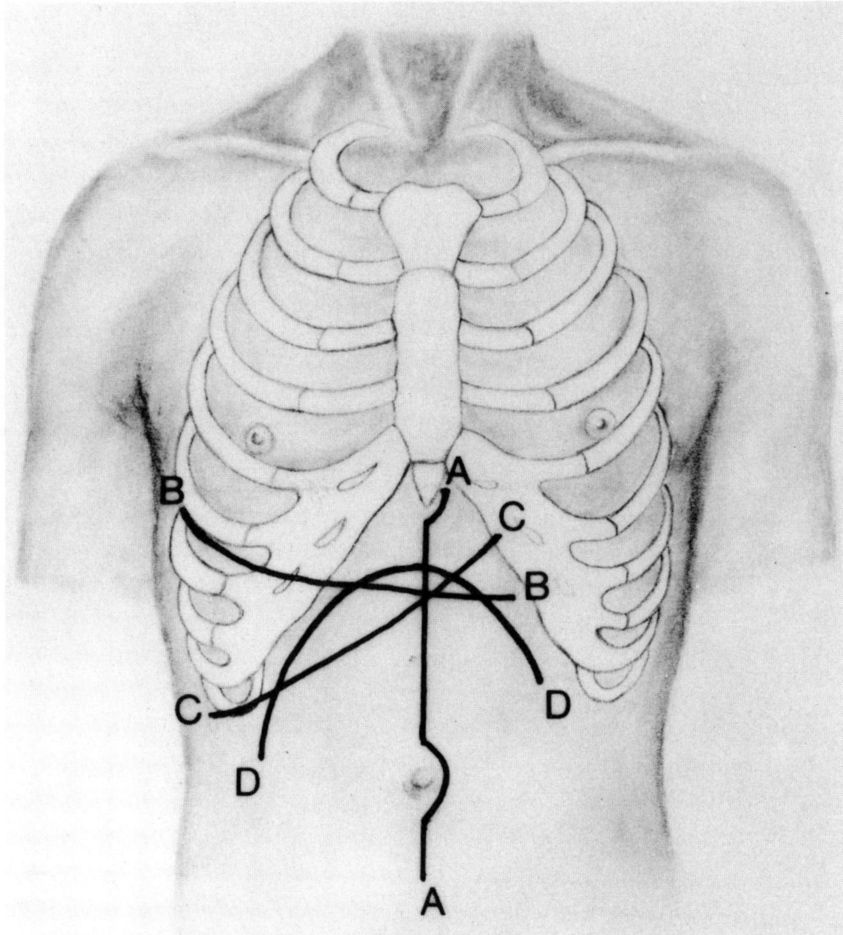

Figure 6.1. Illustrations of incisions used in hepatic resections.
- AA   Midline
- BB   Right thoraco-abdominal
- CC   Right subcostal
- DD   Bilateral subcostal

Kennedy prefer this approach if there is any chance of a caval injury, even for right sided hepatic injuries (1). Certainly, wedge resections of the medial segment of the left lobe can be done through this incision.

As the right side of the liver is somewhat larger than the left, accounting for about 60% by volume, it is a more difficult problem, and really adequate exposure must be obtained for safe resections on this side. For elective surgery the midline does not really give adequate exposure, although in the trauma situation extension towards a sternal split can be life-saving. On the other hand, a right paramedian approach can be used with ease in the Asiatic populations and is preferred by Ong (2).

RIGHT THORACO-ABDOMINAL INCISION

Probably the incision that more easily comes to mind is the right thoraco-abdominal (Figure 6.1). To carry this out for liver surgery, correct placement of the patient on the operating room table is important. The right shoulder must be raised about 50-60° off the table. The hip should be raised no more than 30°. Rotating the patient too far gives an excellent view of the kidney and not rotating the patient far enough hardly makes the chest worth opening. The objective, after all, is to expose the liver, the portal inflow, and the inferior vena cava. Therefore, with the patient in the mid-rotation, an incision is made through the 8th interspace, about equidistant above and below the costal margin. The diaphragm then is also incised antero-posteriorly in a curved manner towards the inferior vena cava, thus avoiding the phrenic nerve, and after rib retractors are placed, good exposure of the right lobe of the liver is achieved. Foster prefers this approach (3). This exposure is particularly useful in deep-chested patients.

The closure of this incision is important and the diaphragm is usually closed first either with #0 Vicryl sutures placed in an interrupted manner or #0 chromic catgut sutures. The closure is taken right up to the costal margin and the costal cartilages themselves are usually closed by placing a #1 Vicryl suture through the actual cartilage in order to get the cut edges face to face. This will avoid gaps in the diaphragm at the point of attachment to the costal cartilages. Following this, the ribs are then pulled together with large #1 Vicryl sutures placed in an interrupted manner until the entire rib incision is closed and the muscle covering, i.e., Serratas anterior, is also closed over the ribs using stitches of interrupted #0 Vicryl.

Other than the fact that the left lobe of the liver is poorly visualized with this incision, its major drawbacks are that the chest must be opened and the costal margin cut. When the chest cavity is open, there is an increased incidence of atelectasis, pneumonia and, in particular, despite routine underwater drainage, pleural effusion. Blood loss also appears to be increased (4). Since the costal margin is cartilagenous, it does not heal well after division and the patient following surgery has a permanent, uncomfortable, "floating" costal margin. This effect can be reduced by cutting away an inch or two of costal margin on either side of the point of division.

On the plus side, not only can the right lobe of the liver be easily visualized through this incision, it can be easily mobilized. The right triangular and coronary ligaments can be divided under vision and the right hepatic vein easily visualized. After the hepatic flexure of the colon is packed down, the portal structures are also easily seen. Further, the inferior vena cava can be controlled above the diaphragm if need be. Also, right thoracotomy allows equilization of abdominal, pleural and room pressure, which minimizes the danger of air embolism. Displacement of the liver into the chest sometimes helps the surgeon to control the difficult hepatic veins draining the caudate lobe. In addition, if another incision has been started, such as the midline, it can be extended laterally into the right thorax should extra measures be required to control bleeding, especially caval bleeding.

THE RIGHT SUBCOSTAL INCISION

The right subcostal incision (Figure 6.1) has many advantages of the right thoraco-abdominal, but without its disadvantages. A subcostal incision is made about 2 finger-breadths below the costal margin from the right flank to the midline, where it may be extended up to, or past, the xiphisternum. It may also be extended across to the opposite costal margin. This incision is probably safer than the thoraco-abdominal if the tumor lies on the dome of the right lobe within the bare area of the liver. The trick with this incision is to adequately mobilize the liver. This is done by dividing the falciform ligament all the way back to the inferior vena cava and then detaching the retroperitoneal hepatic ligaments from below laterally. The lower leaf of the coronary ligament can be divided, and the hand then enters the bare area to protect the inferior vena cava, so that the upper coronary ligaments may be divided. The liver can then be delivered downwards to the incision. A routine closure is used. Starzl prefers this incision for operations on the right side of the liver (5). The disadvantages are the same as all subcostal or Kocher incisions, namely, postoperative numbness below the incision, and the extreme difficulty of repair should infection and a hernia develop.

BILATERAL SUBCOSTAL INCISION

For wedging out bilateral tumors, a bilateral subcostal (Figure 6.1) is now preferred. In fact, at the beginning of this chapter it was pointed out that the upper midline incision was most often used for left sided resections. Experience, however, dictates that the bilateral or left subcostal is just as good. Indeed, for a left trisegmentectomy, Starzl (6) uses the bilateral subcostal incision. Fortner actually prefers this approach even for right sided resections (7). After all, the liver lies transversely, and transverse incisions make sense. Postoperative recovery tends to be faster. Exposure is good, provided the rule of adequate mobilization of the liver is carried out.

CONCLUSIONS

Before deciding on which particular incision to use, however, the surgeon will have studied the patient carefully, and essentially planned exactly what procedure to carry out beforehand. Midline incisions allow access to left sided lesions. Bilateral subcostal incisions allow access to smaller, bilateral, inferiorly placed tumors. With experience, they may also be used in major hepatic resections. Right subcostal incisions allow access to most right sided lesions. Right thoraco-abdominal incisions allow easier access to the back of the liver, particularly in deep-chested individuals.

REFERENCES

1. Madding, GF, Lim, RL, Kennedy, PA: Hepatic and vena caval injuries. *Surg Clin N Am*, 57:275-289, 1977.

2. Ong, GB: Right hemihepatectomy. In *Liver Surgery*, Calne and Della Rovere (Eds.). Philadelphia, PA: W. B. Saunders, 1982, page 23.

3. Foster, JH, Berman, MM: Solid liver tumors. Major problems in clinical surgery. 22:255-303, 1977.

4. Ryan, WH, Hummel, BW, McClelland, RN: Reduction in the morbidity and mortality of major hepatic resections. *Am J Surg, 144:*740-743, 1982.

5. Starzl, TE, Bell, RH, Beart, RW, Putnam, CW: Hepatic trisegmentectomy and other liver resections. *Surg Gynecol & Obstet, 141:*429-437, 1975.

6. Starzl, TE, Iwatsuki, S, Shaw, BW, *et al.*: Left hepatic trisegmentectomy. *Surg Gynecol & Obstet, 155:*21-27, 1982.

7. Fortner, JG, Maclean, BJ, Kim, DK, *et al.*: The Seventies evolution in liver surgery for cancer. *Cancer, 47:*2162-2166, 1981.

W. JOHN B. HODGSON, M.D.

CHAPTER 7
Anatomy

The liver is the anatomical key to the abdomen. Its superficial anatomy was known to the ancient Babylonians in animals 4,000 years ago (1). Although now the internal and external anatomy is clearly defined, still not enough surgeons understand this, even if they are fully cognizant with the liver's anatomical relations to other organs. One of the reasons for this difficulty seems to be that liver anatomy has been presented, not in a dynamic functional manner but as a simple description of the external appearance of the organ. It is the intention of this chapter to take the reader from such a known description into the dynamic variables of liver anatomy.

The liver is the largest organ in the body, weighing approximately 6,600 grams in the adult. It is about 20–23 cms in transverse diameter, 15–17 cms in its greatest vertical diameter and the greatest antero–posterior diameter is about 10–12.5 cms.

The liver is wedge–shaped with a base on the right, the apex on the left and with a superior and inferior surface. Anteriorly, the meeting point of these surfaces is sharp, but elsewhere the remaining margins are rounded.

SURFACE ANATOMY

The liver occupies the entire right hypochondrium, the upper part of the epigastric region and extends a short distance into the left hypochondrium. It lies in contact with the right kidney, the hepatic flexure of the colon, the duodenum, the anterior surface and lesser curvature of the stomach, the tail of the pancreas and spleen, and with the left kidney.

In terms of surface anatomy (Figure 7.1) the liver reaches as far as the 5th intercostal space and in some individuals even as far up as the 4th space. Inferiorly on the right the liver extends down to, or just beyond, the right costal margin. The inferior border then extends from about the middle of the right costal margin

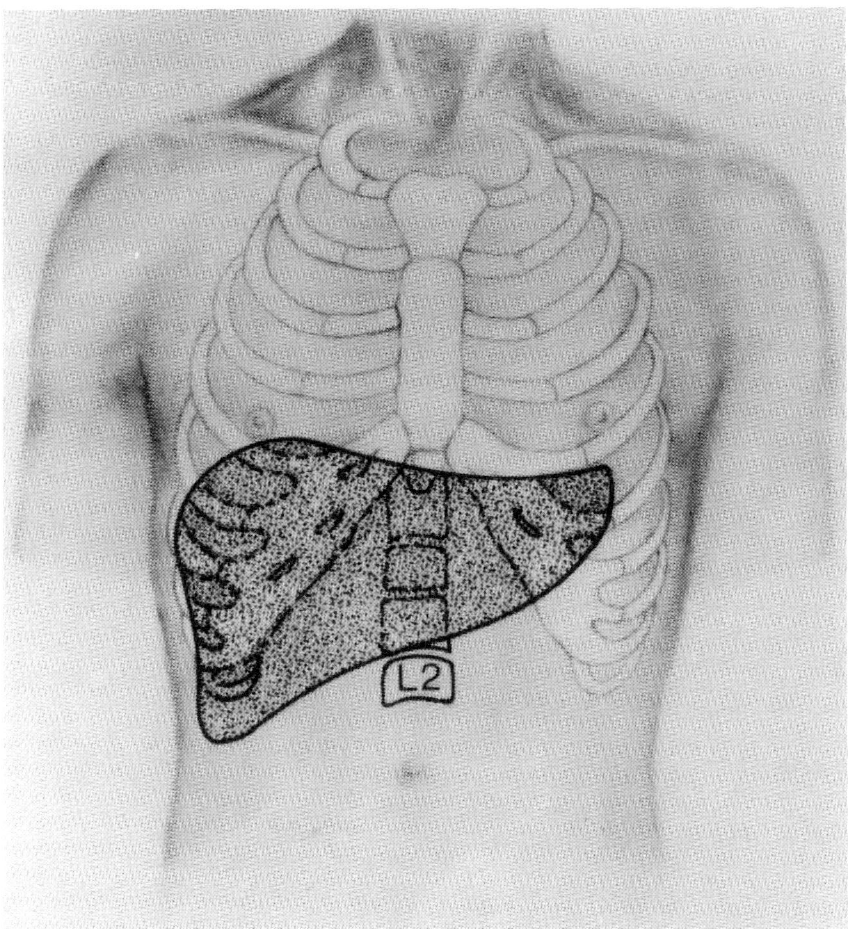

Figure 7.1. Surface anatomy of the liver from the anterior aspect.

across to the tip of the left 8th costal cartilage. The *falciform liga-ment* extends from the anterior surface of the liver to the diaphragm and anterior abdominal wall, just to the right of the midline. It runs from the umbilicus to the right side of the xiphoid process. The *portal vein* runs horizontally and slightly upwards at about the level of the 2nd lumbar vertebra. This is also the surface marking of the *hepatic artery* and the *common bile duct*. The intrahepatic portion of the *inferior vena cava* lies on the right of the first lumbar vertebra and the 12th thoracic vertebra.

PERITONEAL ATTACHMENTS

The peritoneal attachments of the liver (Figure 7.2) are important during liver surgery. They need to be divided carefully to completely mobilize the liver. The *left triangular ligament* is routinely divided to deflect the left lobe of the liver during vagotomy but the *right triangular* and the *upper* and *lower coronary ligaments* need to be divided to expose the *bare area* of the liver and the inferior vena cava.

SUPERFICIAL ANATOMY

The anatomical descriptions of the surface of the liver do not bear any direct relationship to the internal anatomy. First, the falciform ligament divides the liver superficially into right and left sides. These are not the right and left halves of the liver; the left side is actually the *left lateral segment* of the liver and the right side is the whole of the *right lobe* and the *medial segment* of the left lobe.

The surgical approach to the liver will not be posterior as in Figure 7.3 but from the antero–inferior aspect as in Figure 7.4. However, the surgeon familiar with gall bladder anatomy will note that, from standard anatomical texts, the *quadrate lobe* is actually medial to the gall bladder, extending from the right to the falciform ligament. This, in modern parlance, is part of the medial segment of the left lobe of the liver.

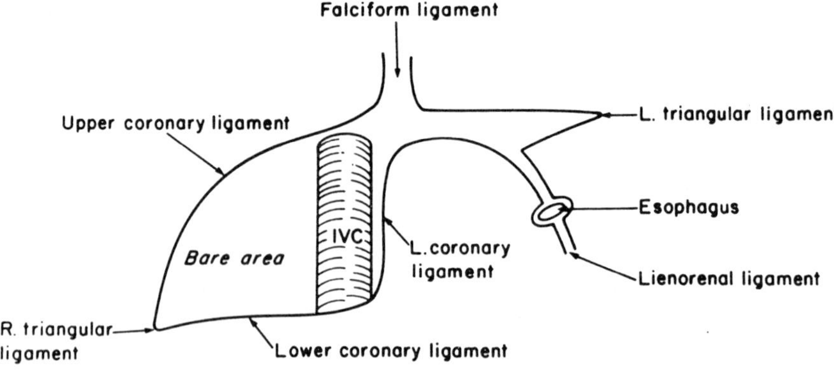

Figure 7.2. The peritoneal attachments and bare area of the liver.

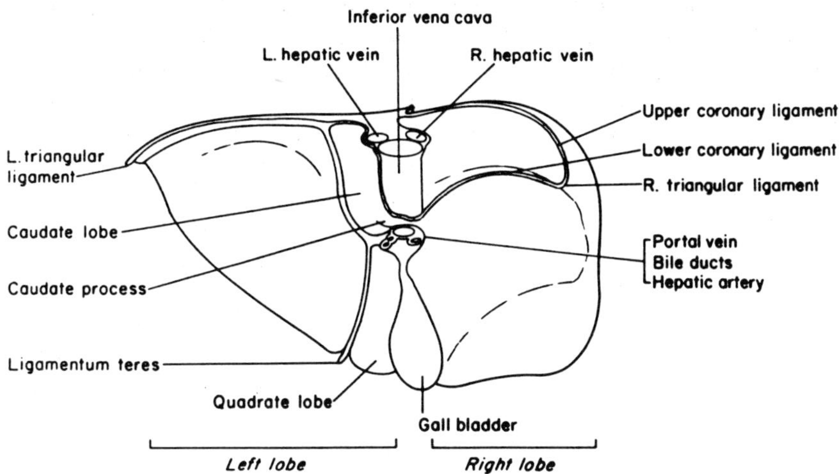

Figure 7.3. The posterior anatomy of the liver.

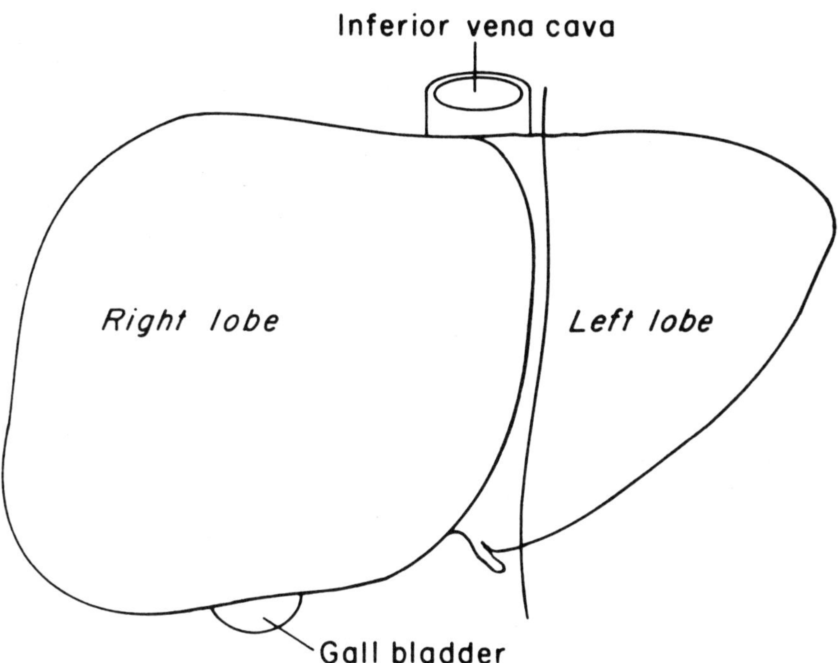

Figure 7.4. The anterior anatomy of the liver.

The *caudate lobe* is closely adherent to the inferior vena cava on its left side and peeks through anteriorly when the lesser omentum is opened. The posterior surface of the caudate lobe is related to the crura of the diaphragm above the aortic opening. The papillary process of the caudate lobe often projects downwards in front of the origin of the *celiac* axis. This lobe is situated to the left of the falciform ligament.

The *fissure* for the ligamentum venosum separates the posterior part of the caudate lobe from the left lobe of the liver. The fissure cuts deeply into the liver in front of the caudate lobe reaching to the *porta hepatis.* The *ligamentum venosum* is the fibrous remnant of the *ductus venosus.* This connected the persisting left *umbilical vein* to the common hepatic vein. The ligamentum venosum passes from the upper border of the left branch of the portal vein, ascends to the floor of the fissure and passes laterally at the upper end of the caudate lobe to join the left hepatic vein near its point of entry into the inferior vena cava. Thus, there is a fibrous connection from the left portal vein to the left hepatic vein.

The *fissure* for the ligamentum teres divides the left medial (quadrate) and the lateral lobes and runs to the porta hepatis where it meets the lower end of the fissure for the ligamentum venosum. It contains the *ligamentum teres* of the liver, the obliterated remains of the *fetal left umbilical vein* which runs from the umbilicus in the free margin of the falciform ligament to the inferior border of the liver, where it joins the left branch of the portal vein opposite to the attachment of the ligamentum venosum.

The *falciform ligament* continues over the dome of the liver backwards to divide into the upper leaf of the coronary ligament and left triangular ligament at the inferior vena cava.

The *porta hepatis* is placed on the inferior surface of the liver between the left medial lobe in front and the caudate lobe behind. The portal vein enters the porta hepatis below and divides into right and left branches. The hepatic artery enters the porta in the intermediate position and the right and left hepatic ducts exit anteriorly.

SEGMENTAL ANATOMY

Hobsley (2) quoted that as long ago as 1888 Rex (3) had noted the proper arrangement of right and left lobes. He also pointed out that Cantlie (4) described the new lobar anatomy in 1897. The bilaterality of the liver remained unrecognized until the work of Martens (5) in 1920 and McIndoe and Counsellor (6) in 1927. Despite this, the "new" or "modern" segmental anatomy had to be re-discovered in the 1940s and 1950s by Donovan and Santulli (7), Hjortsjö (8), Healey and Schroy (9), Healey (10), Couinaud (11) and Goldsmith and Woodburne (12) before wide acceptance began.

The segments of the liver are seen in the illustration (Figure 7.5). However, it must be very clearly understood that although they are based on the anatomical divisions of the inflow blood vessels and the bile ducts, there is much intra-segmental vascularity. This is particularly true of the hepatic veins and represents a major hazard in resection of the liver.

The *main boundary fissure* between the true *right* and *left lobes* of the liver is not apparent superficially but extends from the gall bladder below to the inferior vena cava above. There is a fissure, not apparent superficially, between the *anterior* and *posterior segments* of the right lobe. Anteriorly the falciform ligament marks the boundary division between the medial and lateral segments of the left lobe.

Subsegments are also noted as follows. The caudate lobe has already been described. The *left lateral segment* is divided into a

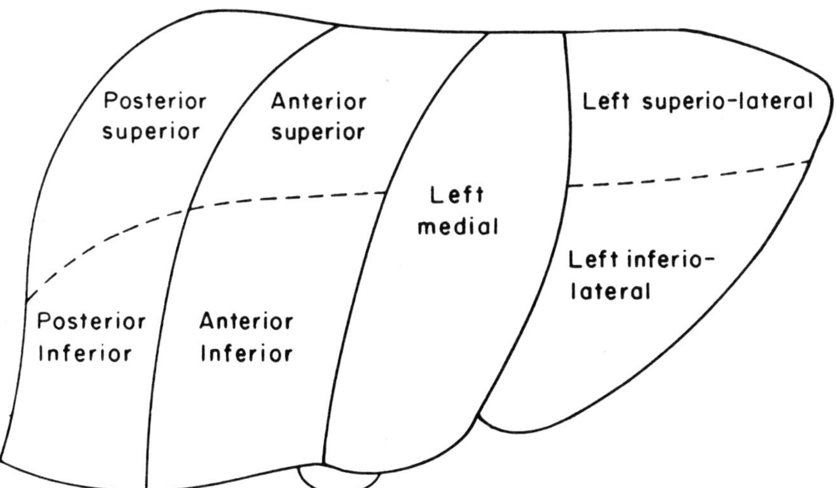

Figure 7.5. The segmental anatomy of the liver.

superior and *inferior* portion. The *left medial segment* is not subdivided although the anterior portion was formerly labelled separately as the quadrate lobe. The right anterior segment is subdivided into an *inferior* portion extending to the lower coronary ligament and a *superior* portion extending to the upper coronary ligament. The right posterior segment is also subdivided. The *postero-inferior* segment is that portion of the liver above the hepatic flexure and right kidney, and can be palpated. The *postero-superior* portion essentially occupies the upper lateral portion of the liver, and extends all the way to the inferior vena cava. This is the position of the bare area which precludes adequate palpation of this segment without full mobilization of the liver.

BLOOD SUPPLY TO THE LIVER

The liver has a double blood supply. The *hepatic artery* supplies only 25% by volume but supplies 80% of the oxygen requirements. The *portal vein* supplies 75% of the blood volume and only 20% of the oxygen requirements.

Hepatic Artery Extrahepatic Distribution

The usual arterial arrangement is that the *celiac axis* gives rise to the *splenic artery*, the *left gastric artery* and the *common hepatic artery*. This divides into right and left branches to supply right and left lobes of the liver (Figure 7.6). The usual position for the hepatic artery is through the *hepatico-duodenal ligament* medial (i.e., to the left) of the common hepatic duct and anterior to the portal vein. The division into right and left branches can occur at any given point between the origin of this artery and the entrance to the liver. The *right hepatic artery* is usually longer than the left and starts off to the left of the common hepatic duct, then passes to the right behind the duct and into the liver parenchyma. It then loses its relationship with the duct and divides rapidly into an *anterior* and *posterior segmental branch*. The cystic artery was derived from the right hepatic artery in half of Healey's studies (13) and in 18 of his 200 cases it actually took origin from the *anterior segmental artery*. Surgeons removing the gall bladder are aware of this fact. In 25% of Michels' dissections (14) the cystic artery had a dual origin. The shorter *left hepatic artery* is

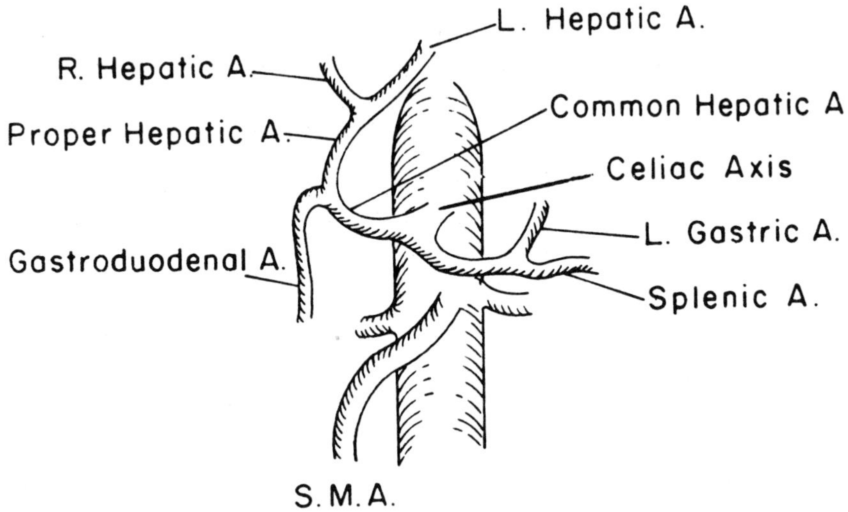

Figure 7.6. "Normal" arterial anatomy of the liver.

usually situated well below the hepatic duct and on entering the liver parenchyma almost immediately gives off segmental branches to the left lobe. It is incorrect to refer to the left middle segmental artery as a middle hepatic artery. Healey demonstrated very clearly that the left hepatic artery divided into *medial* and *lateral* segmental branches in 40% of his cases.

Since 1941, it has been generally accepted that Lander and his colleagues' findings of an anomaly rate of 15% in 100 consecutive dissections (15) was about right. Also, there was general agreement that hepatic arteries are end arteries with no anastomoses in the liver (13). However, these tenets are becoming increasingly difficult to accept.

Michels (14) found a conventional textbook picture of the arterial supply into the liver in only 55% of his dissections. This is in line with our experience. In 25% of his cases the left gastric artery gave rise to the left hepatic artery and in half of these there was an additional left hepatic artery. We have found this situation only occasionally. In 12% of Michels' 200 dissections the superior mesenteric artery was the origin of the entire blood supply to the right lobe of the liver through a separate right hepatic artery whilst the celiac axis gave rise to an independent left hepatic artery entirely supplying the left lobe. We found this situation in 25% of our clinical cases. In 17% of Michels' cases, in addition to the common hepatic artery from the coeliac axis, the superior mesenteric artery gave rise to an additional artery. In Figure 7.7 these anomalous arteries are illustrated (16).

In the clinical situation, arteriography is very necessary for the identification of these vessels preoperatively. Essentially almost any anomalous situation is possible. The entire hepatic arterial supply may originate from the superior mesenteric artery; only the right lobe may be supplied by the superior mesenteric artery; an accessory right hepatic artery may also arise from the superior mesenteric artery when a normal hepatic artery is also present. Bifurcation of the common hepatic artery may occur at the celiac axis leading effectively to duplication of the common hepatic artery. In addition to the entire left lobe being supplied from a branch from the left gastric artery, an accessory left hepatic artery from the left gastric artery may also be found.

This very complicated discussion can be summed up by recalling that the celiac axis and the superior mesenteric artery arise very close to each other embryologically. Convenient branches from either of these two arterial trunks supply the liver. Usually, one or the other becomes dominant. However, the domi-

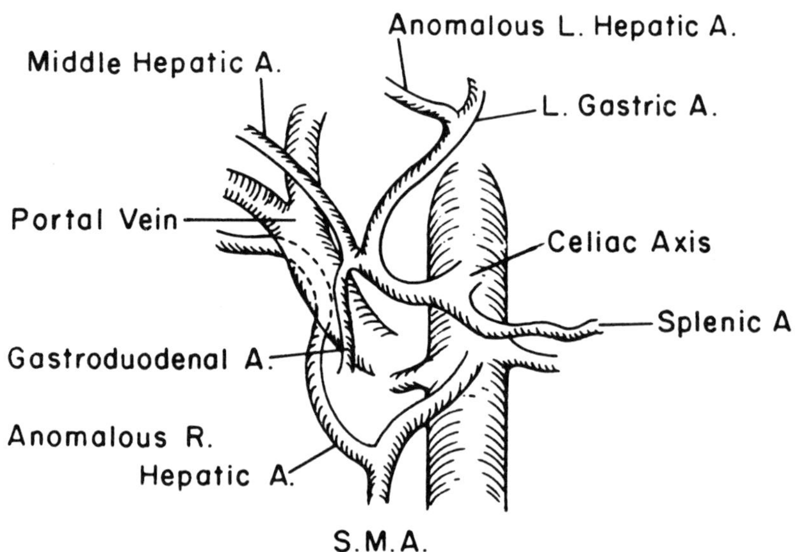

Figure 7.7. Common anomalous variations in arterial anatomy of the liver.

nance may be entirely right-sided, entirely left-sided or may involve a mixture somewhere in between.

In any event, perhaps as a consequence of Michels' work, Lortat–Jacob and Robert (17) were able to perform the first anatomic lobectomy in 1952 which was based on vascular anatomy and in which a preliminary hilar ligation was also performed.

Hepatic Artery Intrahepatic Distribution

The right and left hepatic arteries essentially supply the various segments of the liver which have been previously described. This is particularly marked on the left side where the oblique course of the left hepatic artery extending from the inferior surface superiorly and laterally permits an almost complete resection of the medial segment of the left lobe with preservation of the lateral segment. This usually occurs in extended right hepatic lobectomy or trisegmentectomy. However, in 25% of cases a major portion of the arterial supply to the left lobe is from the right hepatic artery (13) and this of course goes to the medial segment. In general, the arterial vessels follow the prevailing branches of the portal vein and the hepatic duct.

Michels (18) listed 26 possible *collateral arterial pathways* to the liver and recent work by Bengmark and Rosengren (19) has shown that after hepatic artery ligation, these collaterals are more important than first thought. They rapidly develop following hepatic artery ligation in the *phrenico–abdominal* and *inter–costal* arteries as well as by numerous small vessels in the region of the porta hepatis and caudate lobe. Cross-over collaterals occur between right and left lobes after ligation of one or other hepatic arterial trunks in 25% of cases according to Healey *et al* (13). These anastomoses were all small and subcapsular. Those in the fissure for the ligamentum teres connected the medial and lateral segmental arteries; those in the region of the porta hepatis connected the caudate lobe arteries; those to the right of the porta hepatis connected the caudate and the posterior segmental arteries. Kennedy and Madding (20) have a nice demonstration of a true cross-over from right to left lobes via an intrahepatic vessel.

It must be remembered that the pretty pictures demonstrated in the cadaver differ quite markedly from the living anatomy. In this dynamic situation, angiographic studies confirm Bengmark's work and show how quickly arterial collaterals form (21).

The Portal Vein

Anomalies of the *extrahepatic portal vein* are unlikely. The vein returns blood from the gastro–pancreatico–duodenal axis, the spleen and the small bowel mesentery to the liver. It is formed by the junction of the *superior mesenteric* and *splenic veins* posterior to the head and neck of the pancreas. It emerges from behind the duodenum, lies in the free–fold of the gastrohepatic omentum and at the porta hepatis is posterior to the common bile duct and hepatic artery. The problem with the portal vein, of course, is that it has no valves, and if lacerated, bleeding can be disastrous.

The bifurcation of the portal vein, like the hepatic artery, occurs outside the liver itself. Each major branch usually can be dissected 1–3 cms beyond the bifurcation if the surrounding liver is pushed away. The division into right and left branches occurs at the hilum in 75% of patients, but more proximal division occurs in the remaining 25% according to Ryncki (22). The bifurcation is usually in the form of a T, and this transverse part is usually about 3 cms long, with the sharper angle to the left.

Therefore, the *left main branch* of the portal vein is long and curved caudad in the plane of the falciform ligament. The first part is the *umbilical trunk* which has to be avoided in left lateral segmentectomy by keeping the line of resection 1–2 cms lateral to the falciform ligament. The branches to the medial segment originate from the umbilical trunk as it runs in the left lobar segmental fissure, but since this also gives rise to lateral segmental branches, great care must be taken to only ligate these lateral branches if the medial segment of the liver is to be preserved. Further, the umbilical part of the left portal vein or the *left lateral segmental branch* may lie perilously close to the inferior edge of the liver and care must be exercised to avoid entering it right at the commencement of the resection.

The *right branch* of the portal vein is short and *trifurcates* or *bifurcates* almost immediately but can be as long as 3 cms in length. There is considerable variation in the branching of the right portal vein and Elias and Petty felt that no two specimens were alike (23). Kennedy and Madding (20) even noted that in two instances in their studies the portal branch to the right anterior segment originated in the transverse trunk on the left side and therefore ligation of the left main portal trunk would interrupt the portal blood flow to a major portion of the right lobe as well.

Although anastomoses between branches of the portal vein in the normal liver are few, once portal venous obstruction occurs, major circuitous routing of the portal blood does occur. The *coronary veins* are normally absent but in the obstructed portal system do develop and may become major trunks whose origin is in the portal vein itself, the superior mesenteric vein or the splenic vein. In our Institution, ligation of the superior mesenteric vein has resulted in opening channels between the gastro-epiploic veins, the splenic veins, the coronary veins and thence back to the portal veins so that portal blood may get around the obstructed sites. However, in management of hepatic tumors the collateral veins only become really important when obstruction occurs at the hilum from tumor. Then the umbilical vein itself may re-cannalize and allow portal blood into the liver through porto-systemic anastomoses via the umbilicus and retroperitoneal structures such as the colon, the duodenum and pancreas. More commonly, direct porto-systemic connections via the coronary veins through the esophagus to the azygous system occur with disastrous long-term consequences.

Hepatic Veins

The venous return to the liver, except for the caudate lobe, is mostly by way of the right hepatic, middle hepatic and left hepatic veins. These flow into the inferior vena cava below the diaphragm. The *right hepatic vein* is usually single and drains the posterior segment of the right lobe and a major portion of the right antero-superior lobe. Consequently it runs along the inter-segmental plane between the right anterior and posterior segments. The *middle hepatic vein* drains the right antero-inferior segment and the inferior portion of the left middle segment. Therefore it crosses the main boundary fissure and usually joins the left hepatic vein before entering the inferior vena cava. The *left hepatic vein* drains the superior portion of the left middle segment and all the left lateral segment as it runs medially to join the inferior vena cava (Figure 7.8). There are also an indefinite number of *dorsal hepatic veins* draining directly into the inferior vena cava.

This general picture, however, does not describe the pitfalls. Nakamura and Tsuzuki (24) felt that hepatic resection should be based on segmental venous drainage and, in particular, the ability to safely ligate the hepatic veins. They found that 61.4% of the right hepatic veins examined had no branch within 1 cm of the

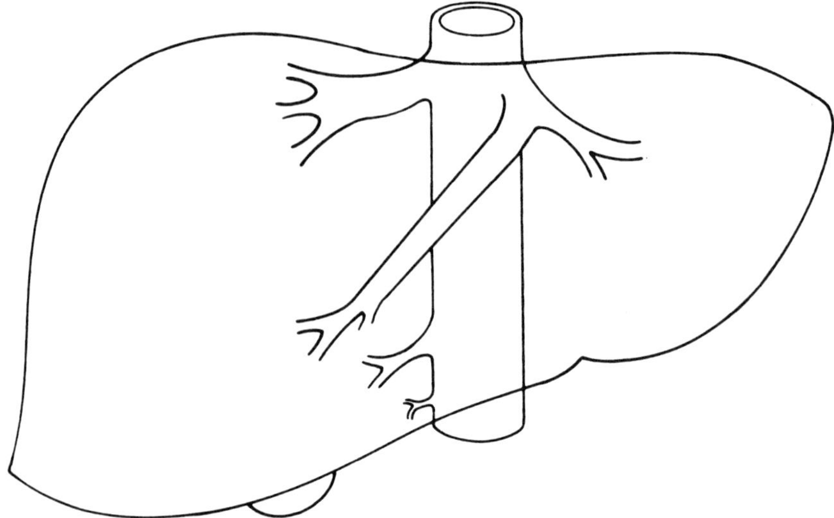

Figure 7.8. "Normal" hepatic venous anatomy.

inferior vena cava and could therefore be ligated safely at the commencement of hepatic lobectomy. However, about 40% would require parenchymal dissection for safe ligation and this therefore should not be done before hepatic lobectomy in these cases.

There are three types of right hepatic veins. *Type I* occurs in about 40% of cases, and in this instance the vein is large and drains the right hepatic lobe. There may also be a small dorsal hepatic vein, the postero-inferior vein, draining a small area of the posterior segment. A further 40% of cases are *Type II*. Here the right hepatic vein is medium-sized and is associated with a separate postero-inferior vein of between 0.5 cms and 1 cm in size draining the postero-inferior segment of the right lobe concomitantly. The remaining 20% are *Type III* where the right hepatic vein is small and short and drains the posterior segment. The postero-inferior segment is drained by a large postero-inferior vein up to 1.8 cm in size. In these cases the superior portion of the right lobe is drained by a large middle hepatic vein (Figure 7.9). In contrast to the right hepatic vein, the middle and left hepatic veins form a common trunk in about 90% of patients, (24, 25) which means that these veins are easily torn if attempts are made to ligate them prior to liver resection. They must be carefully dissected out as part of the procedure in all cases.

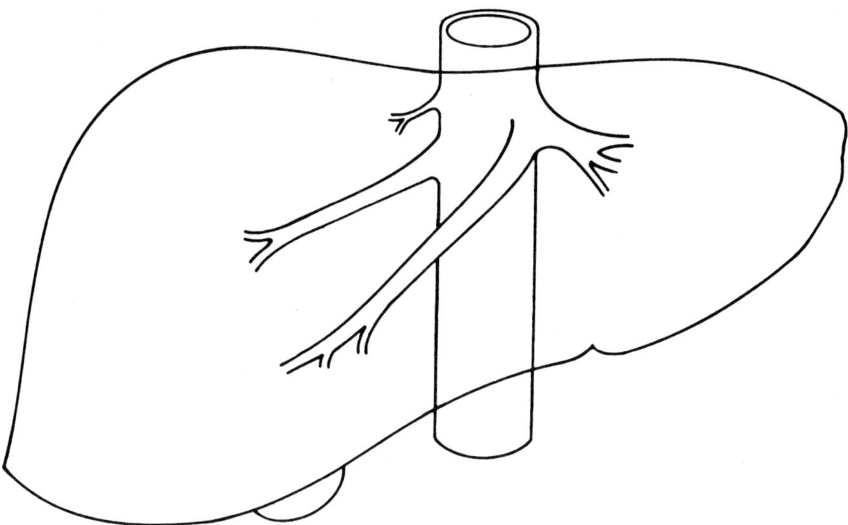

Figure 7.9. Type III hepatic venous drainage showing small right hepatic vein draining only the posterior segment and large postero-inferior vein draining the right postero-inferior segment.

Because there is a common trunk between the middle and left hepatic veins, the variations are more complicated than in the case of the right hepatic vein. The common trunk has essentially five types of patterns. These vary from the simple bifurcation well clear of the inferior vena cava in 10% of cases, to a close bifurcation or a bifurcation with other branches in 40% of the cases, to a trifurcation in 25% of cases to a quadrification in 5% of cases and a complete separation of middle and left hepatic veins in 15% of cases.

The actual area that these veins drain include the right anterior segment, the left medial segment and the left lateral segment. Separate veins drain the right antero-inferior and right antero-superior segments to join the middle hepatic vein. It also has correlating veins on the opposite side draining the left medial segment.

In addition to this relatively stable situation, there is a difficult segment or area lying between the left medial and lateral segments of the liver. This is drained variably. Sixty percent of the time, a large vein runs across the falciform ligament into the left hepatic vein. In about 30% of cases veins drain equally to the left hepatic and left medial veins and in about 10% of cases the drainage is predominantly to the middle hepatic vein.

There are between 3–50 dorsal hepatic veins but most of these are pin–hole sized and only about 10 are of any clinical significance. Of these, only the postero–inferior vein is a constant finding, draining a portion of the right lobe of the liver (Figure 7.10).

Veins draining the caudate lobe are variable. Thirty–six percent of the time there is one vein; 35% of the time two veins are separated longitudinally; 2% of the time there are two veins arranged transversely and 25% of the time there are three or four veins arranged longitudinally.

The right suprarenal veins, the phrenic veins and other anomalies may cause problems from time to time. Essentially the right suprarenal vein may actually drain into the inferior vena cava above the dorsal hepatic vein. Similarly, the phrenic vein may drain into the inferior vena cava within the liver substance itself.

THE BILIARY TREE

The biliary drainage in the liver, like the arterial and portal systems, is variable. Because the extrahepatic tree is one of the

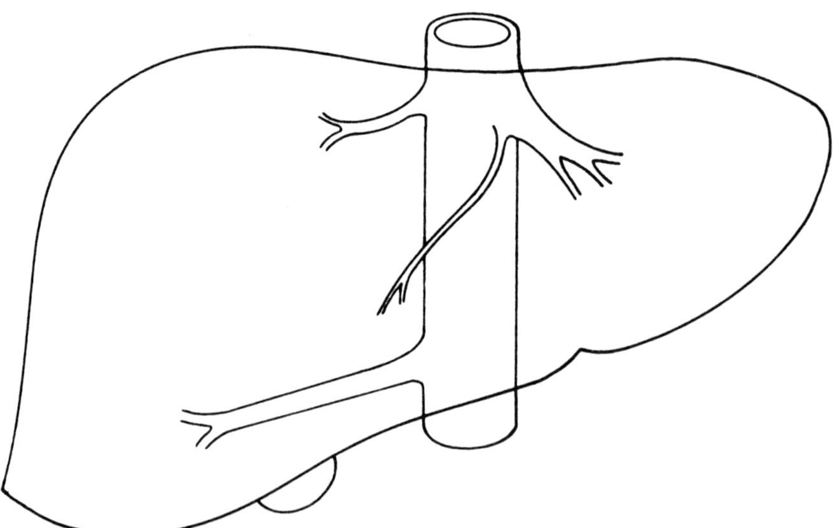

Figure 7.10. Anomalous venous drainage with very large right dorsal vein.

commonest sites of surgical intervention, frequent anatomic anomalies are the most easily understood in hepatic surgery.

The intrahepatic anatomy is segmental, the anterior and posterior segments of the right lobe having separate drainage. The separation to medial and lateral segments on the left side is less clear (13). However, the Longmire procedure (26) is based on the anatomical premise that there is communication, in obstruction of the common hepatic duct, of the biliary tree between segments and also between the right and left sides.

The *right anterior* and *posterior segmental ducts* in 72% of Healey's cases (13) joined near the porta hepatis to form the *right hepatic duct* of approximately 9 mm in length. In the other 28%, either the anterior or the posterior segmental duct cross the lobar fissure to drain into the left hepatic duct. This could present a problem in left lobectomy.

The *left lateral inferior segmental duct* joins the much smaller *left lateral superior segmental duct* at the segmental fissure. The *common left lateral duct* thus formed is joined variably by *ducts* from the *left medial* segment and by *caudate ducts*. However, the caudate may equally well drain into the right hepatic duct.

The right and left hepatic ducts join in the transverse fissure to form the *common hepatic duct*. This varies between 1–5 cms in length. The *cystic duct* is also variable and may be up to 4.5 cms long. It joins the right side of the common hepatic duct to form the common bile duct which varies between 2–7 cms in length (15). This structure consistently lies somewhat to the right of the gastro-hepatic fold and passes behind the duodenum, into the head of the pancreas and empties into the duodenum on its medial aspect at the Ampulla of Vater.

Prinz *et al.* (27) list four extrahepatic ducts or anomalies which may have clinical significance. These are *accessory bile ducts* which can occur as frequently as 18% of the time; a right or left hepatic duct entering directly into the gall bladder is rare but important; a cystic duct entering the right hepatic duct occurs 1% of the time; the right hepatic duct joining the cystic duct is extremely rare. The presence of very thin right hepatic or common hepatic ducts may result in a mistaken identity as accessory ducts. Also, the presence of a *common wall* between the cystic duct and common hepatic duct for a considerable distance, even to the point of a separate entry into the duodenum could result in accidental devitalization of the common duct during dissection.

REFERENCES

1. Foster, JH, Berman, MM: Solid liver tumors. *Major Prob Clin Surg,* 22:9-27, 1977.

2. Hobsley, M: Intrahepatic anatomy. A surgical evaluation. *Brit J Surg,* 45:635-644, 1958.

3. Rex, H: Beiträge Zur Morphologie der Säugerleber. *Morph Jahrb, 14:* 517, 1888.

4. Cantlie, J: On a new arrangement of the right and left lobes of the liver. *Proc Anat Soc Gr Brit and Ire, 32:*4, 1898.

5. Martens, E: Röntgenologische Studien zur arterieelen Gefässversorgung in der Leber. *Arch Klin Chir, 114:*1001, 1920.

6. McIndoe, A, Counsellor, V: Bilaterality of the liver. *Arch Surg, 15:* 589-612, 1927.

7. Donovan, EJ, Santulli, TV: Resection of the left lobe of the liver for mesenchymoma. *Ann Surg, 124:*90-93, 1946.

8. Hjortsjö, C: The topography of the intrahepatic duct system. *Acta Anat, 11:*599-615, 1951.

9. Healey, JE, Jr, Schroy, PC: Anatomy of the biliary ducts within the human liver. *Arch Surg, 66:*599-616, 1953.

10. Healey, JE, Jr: Clinical anatomic aspects of radical hepatic surgery. *J Int Coll Surg, 22:*542-550, 1954.

11. Couinaud, C: Le Foie. *Études Anatomiques at Chirurgicales.* Paris: Masson et Cie, 1957.

12. Goldsmith, NA, Woodburne, RT: The surgical anatomy pertaining to liver resections. *Surg Gynecol Obstet, 105:*310-318, 1957.

13. Healey, JE, Jr, Schroy, PC, Sorensen, RL: The intrahepatic distribution of the hepatic artery in man. *J Int Coll Surg, 20:*133-148, 1953.

14. Michels, NA: The hepatic, cystic and retro-duodenal arteries and their relations to the biliary ducts, with samples of entire celical blood supply. *Ann Surg, 133:*503-524, 1951.

15. Lander, HH, Lyman, RY, Anson, BJ: An anatomic consideration of the structures of the hepatic pedicle. A study of 100 consecutive cadavers. *Quart Bull Northwest Univ Med Sch, 15:*103-109, 1941.

16. Shaw, BW, Jr, Hakala, T, Rosenthal, JT, *et al.*: Combination donor hepatectomy and nephrectomy and early functional results of allografts. *Surg Gynecol Obstet, 155:*321-325, 1982.

17. Lortat-Jacob, JL, Robert, HG: Hepatectomie droite réglée. *Presse Med, 60:*549-551, 1952.

18. Michels, NA: Newer anatomy of liver - variant blood supply and collateral circulation. *J Am Med Assn, 172:*125-132, 1960.

19. Bengmark, S, Rosengren, K: Angiographic study of the collateral circulation of the liver after ligation of the hepatic artery in man. *Am J Surg, 119:*620-624, 1970.

20. Kennedy, PA, Madding, GF: Surgical Anatomy of the liver. *Surg Clin N Am, 57:*233-244, 1977.

21. Mays, ET, Wheeler, CS: Demonstration of collateral arterial flow after interruption of hepatic arteries in man. *N Eng J Med, 290:*993-996, 1974.

22. Ryncki, PV: Anatomie chirurgical du foie. *Helv Chir Acta, 41:*543-574, 1974.

23. Elias, H, Petty, D: Gross anatomy of the blood vessels and ducts within the human liver. *Am J Anat, 90:*59-111, 1952.

24. Nakamura, S, Tsuzuki, T: Surgical anatomy of the hepatic veins and the inferior vena cava. *Surg Gynecol Obstet, 152:*43-50, 1981.

25. Baird, RA, Britton, RC: The surgical anatomy of the hepatic veins; variations and their implications for auxillary lobar transplantation. *J Surg Res, 15:*345-347, 1973.

26. Longmire, WP, Jr, Trout, HH, III, Greenfield, J, Thompkins, RK: Elective hepatic surgery. *Ann Surg, 179:*712-721, 1974.

27. Prinz, RA, Howell, HS, Pickleman, JR: Surgical significance of extrahepatic biliary tree anomalies. *Am J Surg, 131:*755-757, 1976.

W. JOHN B. HODGSON, M.D.

CHAPTER 8
Hepatic Artery Ligation

With a solid grounding in hepatic anatomy, the simplest approach to surgical management of liver tumors is to perform hepatic artery ligation. This will, therefore, be described in this chapter but, since there has been considerable controversy in the literature about the feasibility of this procedure, let alone the results, the chapter will first describe the historical background.

Much of the controversy surrounding hepatic artery ligation was derived from inaccurate conclusions as the result of animal work. There are four major differences in hepatic vascular supply between man and lower animals. These are: 1) the oxygen saturation of blood in the portal vein in man is greater than in dogs. 2) Portal bacteremia does not occur in healthy humans although it is physiologically normal in lower animals. 3) Man has a prodigous capacity to form collaterals in and around the liver, but lower animals do not. 4) The anatomic relations of the portal vein, pancreas and duodenum are different, mainly because these human structures are retroperitoneal but in the cat and dog they lie on a mesentery.

The dogma of death following portal vein ligation in animals was so clearly upheld, that it followed, or so it was thought, that the same thing occurred in hepatic artery ligation. Therefore, nobody noticed Bolognesi's work in 1906 which showed that turkeys quite happily survived portal vein ligation (1). Nor was Child's work (2, 3) given sufficient credance, when in the 1950s he showed that unlike rabbits, cats and dogs, monkeys could survive portal vein ligation.

Furthermore, although survivals have followed ligation of the portal vein in man since it was first reported in 1908 by Brewer (4), controversy continued. Nonetheless, this is an important therapeutic modality in the treatment of lacerations of the portal vein. It is not generally used as a method of tumor treatment.

How was this controversy surrounding hepatic artery ligation able to persist so long? Unfortunately the fear of hepatic artery ligation is based on animal work, although as already indicated in this chapter, humans and animals differ considerably in hepatic

142

vascular anatomy and physiology. In 1949 Markowitz and his associates (5, 6) published their results on experiments over a 20-year period in dogs on the effects of hepatic artery ligation. They confirmed that when the hepatic artery is ligated beyond its lowest tributary in these animals, death occurs in 24–48 hours. The liver effectively becomes a clostridial abscess. In Haberer's earlier experiments, published in 1905, he had concluded that when the hepatic artery was ligated proximal to the right gastric and gastroduodenal arteries, the dogs survived, but died when ligation was done distal to these arteries (7). Hence, the axiom that the closer to the liver the hepatic artery is ligated the greater the risk of hepatic necrosis. Even as recently as 1971, this thinking was promulgated in standard textbooks such as Hillinshead's Surgical Anatomy (8).

Interestingly, physiologists so firmly believed this dogma, that synthetic antibiotics were given to germ-free animals over a 20-year period to study the effects of hepatic artery ligation (9, 10). It resulted in irrefutable dictum that all patients with liver injury needed antibiotics.

Anatomists also supported the idea that hepatic artery ligation killed. In 1923, Segall (11) said that intrahepatic arteries do not anastomose and are therefore end arteries. Sir Gordon Gordon-Taylor (12) left no doubt that in his opinion anastomoses between intrahepatic arterioles were infreqeunt or at best scanty. In 1953, Glauser (13) said there was no communication between right and left hepatic arteries and that in particular on the right side the secondary lobules were each supplied by their own "end artery." In 1960, Michels (14) thought that each hepatic artery was an end artery with a selective distribution so that none could be sacrificed without resultant necrosis of the lobule thus supplied.

Clinically, hepatic artery ligation had come to be regarded as a most radical departure from acceptable medical practice and essentially the practice was forbidden intentionally in the human. Much of this fear was based on a paper published in 1933 by Graham and Connell (15) who reported death in 16 of 28 patients in whom the hepatic artery or its branches were ligated. When their paper is examined, it can be seen that 9 patients survived without adverse sequelae. In only 6 of the patients was there any kind of relationship between ligation of the artery and the death of the patient. Even so, all these patients also had additional factors of primary hepatic disease, grave hepato-cellular dysfunction, concomitant injuries to the biliary tract, sepsis, parenchymal cell damage, hypotension, shock and hypoxia. These did not occur as a result of hepatic artery ligation but were already present at the time. In 6 other patients, hepatic necrosis was not the cause of death anyway. Generally, close inspection of the paper would suggest an entirely different outcome if the concomitant problems could have been dealt with or excluded in some manner. With modern anesthesia, circulatory support, blood transfusions and antibiotics, the mortality might have been quite different.

Unfortunately, because of the development of septic hepatic necrosis in dogs, rabbits and rats after hepatic artery ligation; the dogma concerning the site of ligation of the hepatic artery; the belief that hepatic arteries were end arteries; and the 1933 clinical report of Graham and Connell, the accepted conclusion was that hepatic artery ligation was a dangerous operation.

With this background, Sir Gordon Gordon-Taylor was believed in 1943 when he said "it is an unpalatable truth that, in man, ligature of the hepatic artery or its main branches is an operation fraught with peril to life" (12). Similarly, Jacob Markowitz (5) was believed in 1949 when he said "the ligation of the hepatic artery in the portal fissure beyond the last branches is invariably followed by a fatal outcome usually within 15-50 hours."

However, we now know that this is not the case. Truman Mays successfully used hepatic artery ligation in the 1970s for management of hepatic trauma (16-18). He also demonstrated angiographically in 1974 that after selective ligation of various hepatic arteries, intrahepatic, translobar and subcapsular collaterals can reconstitute blood flow in the ligated system within 24 hours (19). This confirmed the earlier angiographic work of Bengmark and Rosengren (20). Clearly, there is a difference between the cadaveric liver and the living liver.

This was actually appreciated as long ago as 1920 by Martens (21) who indicated that "between the liver arteries there are always fine anastomoses either between the peripheral branches within the liver or by way of the capsular blood vessels. A certain number of cases showed typical high intrahepatic arcades between the right and left ramus located close to the hilus." Then in 1954 Madding (22) pointed out in his review of numerous cases when death occurred after hepatic artery ligation, that this was always associated with extensive surgical procedures producing shock. He felt that if hepatic artery ligation was as bad as claimed, then there should be a high mortality associated with that procedure alone, and this was not the case. Indeed, in the early 1960s, reports of safe hepatic artery ligation began to emerge (23, 24).

The rationale for hepatic artery ligation was to reduce the blood supply to the tumor but at the same time maintain the parenchymal hepatic tissue by means of the portal blood flow.

In benign tumors, the major indication of hepatic artery ligation is in the treatment of hepatic hemangiomas. These produce arterio-systemic venous fistulae which increase venous pressure and filling of the heart, raising the cardiac output and setting up a hyperdynamic state. Left ventricular and diastolic pressure is chronically augmented and this eventually leads to congestive cardiac failure. Where the shunt is large, death can occur in as little as 6 weeks. This is often the case in infancy. In Kunstadter's review of 15 fatal cases (25), hepatomegaly was also present, and occasionally there was a systolic bruit over the liver. There were accompanying multiple cutaneous hemangiomas in most patients. Respiratory distress occurred in about 6 weeks in half the patients.

DeLorimier *et al.* (26) reviewed 25 patients with hepatic hemangiomatosis. Twenty-three had high output congestive cardiac failure because of large arterio-venous shunts. Twenty-two patients died. A diffuse involvement of the liver by hemangio-endothelioma precluded resection as a method of treatment. In this review, one of their cases, a girl, was born with hepatomegaly and multiple cutaneous hemangiomas. She was in congestive cardiac failure which was relieved by hepatic artery ligation and she survived.

There have been consistent reports of spontaneous rupture of the liver in women taking contraceptive pills (27, 28). About one-third of the women who developed primary hepatic tumors secondary to taking "the pill" present with rupture of their tumor. They develop hemorrhagic shock and may first be diagnosed as a ruptured ectopic pregnancy, a ruptured spleen, a perforated ulcer, or acute cholecystitis. However, peritoneal lavage will reveal gross blood indicating the necessity for laparotomy.

An hepatic lobectomy carried out under these conditions has a mortality rate of 50%. The hemorrhage can frequently be stopped by ligating the hepatic artery to the appropriate lobe. The patient's blood volume can be restored and resection performed at a later date. Anderson and Packer successfully treated two patients in this manner (29).

Since rupture of the liver occurs during pseudosiesis, it is not surprising that it can also occur during real pregnancy as well (30–

32). It must be remembered that this potentially fatal complication occurs in normal pregnancies as well as in those in which pre-eclampsia or eclampsia occurs. This is in addition to high risk pregnant patients with periarteritis nodosa and tuberculosis and syphilis.

The usual clinical pattern is that hemorrhagic shock occurs in the immediate post-partum period but it can occur at the onset of labor. When other sources of blood loss such as uterine bleeding are excluded and abdominal signs detected, the peritoneal lavage or culdocentesis will reveal an hemoperitoneum. At laparotomy there may be a rupture of one or both lobes of the liver. In this situation, the liver tissue itself is often very friable and attempts to place sutures across the ruptured area frequently fail. Instead the hepatic artery should be dissected out and ligated as quickly as possible. This can usually be done quickly and safely and will be followed by an uneventful recovery (33).

Bleeding from a percutaneous needle biopsy is not always arterial. In a patient with portal hypertension, ligation of the hepatic artery will not really have a significant effect on bleeding, but will be deleterious to the cirrhotic liver and in these cases, sutures have to be placed in the liver substance itself to try and close the hole and stop the portal venous bleeding. However, if there is continued bleeding proximal to the site of suture placement, then an internal hepatic hematoma may form with the later development of hemobilia (34) or even of actual rupture of the lobe due to intense build-up of intrahepatic pressure (35). As with all surgery, the cause should be determined before the appropriate action can be taken.

Although in 1923 Segall demonstrated in the cadaver that intrahepatic arteries are end arteries, he also showed that hepatic tumors appear to derive most of their blood supply from the hepatic artery (11). This has been used since then as the rationale for hepatic artery ligation in the treatment of malignant tumors. Ackerman has been a prime worker in confirming and adding to these findings (36-39). He shows that experimental tumors are surrounded by a vascular plexus with both arterial and portal input. This might explain the fact that a thin rim of surviving cancer cells can often be found in the periphery of an otherwise totally necrotic tumor after de-arterialization. These anoxic cancer cells appear to be able to survive on portal venous blood alone. Further, Ackerman showed that deposits less than 30 mgs in weight also have a dual blood supply and are less susceptable to de–arterialization. This may explain why de–arterialization alone can not be considered as curative. Nonetheless Nilsson and Zetter-gren found that extensive necrosis of experimental liver tumors after hepatic artey ligation in rats occurred and was accompanied by increased survival (40).

In the clinical situation, Nilsson (41) deliberately ligated the hepatic artery for treatment of liver tumors and since then there have been many reports and studies on the use of hepatic artery ligation (42-58). So, after overcoming years of bad press, hepatic artery ligation does appear to have certain attractions, and the most obvious is simplicity. Unfortunately, the prognosis of patients with hepatic metastases is dismal and intelligent neglect has been the usual approach. Chemotherapy does not appear to have helped (59-61). Resection does not always appear possible, especially with multiple metastases. The surgeon seems to be able to do something with hepatic artery ligation.

PROTOCOL FOR HEPATIC ARTERY LIGATION

As indicated, hepatic artery ligation is simple. However, the patient must fulfill certain criteria. The patient must have a good overall performance status, and should not be jaundiced, nor have ascites or advanced cirrhosis. Renal function should be normal and serum uric acid should be less than 20 mgs%, since sudden necrosis of tumor cells can considerably increase uric acid levels and cause renal failure (62, 63). Hepatic function should be as near normal as possible with no coagulopathy, and between the tumor the liver should have normal areas. The portal vein should be patent. Arterial anatomy must be documented preoperatively.

Widespread metastases should be excluded preoperatively by means of a chest x-ray and in symptomatic patients bone scans should be done. CAT scanning and laparoscopy can be of great value, the laparoscopy particularly to exclude widespread peritoneal metastases.

The most suitable patients for de-arterialization procedures are those with slowly growing tumors like carcinoids and endocrine tumors with symptoms due to hormonal activity (50, 55) but metastatic tumors from colo-rectal cancers also respond well. Gastric and pancreatic cancers when metastatic to the liver seem to respond less well. An occasional good result is obtained with liver metastases of sarcomas and malignant melanomas.

OPERATIVE TECHNIQUES

The operative technique is to start with any incision used for liver resection. I have no particular preference but have used the midline incision or the inter-neural right-sided incision in which the skin incision and muscle incision follows the curve of the abdominal nerve fibers themselves. However, I have not generally used this incision when the intention has been to perform a liver resection. After evaluation of the patient and exclusion of peritoneal carcinomatosis, ascites or unresectable local tumor recurrence at the primary tumor site, then hepatic artery ligation can be done. A rough estimate of percentage of tumor replacement of the liver should always be performed to provide a baseline.

Complete hepatic de-arterialization is a far more extensive procedure than simple hepatic artery ligation. Therefore, since the objective is to describe procedures of increasing difficulty in this book, simple hepatic artery ligation will be described first.

Hepatic Artery Ligation

The hepatic artery in the hepato-duodenal ligament is usually easily palpated. Its course can be traced and the peritoneum over the hepatic artery can be incised, taking care to clip or to cauterize the small peritoneal vessels which often give considerable troublesome bleeding if divided without control. When the peritoneum is dissected off the common hepatic artery, a right angled clamp is taken and used to carefully bluntly dissect around the artery from above and below. When this has been achieved an umbilical tape or vascular sling can be passed around this vessel (Figure 8.1). Once this has been achieved, control is available. Dissection can then be carried out along the artery distal to the placement of the sling and this dissection will usually reveal the gastroduodenal artery and also the right and left hepatic arteries themselves. Further slings can be placed around the arteries as necessary and this will depend on the distance available for ligation between the gastroduodenal artery and the branches of the hepatic artery into right and left sides. When this dissection has been achieved, it is often useful to inject some Fluorescein into the hepatic artery distal to the gastroduodenal artery and then to expose the liver to ultra-violet light. This will indicate whether or not the arterial supply demonstrated by the dissection does indeed run to both lobes of the liver. A simpler but somewhat more messy way of

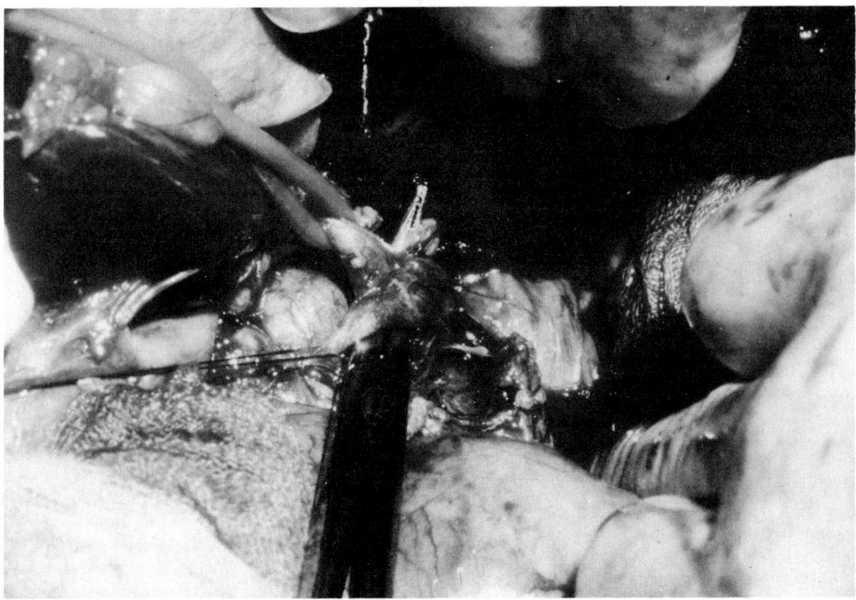

Figure 8.1. Right angled clamp under common hepatic artery with sling under proper hepatic artery and gastroduodenal artery demonstrated in the foreground. (Photograph courtesy of Professor Bengmark, Department of Surgery, Lund, Sweden.)

achieving the same effect is to inject Methylene Blue. When it has been confirmed, using these methods, that the arterial supply to both lobes of the liver has been dissected out, the hepatic artery itself can be ligated in continuity using two ligatures of #00 silk. The abdominal incision can then be closed without drainage. In a slightly more certain way of performing hepatic artery ligation, but with the possibility of the complication of severe bleeding, the artery itself can actually be divided after ligation. This will delay, for a short time, the development of re-canalization of the artery itself and will force the development of collaterals.

Hepatic De-arterialization

Complete hepatic de-arterialization is a different operation entirely. It is carried out using the techniques of Bengmark (46), Balasegaram (53) and Karakousis (64). This should be done through a major incision such as an extended right-sided subcostal incision and is fraught with far more difficulty and hazard than hepatic artery ligation itself. The first step for this procedure is to divide the liver attachments. The falciform ligament can be divided back to the inferior vena cava with a simple thrust of the scissors. The left triangular ligament can also be relatively simply divided by retracting the stomach and cutting the thin filmy tissue of this ligament where it is reflected onto the liver itself (Figure 8.2). As

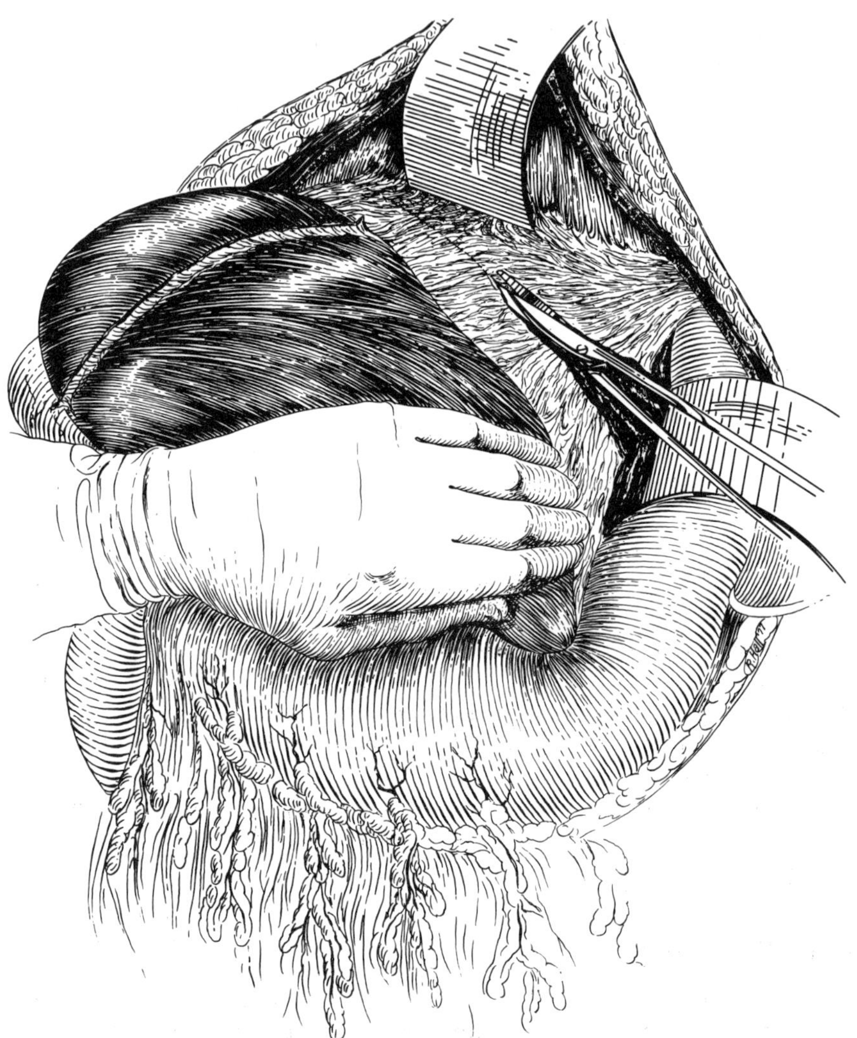

Figure 8.2. Division of left triangular ligament. (*Surgery, Gynecology and Obstetrics, 149:*403, 1979 — With permission.)

it is divided, the liver will easily be reflected from the under-surface of the diaphragm. However, care must be taken posteriorly as there are rather large tributaries from the phrenic veins but since these are usually seen easily, they can be avoided. However, there is a tendency to become too comfortable with this part of the dissection and to dissect too rapidly medially and if this occurs the left hepatic vein can be easily incised with disastrous consequences. An awareness of the anatomy of the hepatic veins will avoid this pitfall. After the dissection of the left triangular ligament the lesser omentum is also divided thus freeing the left lobe of the liver entirely (Figure 8.3).

The right lobe of the liver is also mobilized in a somewhat similar fashion. The right triangular ligament is divided with sharp dissection and then the coronary ligaments themselves are also divided in a medial direction after bluntly dissecting the diaphragm away from the bare area of the liver (Figure 8.4). This combination of blunt and sharp dissection will allow complete exposure of the inferior vena cava on the right side which can then

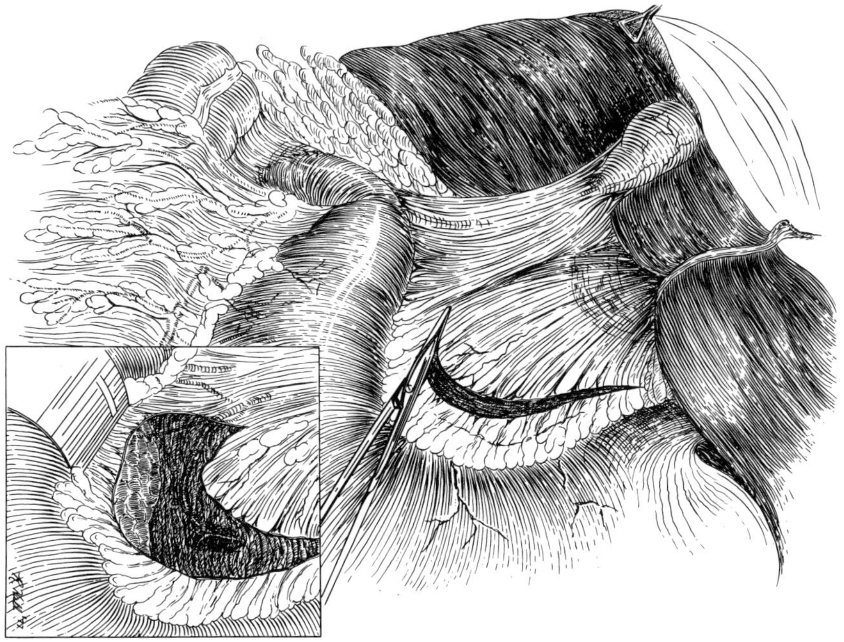

Figure 8.3. Division of lesser omentum and exposure of celiac axis and common hepatic artery. (*Surgery, Gynecology and Obstetrics, 149:*403, 1979 — With permission.)

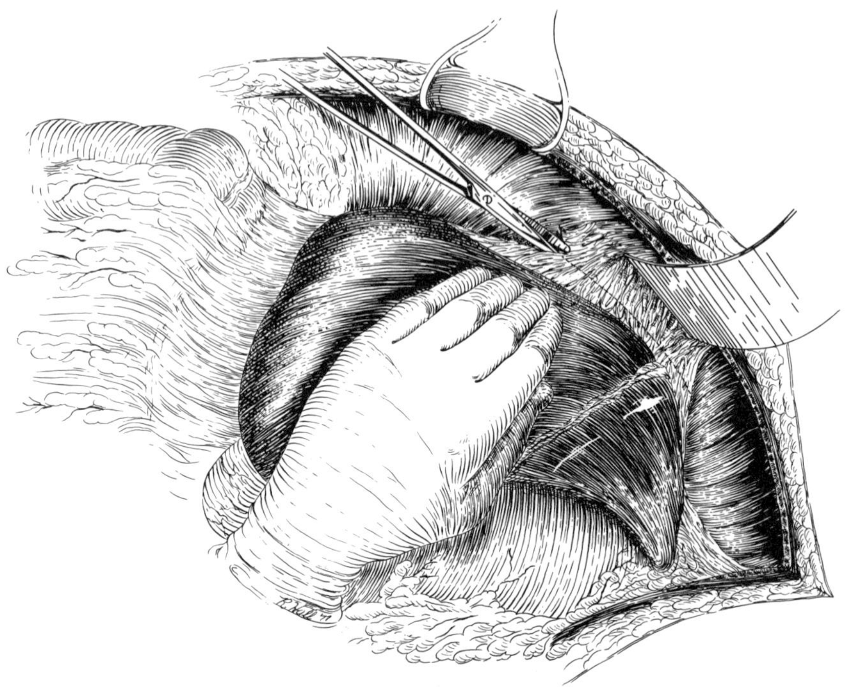

Figure 8.4. Division of the right triangular ligament to expose bare area of the liver. (*Surgery, Gynecology and Obstetrics, 149:*403, 1979 — With permission.)

be matched up with the already achieved exposure of the inferior vena cava on the left. Attention can now be directed to the hepatic artery but in a more detailed manner than in hepatic artery ligation alone. The peritoneum on the ventral aspect of the hepato–duodenal ligament must be incised all the way across. Again, because of the multiple peritoneal vessels which bleed, care has to be taken with each and every one of these in order to avoid continuing troublesome bleeding. When this has been done and the hepatic artery proper has been dissected free using vascular slings, the gastroduodenal artery is again identified and the artery distal to the gastroduodenal artery is dissected free. Similarly, on the right side of this, the common bile duct is isolated and the small lymphatics and blood vessels surrounding it are stripped off, taking great care to individually ligate and divide these lymphatics and vessels. When this has been done, the portal vein is identified beneath the hepatic artery and the common bile duct. Eventually, all structures other than the artery, the common duct and the portal vein are divided.

Where preoperative angiography has demonstrated the presence of aberrant arteries, the vessels must be carefully dissected out during this phase of the operation and identified. When this has been done, all the arterial branches to the liver are ligated and divided. This will leave the portal vein as the sole blood supply to the liver. Unlike simple hepatic artery ligation, this will lead to necrosis of the gall bladder. Therefore, in a complete hepatic de-arterialization, cholecystectomy is mandatory.

The wound can be closed in the usual manner and I prefer to always drain the gall bladder bed usually with a closed drainage system. I also prefer to use interrupted sutures of Polyglycolic acid to close the insicion. A wide spectrum antibiotic has normally been given starting immediately preoperatively and is usually continued for about 48–72 hours postoperatively. This prevents the development of infection in necrotic tumors after the occlusion.

Permanent de-arterialization has an operative mortality of up to 40% and clearly has a higher mortality than simple hepatic artery ligation (51). Abscesses in the necrotizing tumor tissue seem to occur in about 12% of patients (65, 66).

Transient Occlusion of the Hepatic Artery

Bengmark and Fredlund have developed an interesting adjunct to hepatic de-arterialization (56). They consider that there is such rapid re-vascularization of hepatic tumors that after this procedure has been carried out the rim of cancer cells can easily begin to grow again, having survived the basic insult. However, if occlusion could be intermittent, they reasoned, just as the cells are beginning to become dependent on a renewed arterial supply, intermittent occlusion could disrupt cellular division just at the time a good blood supply was needed most. In order to carry out intermittent occlusion, they first de-arterialized the liver. Then, instead of dividing the hepatic artery they placed fine strangulating slings of polyethylene around the isolated vessel. One sling was placed distal to the gastroduodenal artery and the other was placed proximally. Each sling was then threaded through thick catheters and brought out through the abdominal wall (Figure 8.5). With these strangulating slings the arteries could easily be occluded. The thick catheters should have rounded edges at the

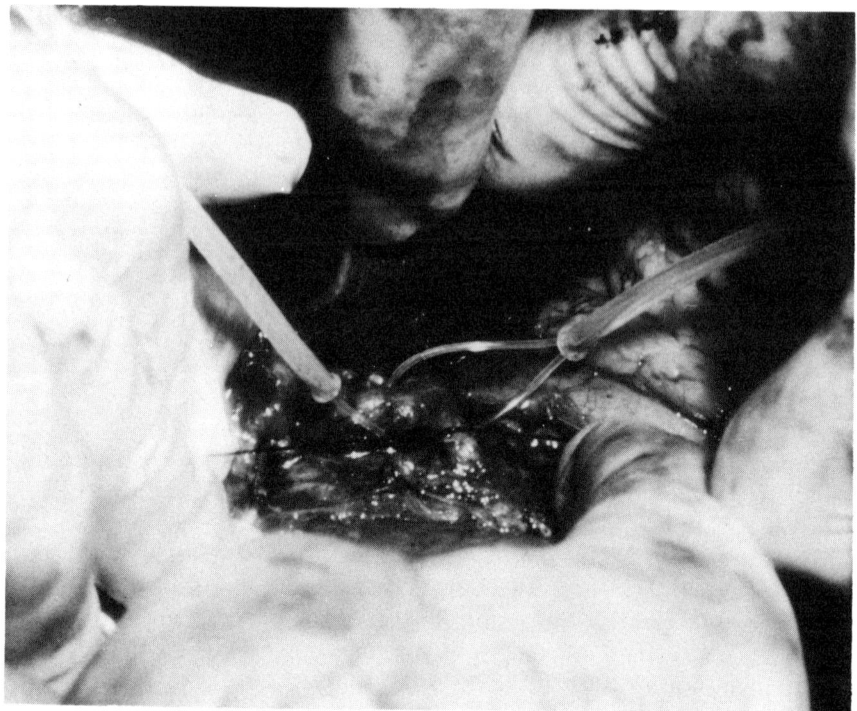

Figure 8.5. Slings around hepatic artery threaded through catheters for subsequent strangulation of vessels. (Courtesy of Professor Bengmark, Department of Surgery, Lund, Sweden.)

lower ends to avoid damaging the vessels when they are pushed down onto them. The slings are then fixed in proper position with skin sutures. The fine slings can be relaxed or pulled up depending on whether it is intended to allow the arterial blood flow to continue or whether to occlude it. Initially, no tension is applied.

Before the planned occlusion a strong analgesic should be given. Occlusion is normally maintained for 16 hours. This causes a moderate lesion of the liver cells which will be demonstrated by an increase in liver transaminases in the circulation. Nonetheless, Bengmark and Fredlund thought the patients seemed to be less affected by a transient occlusion of the hepatic artery than by permanent arterial ligation. They felt that this was because the operative trauma and liver damage did not coincide and they thought that a physiologic adjustment of the liver flow and metabolism may also occur (56). Experimental studies in pigs have confirmed this reasoning (66).

Bengmark and Fredlund also place an indwelling hepatic artery catheter at the same time (56) but this type of therapy will be discussed in the next chapter.

Vessel Ligation as an Adjunct to Resection

In 1970 Bengmark *et al.* described an interesting patient with a leiomyosarcoma (67). The initial mass in the upper abdomen weighing 2,000 grams had been extirpated but the problem remained as to how to treat the metastatic disease of the liver. The left lateral lobe was totally replaced by tumor and from his drawings it would appear that there was a 10 cm tumor involving the left medial lobe together with the right medial lobe and in addition there were three small tumors on the diaphragmatic surface of the right lobe. The porta hepatis was compressed between the two major tumors making a radical operation impracticable. The hepatic artery was, therefore, ligated and transected distal to the gastroduodenal artery and de–arterialization was also carried out. Five weeks later a second laparotomy was performed and it was noted that the tumors on the diaphragmatic surface had disappeared and the other two had diminished considerably in size. Therefore, a left lateral lobectomy was carried out together with a wedge resection of the centrally situated tumor. Altogether 500 grams of this tumor was resected which on microscopy was shown to be necrotic. Small patches only of viable tumor cells were seen at the periphery. The postoperative follow up was only for three months but was uneventful.

As an aside, in Kyoto University Medical School in Japan, in 1975, a branch of the portal vein to the side of the liver involved with tumor was ligated (68). The morbidity associated with this procedure was minimal and in some of their patients, the portal vein ligation had been carried out in association with partial resection on the other side. A median survival of 10 months was claimed for metastatic colon carcinoma to the liver. As with the work done by Kim *et al.*, tumor vascularity appeared to play an important part in survival rates (69). Generally the results are that the more vascular the hepatic tumor on angiogram the better the prognosis following hepatic artery ligation and infusional therapy.

In one of our patients with massive tumor of the right lobe of the liver, we divided the right portal vein and right hepatic artery and placed a catheter from an Infusaid pump to his left hepatic artery. He had much pain and discomfort postoperatively and three months later, having had significant shrinkage of the remaining normal liver tissue, but only a little shrinkage of the tumor, we removed a 19 x 12 x 10 cm tumor. He is alive eight months after his initial surgery but has recurrent tumor on his right chest wall.

Results

This brings up the question as to whether or not it is all worth it. Since 50-70% of patients dying of cancer have liver metastases (70) and the median survival time overall of the patients with untreated disease is only 75 days after diagnosis (71), it would seem that almost anything would improve the situation. In one autopsy series, hepatic metastasis was the only malignancy present in 19% of the patients who died from cancer of the colon (72). Gastrointestinal cancers are particularly likely to metastasize to the liver and at the time of initial laparotomy, liver metastases are present in about 20% of patients with cancer of the stomach, 25% of patients with cancer of the colon and rectum, 50% of patients with cancer of the pancreas and 63% of patients with cancer of the gall bladder (73).

Median survival of the best group of patients, that is those with cancer of the colon, is about 6 months and only around 10% of patients survive one year and 3% survive two years. A few patients survive more than 2 years after the diagnosis if untreated (71). It has already been indicated that systemic chemotherapy given intravenously does not appear to have any effect on the prognosis of this disease (59-61).

What then, is the result of hepatic artery ligation? Swedish surgeons seemed to have been in the forefront of managing tumors by hepatic artery ligation. Nilsson (41) has a survival time of 1-4 months in his group whereas Larmi *et al.* were able to show survivals of between 2-8 months (74). Patients with carcinoid syndrome from metastatic lesions in the liver appear to derive definite benefit from ligation of the hepatic artery alone (47, 55).

Lee summarized the situation and pointed out that complete de-arterialization of the liver increased the risk of liver necrosis without improving the response rate of the tumor (73). For example, Almersjö *et al.* found no correlation between the extent of de-arterialization and survival time (44). Generally, Lee felt that hepatic artery ligation for metastatic tumors in the liver could be well tolerated unless far advanced hepatic decompensation had occurred or the portal circulation was impaired. She felt that cirrhosis of the liver should be considered a contra-indication for hepatic artery ligation since the liver in this disease is progressively arterialized (75). Lee also reported an overall mortality rate associated with hepatic artery ligation of about 19% with 4% directly attributable to ligation of the artery. She also felt that patients with carcinoid syndrome from metastatic lesions in the liver derived definite benefit from ligation of the hepatic artery alone but for other lesions she felt the benefit was far less certain (73). Mays was much more enthusiastic although he agreed that life was not prolonged. His therapeutic approach, however, was based on the quality of life that the patients enjoyed. He felt that after hepatic artery ligation, symptoms of liver failure and the undulating fever often associated with tumor may be eliminated. He also felt strongly that chemotherapy tied the patient to a schedule of laboratory leukocyte and platelet counts with hair loss, uncomfortable glossitis and stomatitis befouling the last weeks of these patients' lives and all of this could be avoided by simple hepatic artery ligation (76).

REFERENCES

1. Bolognesi, G: La ligature de la veine porte chez des animaux avec circulation de Jacobson. *Arch Ital Biol, 46:*51, 1906-1907.

2. Child, CG, III, Milnes, RF, Holswade, GR, Gore, AL: Sudden and complete occlusion of the portal vein in the Macaca Mulatta monkey. *Ann Surg, 132:*475-495, 1950.

3. Child, CG, III, McClure, RD, Hays, DM: Studies on the hepatic circulation in the Macaca Mulatta monkey and in man. *Surg, Forum 2:*140-146, 1957.

4. Brewer, GE: Hydatid cyst of the liver with ligature of the portal vein. *Ann Surg, 47:*619-622, 1908.

5. Markowitz, J: The function of the hepatic artery in the dog. *J Digest Dis, 16:*344, 1949.

6. Markowitz, J, Rappaport, A, Scott, AC: Prevention of liver necrosis following ligation of hepatic artery. *Proc Soc Exp Biol, 70:*305, 1949.

7. Haberer, H: Experimental ligation of the hepatic artery. *Arch Klin Chir, 78:*557, 1905.

8. Hollinshead, WH: *Anatomy for Surgeons*, 2nd Ed. New York: Harper and Row, 1971.

9. Fitts, WT, Scott, R, Mackie, JA: Effect of antibiotics on ligation of the hepatic artery. *Surgery, 28:*458, 1950.

10. Crook JN, Paris, MF, Nance, FC: Studies of the hepatic blood flow and hepatic function after ligation of the hepatic artery and portal vein. *Am Surg, 36:*724-727, 1970.

11. Segall, HN: An experimental anatomical investigation of the blood and bile channels of the liver. *Surg Gynecol Obstet, 37:*156, 1923.

12. Gordon-Taylor, G: A rare cause of severe gastrointestinal hemorrhage with a note on aneurysm of the hepatic artery. *Brit Med J, 1:*504-505, 1943.

13. Glauser, F: Studies on intrahepatic arterial circulation. *Surgery, 33:* 333-340, 1953.

14. Michels, NA: Newer anatomy of the liver - variant blood supply and collateral circulation. *J Am Med Assn, 172:*125-132, 1960.

15. Graham, RR, Connell, D: Accidental ligation of the hepatic artery. *Brit J Surg, 20:*566-578, 1933.

16. Mays, ET: Lobar de-arterialization for exsanguinating wounds of the liver. *J Trauma, 12:*397-407, 1972.

17. Mays, ET: Hepatic trauma. *N Eng J Med, 288:*402-405, 1973.

18. Mays, ET: The hepatic artery. *Surg Gynecol Obstet, 139:*595-596, 1974.

19. Mays, ET, Wheeler, CS: Demonstration of collateral arterial flow after interruption of hepatic arteries in man. *N Eng J Med, 290:*993-996, 1974.

20. Bengmark, S, Rosengren, K: Angiographic study of the collateral circulation of the liver after ligation of the hepatic artery in man. *Am J Surg, 119:*620-624, 1970.

21. Martens, E: Röntgenologische studien zur arteriellen Gefassversorgung in der Leber. *Arch F Klin Chir, 114:*1001, 1920.

22. Madding, GF, Smith, WL, Hershberger, LR: Hepato-portal arteriovenous fistula. *J Am Med Assn, 156:*593-596, 1954.

23. Andreassen, M, Lindenberg, J, Winkler, K: Peripheral ligation of the hepatic artery during surgery for non-cirrhotic patients. *Gut, 3:*167-171, 1962.

24. Brittain, RS, Marchioro, TL, Hermann, G, *et al.*: Accidental hepatic artery ligation in humans. *Am J Surg, 107:*822-832, 1964.

25. Kunstadter, RH: Hemangioendothelioma of liver in infancy: Case report and review of literature. *Am J Dis Child, 46:*803-910, 1933.

26. DeLorimier, AA, Simpson, EB, Baum, RS, Carlsson, E: Hepatic artery ligation for hepatic hemangiomatosis. *N Eng J Med, 277:*333-337, 1967.

27. Mays, ET, Christopherson, WM, Barrows, GH: Focal nodular hyperplasia of the liver. *Am J Clin Path, 61:*735-746, 1974.

28. Mays, ET, Christopherson, WM, Mahr, MM, William, HC: Hepatic changes in young women ingesting contraceptive steroids. *J Am Med Assn, 235:*730-732, 1976.

29. Anderson, PH, Packer, JT: Hepatic adenoma observation after estrogen withdrawal. *Arch Surg, 111:*898-900, 1976.

30. Sanes, S, Kaminski, CA: Spontaneous rupture of the liver during pregnancy into peritoneal cavity. *Am J Obstet Gynecol, 52:*325-329, 1946.

31. Kramish, D, Auer, ES, Reckler, SM: Spontaneous rupture of the liver during pregnancy. *Obstet Gynecol, 4:*21-28, 1954.

32. Haller, AP, *et al.*: Spontaneous rupture of the liver with non-conclusive exlampsia. *Am J Obstet Gynecol, 62:*1170, 1961.

33. Mays, ET, Conti, S, Fallahzedeh, H, Rosenblatt, M: Hepatic artery ligation. *Surgery, 86:*536-543, 1979.

34. Cox, EF: Hemobilia following percutaneous needle biopsy of the liver. *Arch Surg, 95:*198, 1967.

35. Carey, LC, Worman, LW: Explosion injury of the liver from intra-parenchymal hemorrhage. *J Trauma, 6:*48-49, 1966.

36. Ackerman, NB, Lien, WM, Kand, ES, Silverman, NA: The blood supply of experimental liver metastases. I. The distribution of hepatic artery and portal vein blood to "small" and "large" tumors. *Surgery, 66:*1067-1072, 1969.

37. Lien, WM, Ackerman, NB: The blood supply of liver metastases. II. A micro-circulatory study of the normal and tumor vessels of the liver with the use of perfused silicone rubber. *Surgery, 68:*334-340, 1970.

38. Ackerman, NB, Lien, WM, Silverman, NA: The blood supply of experimental liver metastases. III. The effects of acute ligation of the hepatic artery or portal vein. *Surgery, 71:*636-641, 1972.

39. Ackerman, NB: The blood supply of experimental liver metastases. IV. Changes in vascularity with increasing tumor growth. *Surgery, 75:*589-596, 1974.

40. Nilsson, LAV, Zettergren, L: Effect of hepatic artery ligation on induced primary liver carcinoma in rats. *Acta Pathol Microbiol Scand, 71:*187-193, 1967.

41. Nilsson, LAV: Therapeutic hepatic artery ligation in patients with secondary liver tumors. *Rev Surg, 23:*374-376, 1966.

42. Madding, GF, Kennedy, PA, Sogemeier, E: Hepatic artery ligation for metastatic tumor of the liver. *Am J Surg, 120:*95-96, 1970.

43. Murray-Lyon, IM, Dawson, JL, Parsons, VA, *et al.*: Treatment of secondary hepatic tumors by ligation of the hepatic artery and infusion of cyto-toxic drugs. *Lancet, 2:*172-175, 1970.

44. Almersjö, O, Bengmark, S, Rudenstam, CM, *et al.*: Evaluation of hepatic de-arterialization in primary and secondary cancer of the liver. *Am J Surg, 124:*5-9, 1972.

45. Fortner, JG, Mulcare, RJ, Solis, A, *et al.*: Treatment of primary and secondary liver cancer by hepatic artery ligation and infusion chemotherapy. *Ann Surg, 178:*162-172, 1973.

46. Bengmark, S, Fredlund, P, Hafstrom, LP, Vang, J: Present experience with hepatic de-arterialization in liver neoplasm. *Progr Surg, 13:*141-166, 1974.

47. McDermott, WV, Jr, Hensle, TW: Metastatic carcinoid to the liver treated by hepatic de-arterialization. *Ann Surg, 180:*305-308, 1974.

48. Plengvanit, U, Viranuvatti, V, Chearanai, O: Treatment of primary liver carcinoma. *Med Chir Dig, 3:*301-306, 1974.

49. Fredlund, P, Bengmark, S: De-arterialization procedures in the treatment of liver tumors "Il fegato" XXI, 475, 1975.

50. Jugdutt, BI, Watanabe, M, Turner, F: Hepatic artery ligation in treatment of carcinoid syndrome. *Can Med Assn J, 112:*325-327, 1975.

51. Sparks, FC, Misher, MB, Hallauer, WC, *et al.*: Hepatic artery ligation and postoperative chemotherapy for hepatic metastases: Clinical and pathophysiological results. *Cancer, 25:*1074-1082, 1975.

52. Zike, WL, Safaie-Shirazi, S, Gulesserian, HP: Hepatic artery ligation and toxic infusion in treatment of liver neoplasms. *Arch Surg, 110:*641-643, 1975.

53. Balasegaram, M: Management of primary liver cell carcinoma. *Am J Surg, 130:*33-37, 1975.

54. Nagasue, N, Inokuchi, K, Kobayashi, M, *et al.*: Hepatic de-arterialization for non-resectable primary and secondary tumors of the liver. *Cancer, 38:*2593-2603, 1976.

55. Fardon, JR: The carcinoid syndrome. Methods of treatment and recent experience with hepatic artery ligation and infusion. *Clin Oncol, 3:* 365, 1977.

56. Bengmark, S, Fredlund, PE: Temporary de-arterialization combined with intra-arterial infusion of oncolytic drugs in the treatment of liver tumors. *Progress in Clinical Cancer, VII,* Ariel, IM (Ed.). New York: Greene and Stratton, 1978, page 207.

57. McDermott, WV, Jr, Paris, AL, Clouse, ME, Meissner, WA: De-arterialization of the liver for metastatic cancer. *Ann Surg, 187:*38-46, 1978.

58. Dahl, EP, Fredlund, PE, Tylen, U, Bengmark, S: Transient hepatic de-arterialization followed by regional intra-arterial 5-Fluorouracil infusion as treatment for liver tumors. *Ann Surg, 193:*82-88, 1981.

59. Moertel, CG: Clinical management of advanced gastrointestinal cancer. *Cancer, 36:*675-682, 1975.

60. Schein, PS. Kirner, D, Macdonald, JS: Chemotherapy of large intestinal cancer. *Cancer, 36:*2418-2420, 1975.

61. Taylor, I: A critical review of the treatment of colorectal liver metastases. *Clin Oncol, 8:*149-158, 1982.

62. Rieselbach, RE, Bentzel, CJ, Cotlove, E, *et al.*: Uric acid excretion and renal function in the acute hyperurecemia of leukemia. *Am J Med, 37:* 872, 1974.

63. Kim, DK, Penneman, R, Kallum, B, *et al.*: Acute renal failure after ligation of the hepatic artery. *Surg Gynecol Obstet, 143:*391-394, 1976.

64. Karakousis, CP, Douglass, HO, Jr, Holyoke, ED: Technique of infusion chemotherapy, ligation of the hepatic artery and de-arterialization in malignant lesions of the liver. *Surg Gynecol Obstet, 149:*403-407, 1979.

65. Jochimsen, PR, Zike, WL, Shirazi, SS, Pearlman, NW: Iatrogenic liver abscesses. *Arch Surg, 113:*141-144, 1978.

66. Bengmark, S, Fredlund, PE: Palliative treatment of primary and secondary malignant liver neoplasms. In *Liver Surgery*, Calne and Della Rovere (Eds.). Philadelphia, PA: WB Saunders, 1982, pages 156-158.

67. Bengmark, S, Brix, M, Börgisson, B, *et al.*: Treatment of hepatic tumors. *Digestion, 3:* 309-317, 1970.

68. Honjo, I, Suzuki, T, Ozawa, K, *et al.*: Ligation of a branch of the portal vein for carcinoma of the liver. *Am J Surg, 130:* 296-302, 1975.

69. Kim, DK, Caird Watson, R, Pahnke, LD, Fortner, JG: Tumor vascularity as a prognostic factor for hepatic tumors. *Ann Surg, 185:* 31-34, 1977.

70. Ariel, IM, Pack, GT: Intra-arterial chemotherapy for cancer metastatic to liver. *Arch Surg, 91:* 851-862, 1965.

71. Jaffe, BM, Donegan, WL, Watson, F, *et al.*: Factors influencing survival in patients with untreated hepatic metastases. *Surg Gynecol Obstet, 127:* 1-11, 1968.

72. Willis, RA: *The Spread of Tumors in the Human Body*. London: Butterworths, 1952, page 180.

73. Lee, Y-TN: Non-systemic treatment of metastatic tumors of the liver - A review. *Med Pediat Oncol, 4:* 185-203, 1978.

74. Larmi, TKI, Karkola, P, Klintrupp, II, *et al.*: Treatment of patients with hepatic tumors and jaundice by ligation of the hepatic artery. *Arch Surg, 108:* 178-181, 1974.

75. Hulten, O: Arterialization of the liver in cirrhosis. *Scand J Clin Lab Invest, 92:* 42-43, 1966.

76. Mays, ET: Vascular occlusion. *Surg Clin N Am, 57:* 291-323, 1977.

W. JOHN B. HODGSON, M.D.

CHAPTER 9
Technical Aspects
of Intrahepatic Chemotherapy

Having mastered the technique of hepatic artery ligation, the next advance concerns the rationale, placement and management of vascular catheters for intrahepatic chemotherapy.

Since 50-75% of patients who die of cancer have liver metastases (1) and the median survival time is only 75 days after diagnosis (2) an aggressive approach is rational. There is much evidence, as discussed in the previous chapter, to support the theory that hepatic artery ligation causes selective necrosis of the tumor with preservation of the normal parenchyma. However, there is almost always a margin or shell of viable malignant cells at the periphery of the devascularized nodule, so that, in the end, survival is unchanged.

Clearly there is a definite place for chemotherapy. But, systemic chemotherapy using the Pyrimidine antagonist fluorouracil (5FU) has not had any significant effects on survival once the tumor has reached the liver (3). Therefore, regional and continuous chemotherapy to the liver has been advocated. The object is to achieve a higher local concentration of the drug, which will hopefully prolong the contact of the drug and tumor cells, and also reduce systemic toxicity. It was also hoped that the long-term infusion chemotherapy would sequentially destroy tumor cells as they randomly entered their vulnerable metabolic phase.

Intra-arterial hepatic chemotherapy was initiated in the 1950s by Bierman (4) and later by Klopp (5). Then it was re-popularized in the 1960s by Sullivan (6, 7), Clarkson (8) and Brennan (9) and their co-workers.

It is not the place at this time to consider chemotherapeutic details as there is a separate chapter on this subject. However, in summary, the initial approach was to use intra-arterial Methotrexate with Citrovorum rescue as this gave better responses than systemic Methotrexate alone (6). Later, Floxuridine (FUDR) was used because it was completely metabolized in the liver and had

162

very little systemic toxicity (10-12). 5FU was thought to be more effective and this was used by most workers at this time (1, 9, 11-23). Although some reports indicated little difference between hepatic infusion and systemic chemotherapy, more extensive pharmacological studies by Brennan (9) and clinical studies by Burrows (15) indicated at least a 2:1 superiority of hepatic artery infusion over systemic chemotherapy for hepatic metastases.

A satisfactory objective response has been defined as a decrease in size by more than 50% and the return to normal, or nearly normal, of liver function tests. Various series have shown a response rate of between 35-85% with doubling or tripling of survival time compared with all non-responders (24).

The best responses seem to have been obtained in patients with primary breast and colorectal tumors (12, 23) and lesions of the stomach, lung and esophagus have had a fair response (12). Although melanoma is said to respond poorly, anecdotal cases do occur, such as that reported by Kondi *et al.* which had a 14-month objective response to intra-arterial Bleomycin to the liver and oral Hydroxyurea (25). FUDR infusion therapy seems to have some effect on metastatic carcinoma from the gall bladder or biliary tract to the liver.

Patients selected for this procedure should include those in whom it is not possible to excise the tumor. Therefore, patients with significant disease are usually chosen. However, if it is advanced or hepatic decompensation is pending, then arterial catheterization by laparotomy should not be carried out.

These patients may respond to percutaneous placement of the catheter passed via the brachial artery to the hepatic artery.

Gulesserian *et al.* (26) performed hepatic artery ligation and distal hepatic artery infusion with minimum morbidity and mortality in 38 patients with a median survival of 13.3 months. Similar results were obtained by Sparks *et al.* (27) and Ramming *et al.* (28).

Fortner also infused the portal vein, and in one of his groups consisting of 24 patients he performed hepatic artery ligation and arterial and portal venous infusion. These were placed among an adequately treated group of 77 patients using similar but not identical methods and he achieved a 2-year survival rate of 18%.

Donegan *et al.* (17) felt that the hepatic artery must be infused to obtain a response and in his group there was no effect when the portal vein was used. Ariel (1) agreed. This was thought to be due to greater concentration of the chemotherapeutic agents that could be delivered through the hepatic artery than by the portal vein. Murray-Lyon *et al.* (30) tried hepatic artery ligation and portal vein infusion, but were beset by technical difficulties. However, Almersjö (31) succeeded and his patients had a median survival of 11 months. Taylor (32) divided his patients into groups depending on the extent of the tumor, using the same technique. For those with less than 20% tumor volume, median survival was 15 months; for those between 20–70% it was 10.5 months; for those with more than 70% it was 5.5 months. Although Taylor felt the benefit was only marginal, this combined approach actually gives a better survival than historical Duke's C colon cancer patients without liver metastases.

Chuang and Wallace (33) in a group of patients with failed hepatic artery infusion, used trans–catheter embolization of the hepatic artery and achieved a median survival of 11.5 months for their group. There is a post-embolization syndrome of nausea, vomiting, paralytic ileus, right upper quadrant pain and fever which lasts a few days which we have also seen in our Institution.

El Domeiri (34) was concerned about the deleterious effects of sudden ligation of the hepatic artery and he wanted to achieve central tumor necrosis and destroy the rapidly proliferating peripheral cells by infusional chemotherapy. So he used a catheter with an inflatable balloon inserted surgically. The balloon was inflated twice daily for an hour during which time chemotherapy was infused. This continued for a mean of three weeks and appeared more effective than systemic chemotherapy or intra-arterial chemotherapy alone. Bengmark and Fredlund (35) used a similar technique with slings placed around the artery which could be closed by tightening the sling. A median survival time of 11 months was achieved, but these techniques remain difficult and time–consuming.

The long-term regional infusion approach using an external pump appears to have given the best overall results with a claimed 70–80% objective response rate and prolongation of life for an average of 14–16 months in responders (11, 19, 24, 36). This continuous method of delivering chemotherapy appears to be superior to the induction approach followed by weekly intravenous injections. In fact, induction through the hepatic artery or induction through a systemic vein is about the same (37).

Conventional treatment with either 5FU or FUDR administered on an outpatient basis by bolus injection into a peripheral vein (8–10 mgs/kg intravenously every 1–2 weeks) or as an in-patient by short-term continuous infusions through a peripheral vein at about 20–30 mgs/kg per day for 5 days in one month cycles results in a wildly fluctuating effect on plasma drug concentrations. These variations clearly swing from toxic levels to sub-therapeutic levels. Furthermore, inadequately placed hepatic artery catheters also cause difficulties and problems in maintaining a sub-toxic but therapeutic level of drug.

The major problem with intra–arterial hepatic chemotherapy has been maintenance of the catheter. Clearly, problems with the catheter have reduced continuing popularity of this method. Catheters placed during laparotomy can theoretically be left for months. Catheters placed percutaneously have been less successful, and have only been maintained in place for a few weeks (10). Not surprisingly, these catheters have a high rate of infection, catheter extravasation and leakage. Septicemia has been reported, even when the catheter was placed by the operative approach (10). The complications of operative placement were severe enough to raise the 30–day mortality rate to 6–14% (11, 23). Morbidity was so high that in 32% of cases it was not possible to complete the course of infusion because of early complications (12). Long–term complications included catheter migration (10%), peptic ulcer disease (11%), and thrombosis of the hepatic artery (20–40%) (11, 24). Sullivan (24) suggested that thrombosis of the hepatic artery only occurred in those cases where the artery was not tied off although this is no longer thought to be the case. Indeed it seems that the converse is true. Actually ligation of the hepatic artery results in thrombosis about the catheter as there is no flow other than that produced by the catheter fluid. Eventually thrombosis will prevent further infusion of solution.

The most ideal approach is to place the catheter in such a way that it would not interfere with the arterial blood flow through the hepatic artery. Moreover, the tip of the catheter should be placed at the hepatic artery so that a continuous slow drip of chemotherapy can be mixed in the arterial blood and swept straight through to the liver, thus reducing destructive effects on the arterial wall.

As indicated in the chapter on the anatomy of the liver, there are many variations on the arterial inflow to the liver. This affects placement of the catheter. Watkins *et al.* (12) preferred to use a single catheter placed at laparotomy into the gastroduodenal artery. Anatomic variants were overcome by judicious ligation of the appropriate vessels. We also use this method (Figure 9.1).

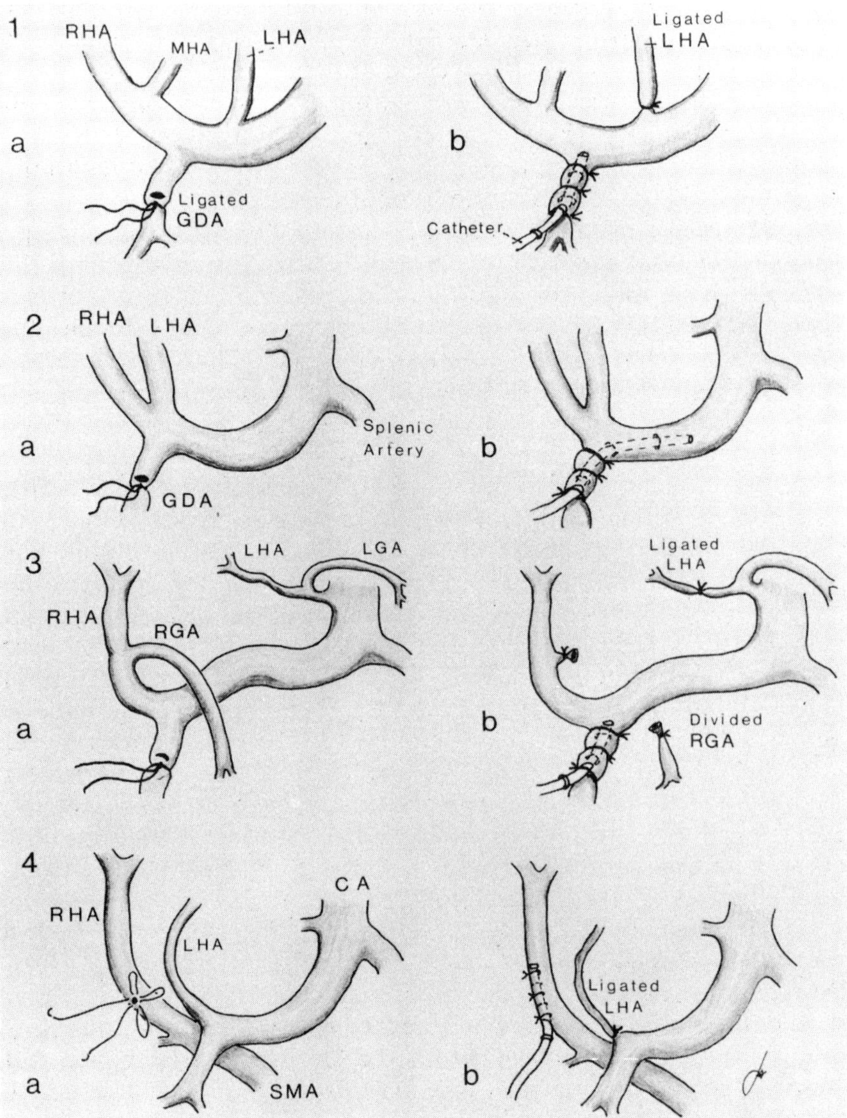

Figure 9.1. Catheter placement in anomalous arterial variations.
1. When the left hepatic artery (LHA) is given off proximal to the gastro-duodenal artery (GDA), which usually occurs because of the presence of a middle hepatic artery (MHA), the catheter is placed normally in the GDA after the LHA is tied off. Intrahepatic arborization will allow full perfusion of the liver via the right hepatic artery (RHA) and MHA.

Figure 9.1 (continued). Catheter placement in anomalous arterial variations.
2. Where the right hepatic artery (RHA) and left hepatic artery (LHA) are given off opposite, or very close to, the gastroduodenal artery (GDA), the catheter should be pushed upstream to ensure even distribution of chemotherapy to both lobes of the liver.
3. Where the right gastric artery (RGA) arises from the right hepatic artery (RHA), beyond the origin of the gastroduodenal artery (GDA), it should be divided to avoid peptic ulceration. When the left hepatic artery (LHA) arises from the left gastric artery (LGA), it should be tied off so that only one catheter is required to completely perfuse the liver.
4. In a situation where the celiac axis (CA) only gives rise to a small left hepatic artery (LHA) and the superior mesenteric artery (SMA) gives rise to a large right hepatic artery (RHA), it is preferable to tie off the smaller vessel, the LHA in this case, and to cannulate the larger vessel, in this case, the RHA.

Since 1967 Watkins *et al.* (38) have aggressively pursued the percutaneous transbrachial route (Figure 9.2) with a successful placement in 97.4% of attempts. In both their series they used an external pump for continuous delivery of the drugs. They claimed that the 15% rate of upper gastrointestinal tract ulceration as quoted by Cady (11) was due to nutritional factors rather than any influence of anti-cancer drug on the gastrointestinal mucosa.

Continuous hepatic artery infusions using external pump devices have represented a major step forward but have also been limited by frequent problems related to the external catheter. This includes the use of bulky external pump devices; significant infection including intra-abdominal infections because of the transcutaneous placement of the catheter and also, of course, thrombosis of the hepatic artery, malfunction of the catheter and migration of the catheter.

HEPATIC ARTERY INFUSIONS

The Infusaid Pump

Ensminger (39) carried out a pharmaco-kinetic study in 1978 which demonstrated that almost all FUDR is extracted by hepatic artery infusion whereas only about 50% of 5FU is extracted by the liver. Therefore, he concluded that FUDR is probably a preferable drug for hepatic artery infusion.

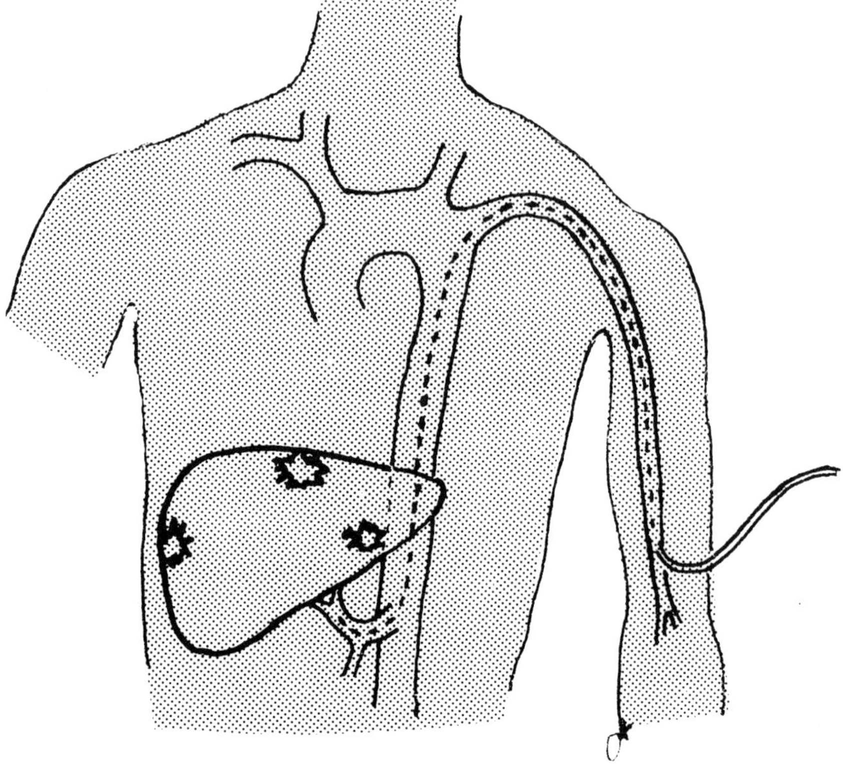

Figure 9.2. Percutaneous transbrachial hepatic arterial catheter.

This discovery, following on the use of silastic catheters, was linked with a major technologic advance which was the recent development of the totally implantable drug infusion system, the Infusaid pump. (Infusaid Corp., Norwood, Mass.). This Infusaid implantable pump is about the size of a hockey puck and is, therefore, clearly substantial (Figure 9.3). It approximates the size of the original pacemaker. It is constructed of titanium in the shape of a dish and is separated into two chambers by a welded diaphragm which is actually an expandable metal bellows. This encloses a precise quantity of freon which exists either as a liquid or a gas depending on its state of compression against the bellows and the outer shell of the pump. The inside of the bellows (Figure 9.4) serves as a refillable drug reservoir. The act of refilling this reservoir compresses the enclosed freon which constantly is

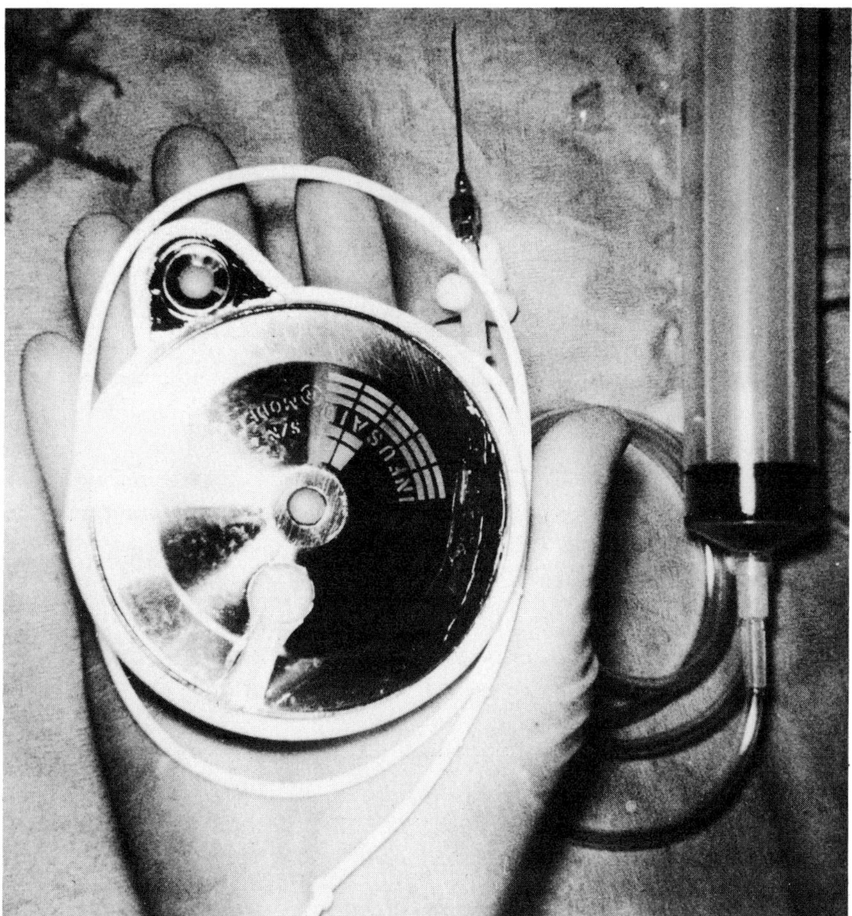

Figure 9.3. The Infusaid implantable pump and Huber needle.

attempting to change back to its gaseous phase. This is regardless
of the compressed chamber volume. The pressure thus produced
forces the drug out from the reservoir through a micropore filter
and a flow-restricting capillary tube assembly into a soft silastic
catheter for delivery to the selected body site. Because the whole
pump is sealed the drug can only be placed in the reservoir by
means of a percutaneous needle injection which penetrates the
self-sealing entry port (Figure 9.4). The needle is a Huber-type
with the opening on the side so that the end is not burred over by
the needle stop after penetration. Hence, when the drug is injected

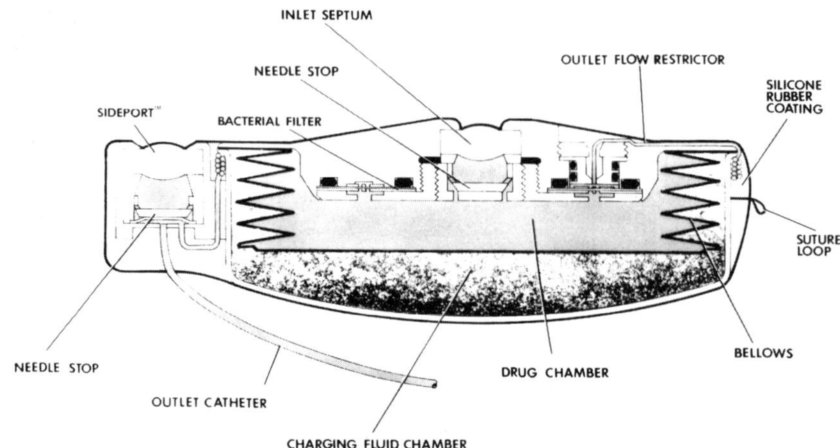

Figure 9.4. Diagramatic representation of the implantable Infusaid pump in cross section.

in a quantity of 50 cc into the reservoir the chamber itself is expanded. This simultaneously decreases the freon volume which condenses from vapor to liquid so storing energy for the next flow cycle.

The infusion rate is dependent on the size of the capillary tubing allowing the drug to flow out into the silastic catheter. Since the pump is completely self–contained and the energy is supplied in the form of renewed doses of drug, it can be permanently implanted for extended chemotherapeutic use.

The pump has a high structural integrity and is made of materials which are biologically and chemically compatible for safe implantation. It produces a pressure of approximately 428 mms of mercury and only has one moving part with no rubbing surfaces to wear out or stick or produce particle contamination. Dosage rates are manipulated for each patient by altering the concentration of the drug placed in the infusion chamber.

One of the most important aspects of the pump itself is the integration of the silastic catheter. This has overcome many of the problems previously associated with implantation of catheters into the hepatic artery. Because it is soft, it is possible to place it into a short branch of the hepatic artery and fix it to surrounding tissue. More rigid catheters have produced problems because it has not been possible to stabilize them and movements of one part of the body have been transmitted through the catheter to its tip which has subsequently worked out of the hepatic artery or even through its wall. Conversely, with the advent of the silastic catheter and techniques involved, it has been possible to maintain hepatic artery flow without any compromise of this vessel after implantation of the catheter.

Techniques of Catheter Implantation

Because of the wide variability of the hepatic arterial system, it is mandatory to carry out an arteriogram before placing the catheter in order that the exact blood supply can be seen to the liver. Then a decision can be made as to which vessels can be used for implantation preoperatively.

The commonest vessel and easiest vessel to use is the gastroduodenal artery (Figure 9.5). The catheter can be placed in this vessel with its tip at but not into the hepatic artery but no compromise to the duodenum or stomach is noted because of the rich associated blood supply of these areas. At the time of surgery, I prefer to use Methylene Blue injected into the catheter to check that both sides of the liver indeed are being infused. The use of Methylene Blue also has another major advantage and that is that it is very easy to see any blush on the duodenum or stomach which can be caused by secondary or tertiary arterioles leading from the hepatic artery to these organs. Clearly, peptic ulceration will occur if nothing is done to avoid this. We then, if we do see a blue blush on the stomach or duodenum, take great care to separate all the peritoneum from the hepatic artery and to completely denude the hepatic artery for a distance of 2–3 cms away from the site of implantation of the catheter into the gastroduodenal artery. Having done this we then reinject Methylene Blue and once again check. We usually find this is sufficient but occasionally a smaller area remains involved. A further search will indicate that the culprits are tiny vessels stained with Methylene Blue and these can all be divided and once again an injection can be given. At this point no further blushing should be seen. In other words, it is quite important to consider as part of the implantation procedure, de–vascularization of the lesser curve of the stomach. Obviously, using the gastroduodenal artery as the point of implantation means that the right gastric artery must be ligated.

When the right and left hepatic arteries originate too close to the gastroduodenal artery to permit mixing of the drug and equal

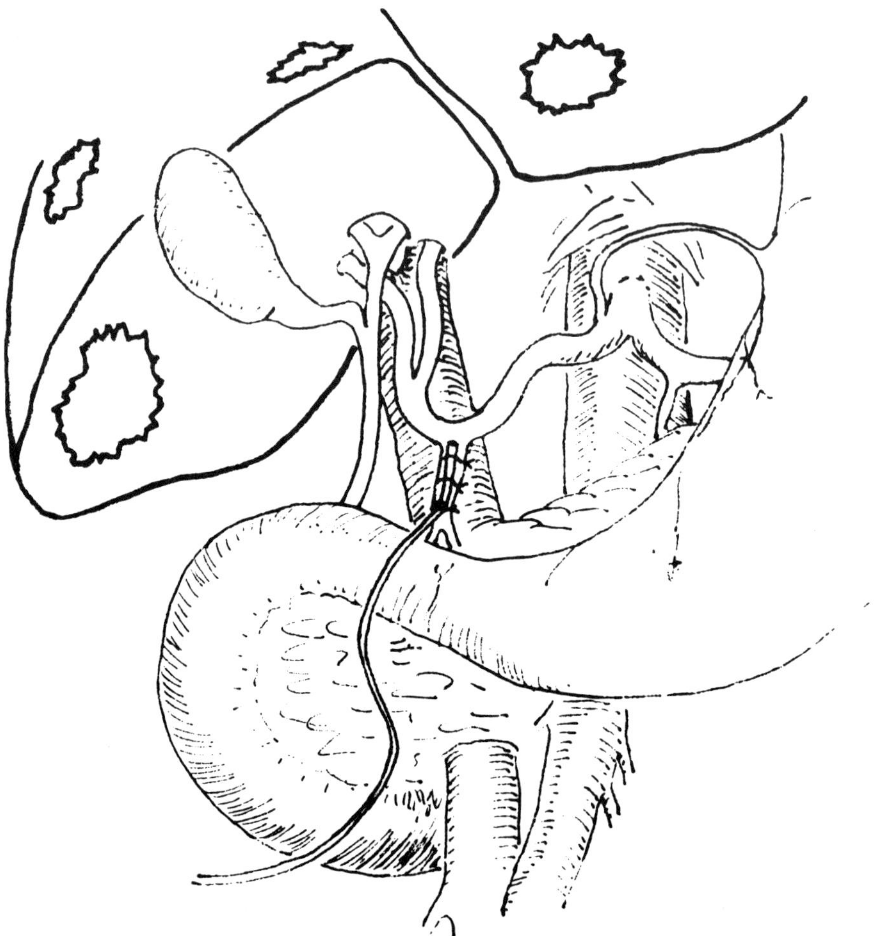

Figure 9.5. Implantation of the arterial catheter into the gastroduodenal artery when "normal" anatomy is present (after Niederhuber).

distribution to all areas of the liver the splenic artery can be used as a point of implantation of the catheter (Figure 9.6). After the catheter has been placed again with its tip at but not into the hepatic artery it should be held in place using two #000 silk ties. This will ligate the splenic artery. Further the gastroduodenal artery should also be ligated. The same technique should be used if there is a trifurcation to the liver from the celiac axis. The spleen will not infarct with a ligation at the proximal end of the

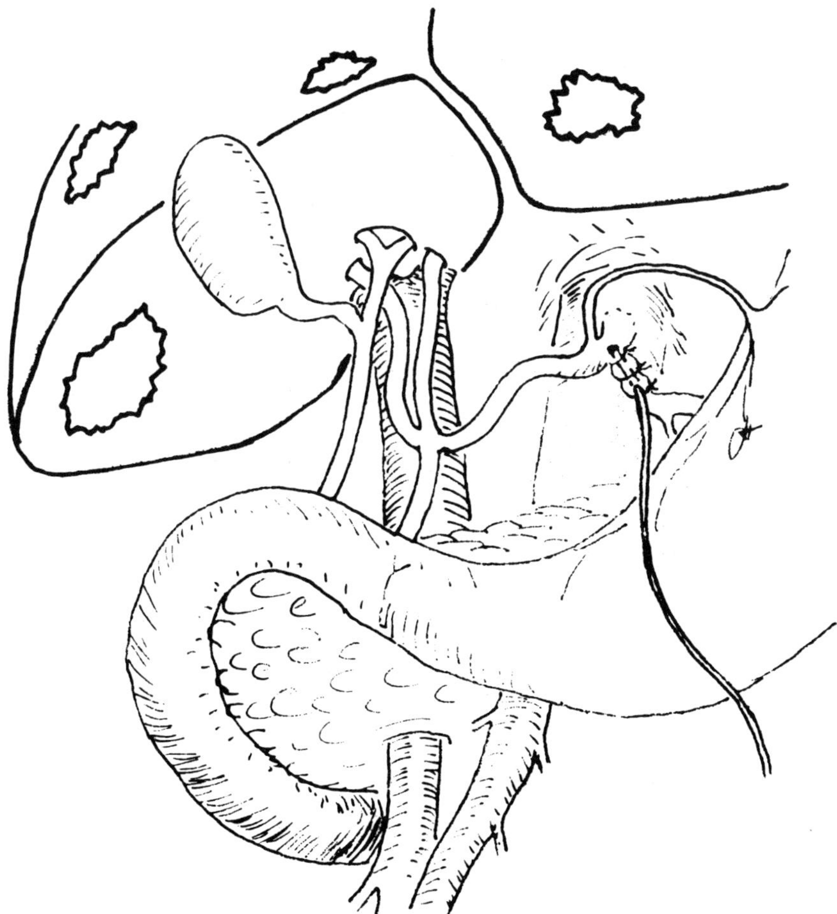

Figure 9.6. When a trifurcation of right and left hepatic arteries together with the gastroduodenal artery arises from the common hepatic artery, the splenic artery can be used as a point of implantation of the catheter.

artery as it will pick up a blood supply through the short gastric arteries or other vessels of the richly anastomosing gastric and pancreatic arterioles.

When the left side of the liver is supplied independently, then the left gastric artery can be cannulated independently from the gastroduodenal artery (Figure 9.7). However, this can be difficult mainly because these vessels are small. Under these circumstances, I tend to prefer to place a single catheter into the gastroduodenal

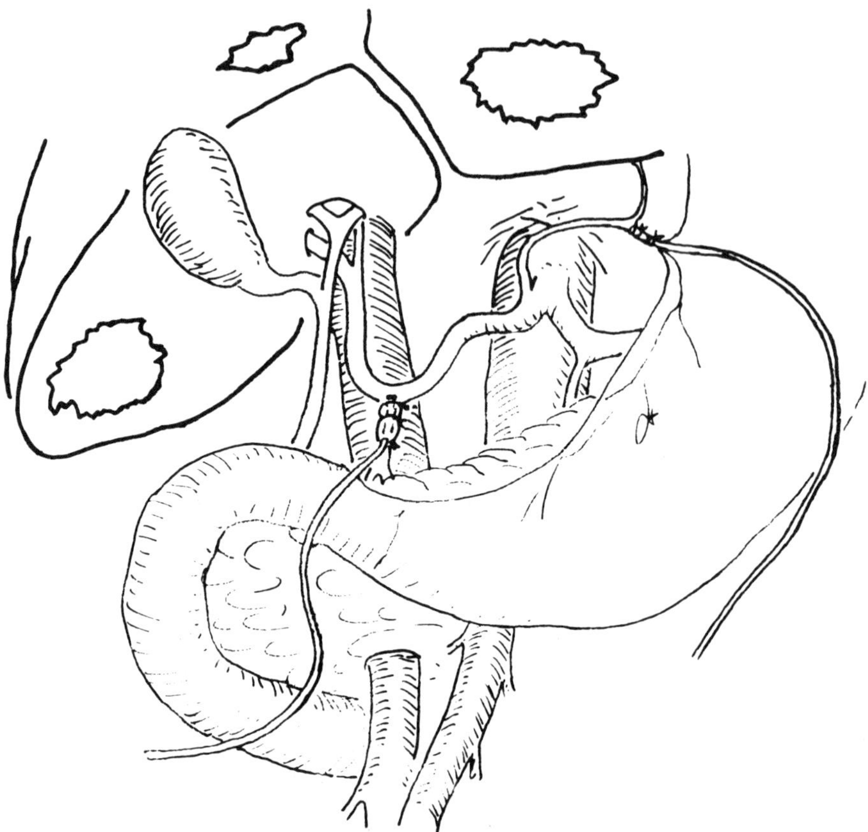

Figure 9.7. When the left hepatic artery arises independently from the left gastric artery it can be cannulated independently through the left gastric artery to supply chemotherapy directly to the left lobe. In addition, the gastroduodenal artery is cannulated in the usual way to supply the chemotherapy to the right lobe and left middle lobes.

artery and to ligate and divide the separate small left hepatic artery so that intra-arterial anastomoses will occur and provide distribution of the drug in that way.

Where the patient has a replaced right hepatic artery or if the entire hepatico-arterial system is derived from the superior mesenteric artery, then the catheter has to be placed into the side wall of the hepatic artery itself (Figure 9.8). This is done using a small pursestring of #5-0 prolene about an arteriotomy and through which the catheter is then passed. The pursestring is tied and then

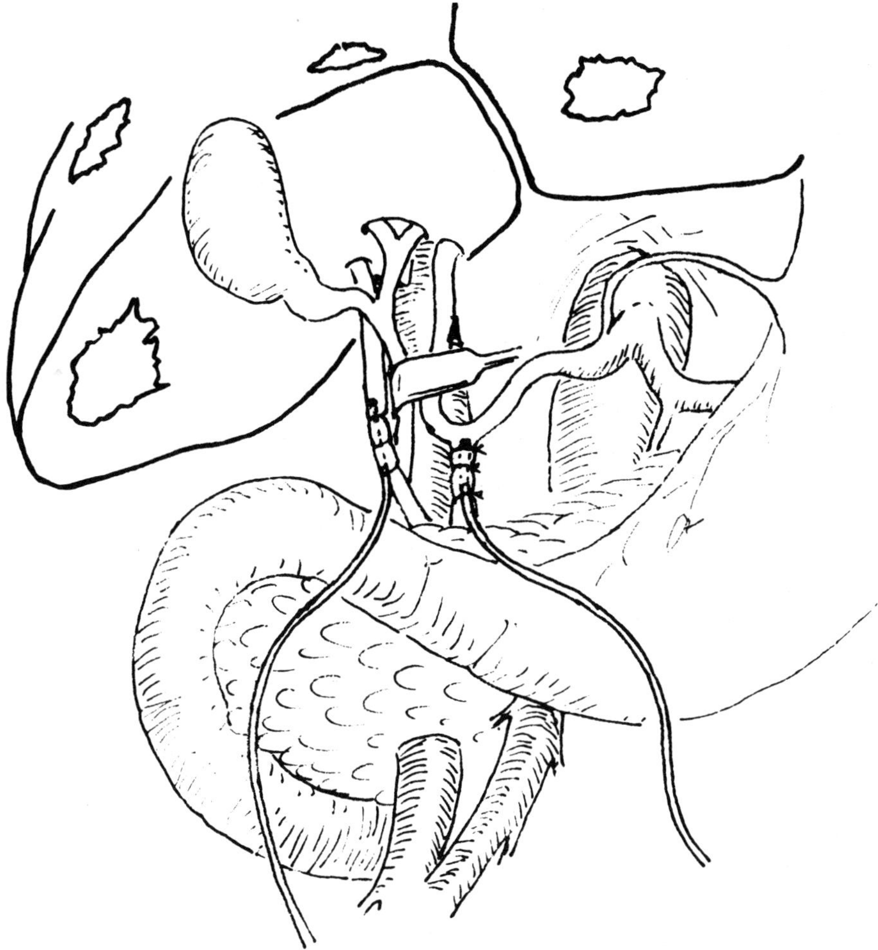

Figure 9.8. In a patient with a replaced right hepatic artery from the superior mesenteric artery, the catheter has to be placed into the side wall of the hepatic artery itself. The illustration demonstrates the left hepatic artery being supplied independently by a second catheter through the gastroduodenal artery.

a separate stitch is placed through the wall of the vessel to hold the catheter against the side wall of the artery so as not to occlude it.

Where the patient has so much liver involvement that it is too stiff to allow reflection in order to obtain adequate dissection of the hepatic arterial system (40), or with some of the vascular anomalies described above which would mean the use of two pumps in some of the patients, I have used the portal system for access. Occasionally, there is a very large gastroduodenal vein running straight into the portal system which is easy to cannulate and again the Methylene Blue indicates the position of the tip of the catheter which can be correctly placed so that both sides of the liver are perfused. Furthermore, the omentum is also extremely useful as omental veins all lead directly to the portal system and any one of these can be cannulated and the catheter passed down and its position checked by Methylene Blue to see if both sides of the liver are perfused.

Subcutaneous Implantation of the Pump

Having placed the catheter, it is brought out through the anterior abdominal wall and attached by means of a small connector to the catheter originating directly from the Infusaid pump. The pump will be placed in a pump pocket prepared subcutaneously on the anterior abdominal wall just above the fascia. I have found that the pump with the side port is best placed with the side port in a central position so that if the pump pocket is on the right-hand side the side port would be placed in the 2 o'clock position and if the pump pocket is on the left-hand side then the side port would be placed in the 10 o'clock position. Originally, I placed the side port the other way around but found so many patients complained of discomfort from the side port stretching the skin that I switched.

Preparation of the pump before implantation is also important as a technique. The previously sterilized pump is taken and placed on a heating pad or else placed in a bowl of hot water. The surgeon should be able to hold his hand in the water. A 10 cc syringe with bacteriostatic water is taken and connected to a Huber needle. The Huber needle is then pushed through the inlet septum and usually a few bubbles of air will escape. The 10 cc is injected into the chamber of the pump. The end of the tubing emanating from the pump is cut so that free-flow can be assured. Pressure from the freon forces air out of the drug chamber and after waiting for a few minutes, almost all of the 10 cc initially injected will be returned. When this has occurred, the syringe and needle are removed and the side port flushed. This removes all air from the system. A 50 cc syringe is then taken and filled with bacteriostatic water containing Heparin 20,000 units. An extension line from an intravenous set is attached and the other end is connected to a 3-way stopcock. A filled 10 cc syringe is placed on the side port of the stopcock for use as a reservoir should any of the fluid be lost from the 50 cc syringe during injection. If all goes well, 50 cc can be injected directly into the drug chamber of the pump after the Huber needle once again has penetrated the inlet septum. Once this has occurred, the stopcock is closed and the needle is withdrawan and the pump observed. A bead will be seen to be emanating from the tip of the catheter. This is confirmation that the pump is working and it can be implanted in its prepared pocket. The prolene loops are there to be used to fix the pump in place. As many of these as practicable should be used to stitch the pump to the fascia. The pump pocket should be big enough to take the pump without any compromise of skin and should be clear of the incision through which the surgery has been carried out.

Refilling the Pump

After a week to ten days, the pump is usually emptied and then refilled with FUDR 100 mgs diluted to 50 cc with bacteriostatic water and Heparin. The dosage of FUDR is increased as the patients progress to a maximum of 400 mgs every two weeks.

Results

In the 1980s the expected response with intrahepatic treatment with 5FU seems to be quoted as between 15-50% (41, 42). This is probably a more realistic response rate than the earlier quotes as these newer trials were done in carefully controlled surroundings with carefully monitored methods. This is not surprising when technical failures are taken into account.

However, when patients with liver tumors, either primary or secondary to the liver, had Infusaid pumps implanted and connected via the hepatic artery, in all the early experience, except at the Sloan-Kettering Memorial Hospital in New York City, there seems to have been greater than expected response with infusion of Fluoroxidine.

In the earliest published paper Buchwald *et al.* (43) from Minnesota in 1980 used the pump in 5 patients and obtained a 50% response rate. Four of their patients received infusions with FUDR at rates of 0.2-0.5 mgs/kg per day for periods of 3-29 weeks. The fifth patient had a defective pump and this was removed. All catheters were placed into the hepatic artery under direct vision at laparotomy. Although all patients have subsequently died, this study did indicate that continuous long-term intra-arterial infusion therapy was a practical proposition. The patients continued their normal daily activities and demonstrated that they were able to be managed entirely on an outpatient basis.

McKinstry (44) reported on the work of Ensminger and Niederhuber from Michigan General Clinic Research Center in Ann Arbor. In 1981 they already had 33 patients in whom the Infusaid pump had been tested and they had an 85% response in their first 13 patients. Ensminger felt that the Infusaid pump allowed levels of FUDR in the liver to reach 100–400 times greater than levels in other tissues. Therefore, the systemic effects of the drug are kept low so that the undesirable side-effects are minimized and the patient's general health is maintained. Further, because of the increased exposure in the end organ i.e., the liver, there is a greater likelihood that there will be a favorable response. Also, it would be hoped that once the response has been obtained it would be greater once it had occurred.

Ensminger found that he could send patients back to referring physicians who were able to refill the pump for him. With its capacity of 50 ml the pump could deliver between 3–6 ml of fluid at a set flow rate per day. Refills are usually necessary once every two weeks.

In Alabama, Balch *et al.* (45) had a similar viewpoint. They also made the point that patients with untreated bilateral liver metastases survive only 3–4 months whereas those with solitary metastases may survive two years. With this in mind, they treated 50 cases with a response rate of 83%.

Chemical hepatitis was a problem as it occurred in almost all their patients, although FUDR was alternated every two weeks with saline. They attempted to overcome this difficulty by halving the dose at each refill until the liver enzymes improved, and then incrementally increasing the dosage as tolerated.

There was 1 death from a myocardial infarction in the postoperative phase. Otherwise there was no incidence of thrombosis, catheter occlusion, catheter migration or infection. A few patients had transient seromas of the pump pockets but there were no infections.

Median follow up was more than 6 months and there were only 2 patients who had tumor progression in the liver. Seven of them had relapse in extrahepatic sites such as the lung, pelvis, the incision and in the bone. These patients were given Mitomycin C through the side port of the pump. Of the 4 patients that died, 2 had no response to chemotherapy.

At the Massachusetts General Hospital, Cohen *et al.* (40) have also had experience in 50 cases but their approach has been to place the catheter trans-brachially to the hepatic artery. The approach is used because in patients with extensive liver metastases, recovery from laparotomy may be slow. Also, in patients with marked hepatomegaly, it can be exceedingly difficult to visualize the hepatic artery because the stiff liver does not allow exposure of the gastrohepatic ligament. Essentially, when the catheter has been placed angiographically via the axillary artery, the percutaneous portion was cut off and connected to a subcutaneous catheter which was attached to the Infusaid pump placed in a subcutaneous pocket under local anesthesia.

They had 41 patients with colorectal cancer metastatic to the liver and 8 of these had concomitant lung metastases. The other patients had primary hepato-cellular carcinoma or other metastatic cancers to the liver. In 11 of their 50 patients laparotomy was actually done for catheterization and in 9 of these the catheter was implanted into the hepatic artery. Two patients had the catheter implanted into the portal vein.

They did have 1 infection in a pump pocket a year after implantation of the pump. Of the 38 patients who had trans-axillary hepatic arterial catheter placement, 7 had withdrawal of the catheter which required replacement. There were episodes of cracking of the polyethylene catheter which required exchanges and in 2 patients it was not possible to replace the catheter successfully into the hepatic artery.

The overall response rate was 70% with a minimum follow up of 6 months. Some of their patients survived as long as 21 months after implantation.

Chemical hepatitis was said to only occur in 5 of their patients and 1 of these remained grossly jaundiced for a year despite discontinuation of the FUDR. Their most significant side-effects were symptomatic ulcers or gastritis and 8 of their patients had to have partial gastrectomy.

In a more recent paper by Cohen *et al.* (46), studying 69 patients with colorectal carcinoma, a 3-drug regime was used with the Infusaid pump. These drugs were Fluoroxidine, Mitomycin C and Carmustine (BCNU). This time, only a 51% response was obtained, with a median survival of one year. Worse still, one third of their patients had less than 25% of hepatic involvement and therefore would be placed in Stage I. Patients placed in Stage I would normally expect to have resectable tumor.

When Schwartz *et al.* (47) published their results from Rochester, they felt that there had been no benefit at all from the use of the Infusaid pump.

In our group of over 40 patients followed for up to 18 months, we found that the Infusaid pump on its own made no difference to survival time, but when further modalities such as arterial embolization and portal vein branch ligation were added, median survival time could be doubled to 12 months in patients of at least Stage II involvement of the liver.

Kemeny *et al.* (48) reported to the American Society of Clinical Oncologists that the side-effects with implantation of the Infusaid pump were significant. In fact the major problem at the Sloan-Kettering Memorial Hospital seemed to have been peptic ulceration. Also, the response rate was only 39% in her group of 23 patients. However, in a subsequent paper from Durante California, her sister Margaret reported that the major complication of the use of intra-arterial chemotherapy supplied by the Infusaid pump was sclerosing cholangitis (49).

Chemical hepatitis is a problem which we found increases as intrahepatic chemotherapy continues but it has also been reported to be irreversible and fatal (50). Our experience was similar to Balch *et al.* (45) in that we were able to overcome the problem in many instances by alternating FUDR every two weeks with saline and then halving the dose at each refill until the liver enzymes improved. However, unlike Ensminger (44), we have not always been successful in sending patients back to the referring physicians as not all oncologists are capable of refilling this pump.

CONCLUSION

Provision of methods for direct intrahepatic infusion of chemotherapy is a step forward from simple ligation of the hepatic artery and does seem to improve the survival rate significantly. The place of treatment using FUDR continuously infused from an Infusaid pump has still not been clarified as the great survival rates claimed in the earlier studies may well simply include those patients who would have survived anyway or in whom the disease was resectable. We have been reserving the use of the pump to patients with unresectable disease and have been disappointed with the results. We have, therefore, combined the Infusaid pump with resection and have come to the conclusion that whenever possible the tumor should be removed as the survival rate in our group of patients was much improved with this method.

REFERENCES

1. Ariel, IM, Pack, GT: Intra-arterial chemotherapy for cancer metastatic to the liver. *Arch Surg, 91:*851–862, 1965.

2. Jaffe, BM, Donegan, WL, Watson, F, *et al.*: Factors influencing survival in patients with untreated hepatic mestatases. *Surg Gynecol Obstet, 127:* 1–11, 1968.

3. Moertel, CG: Clinical management of advanced gastrointestinal cancer. *Cancer, 36:*675–682, 1975.

4. Bierman, HR, Byron, RI, Miller, ER, *et al.*: Effects of intra-arterial administration of nitrogen mustard. *Am J Med, 8:*535, 1950.

5. Klopp, CT, Bateman, J, Berry, N, *et al.*: Fractionated regional cancer chemotherapy. *Cancer Res, 10:*229, 1950.

6. Sullivan, RD, Miller, E, Sikes, MP: Anti-metabolite/metabolite combination cancer chemotherapy. *Cancer, 12:*1248–1261, 1959.

7. Sullivan, RD, Zurek, WZ: Chemotherapy for liver cancer by protracted ambulatory infusion. *J Am Med Assn, 194:*481–486, 1965.

8. Clarkson, B, Young, C, Dierick, W, *et al.:* Effects of continuous hepatic artery infusion of anti-metabolites on primary and metastatic cancer of the liver. *Cancer, 15:*472–488, 1962.

9. Brennan, MJ, Talley, RW, Drake, EL, *et al.*: 5-Fluourouracil treatment of liver metastases by continuous hepatic artery infusion via Couinaud catheter. *Ann Surg, 158:*405–419, 1963.

10. Labelle, JJ, Lucas, RJ, Eisenstein, B, *et al.*: Hepatic artery catheterization for chemotherapy. *Arch Surg, 96:*683–693, 1968.

11. Cady, B, Oberfield, RA: Regional infusion chemotherapy of hepatic metastases from carcinoma of the colon. *Amer J Surg, 127:*220–227, 1974.

12. Watkins, E, Khazii, AM, Nahra, KS: Surgical basis for arterial infusion chemotherapy of disseminated carcinoma of the liver. *Surg Gynecol Obstet, 130:*581–605, 1970.

13. Rochlin, DB, Smart, CR: An Evaluation of 51 patients with hepatic artery infusion. *Surg Gynecol Obstet, 123:*535–538, 1966.

14. Gorgun, B, Watne, AL: Infusion chemotherapy in hepatoma and metastatic liver tumors. *Am J Surg, 113:*363–368, 1967.

15. Burrows, JH, Talley, RW, Drake, HH, *et al.*: Infusion of fluourinated pyrimidines into hepatic artery for treatment of metastatic carcinoma of the liver. *Cancer, 20:*1886–1892, 1967.

16. Donegan, WL, Harris, HS: Metastatic colorectal carcinoma – response to hepatic infusion. *Missouri Med, 67:*163–168, 1970.

17. Donegan, WL, Harris, HS, Spratt, JS: Prolonged continuous hepatic infusion. *Arch Surg, 99:*149–157, 1969.

18. Massey, WH, Fletcher, WS, Judkins, MP, *et al.*: Hepatic artery infusion for metastatic malignancy using percutaneously placed catheters. *Am J Surg, 121:*160–164, 1971.

19. Ansfield, FJ, Ramirez, G, Skibba, JC, *et al.*: Intrahepatic arterial infusion with 5-fluourouracil. *Cancer, 28:*1147–1151, 1971.

20. Freckman, HA: Chemotherapy for metastatic colorectal liver carcinoma by intra-aortic infusion. *Cancer, 28:*1152–1160, 1971.

21. Tandon, RN, Bunnell, IL, Copper, RG: The treatment of metastatic carcinoma of the liver by the percutaneous selective hepatic artery infusion of 5-fluourouracil. *Surgery, 73:*118–121, 1973.

22. Davis, HL, Ramirez, G, Ansfield, FJ: Adenocarcinoma of the stomach, pancreas, liver and biliary tract. *Cancer, 33:*193–197, 1974.

23. Stehlin, JS, Hafstrom, L, Greeff, PJ: Experience with infusion and resection in cancer of the liver. *Surg Gynecol Obstet, 138:*855–863, 1974.

24. Sullivan, RD: Systemic and arterial infusion chemotherapy for metastatic liver cancer. *Int J Rad Oncol Biol Phys, 1:*973–976, 1976.

25. Kondi, ES, Gallitano, AL, Evjy, JT, *et al.*: Prolonged survival in patients with hepatic malignant melanoma treated by intra-arterial Bleomycin and later oral Hydroxyurea. *Am J Surg, 128:*85–87, 1974.

26. Gulesserian, HP, Lawton, RL, Condon, RE: Hepatic artery ligation and cytotoxic infusion in treatment of liver metastases. *Arch Surg, 105:*280–285, 1972.

27. Sparks, FC, Misher, MB, Hallauer, WC, *et al.*: Hepatic artery ligation and postoperative chemotherapy for hepatic metastases: Clinical and pathophysiological results. *Cancer, 35:*1074–1082, 1975.

28. Ramming, KP, Sparks, FC, Eilber, *et al.*: Hepatic artery ligation and 5-fluourouracil infusion for metastatic colon cancer and primary hepatoma. *Am J Surg, 132:*236–242, 1976.

29. Fortner, JG, Pahnke, LD: A new method for long-term intrahepatic chemotherapy. *Surg Gynecol Obstet, 143:*979–980, 1976.

30. Murray-Lyon, IM, Dawson, JL, Parsons, BA, *et al.*: Treatment of secondary hepatic tumors by ligation of the hepatic artery and infusion of cytotoxic drugs. *Lancet, 2:*172–175, 1970.

31. Almersjö, O, Bengmark, S, Hafstron, L, *et al.*: Liver resection for cancer. *Acta Chir Scand, 142:*139–144, 1976.

32. Taylor, I: Cytotoxic perfusion for colorectal liver metastases. *Brit J Surg, 65:*109–114, 1978.

33. Chuang, VP, Wallace, S: Hepatic artery embolization in the treatment of hepatic neoplasms. *Radiology, 140:*51–58, 1981.

34. El-Domeiri, AA: A method of intermittent occlusion and chemotherapy infusion of the hepatic artery. *Surg Gynecol Obstet, 143:*107–109, 1976.

35. Bengmark, S, Fredlund, PE: Temporary de-arterialization combined with intra-arterial infusion of oncolytic drugs in the treatment of liver tumors. *Prog Clin Cancer, 7:*207-216, 1978.

36. Reed, ML, Vaitkevicius, VK, Al-Sarraf, M, *et al.*: The practicability of chronic hepatic artery infusion therapy of primary metastatic hepatic malignancies: 10-year results of 124 patients in a prospective protocol. *Cancer, 47:*402-409, 1981.

37. Grage, TB, Vassilopoulos, PP, Shingleton, WW, *et al.*: Results of a prospective randomized study of hepatic artery infusion with 5-fluorouracil vs intravenous 5-fluorouracil in patients with hepatic metastases from colorectal cancer: A Central Oncology Group study. *Surgery, 86:*550-555, 1979.

38. Watkins, E, Oberfield, RA, Cady, B, Clouse, ME: Arterial infusion chemotherapy of diffuse hepatic malignancies. *Prog Clin Cancer, 7:*235-245, 1978.

39. Ensminger, WD, Rosowsky, A, Raso, V, *et al.*: A clinical pharmacological evaluation of hepatic arterial infusion of 5-fluouro 2-deoxyuridine and 5-fluourouracil. *Cancer Res, 38:*3784-3792, 1978.

40. Cohen, AM, Kaufman, SD, Wood, WC, Greenfield, AJ: Regional hepatic chemotherapy using an implantable drug infusion pump. *Am J Surg, 145:*529-532, 1983.

41. Sugarbaker, PH, Macdonald, JS, Gunderson, LL: Colorectal cancer. In *Cancer, Principals and Practice of Oncology*, Devita, VT, Jr., Hellman, S, Rosenberg, SA (Eds.). Philadelphia: JP Lippincott, 1982, pp. 643-723.

42. Engstrom, PF, Macintyre, JM, Douglass, HO, Jr., *et al.*: Combination chemotherapy of advanced colorectal cancer utilizing 5-fluorouracil, semustine, decarbazine, vincristine and hydroxyurea. A Phase III trial by the Eastern Cooperative Oncology Group (E.S.T. 4275). *Cancer, 49:*1555-1560, 1982.

43. Buchwald, H, Grage, TB, Vassilopoulos, PP, *et al.*: Intra-arterial infusion chemotherapy for hepatic carcinoma using a totally implantable infusion pump. *Cancer, 45:*866-869, 1980.

44. McKinstry, DW: Implanted drug delivery system for regional cancer chemotherapy. *Res Resource Rep, 5:*1-5, 1981.

45. Balch, CM, Urist, MM, McGregor, ML: Continuous regional chemotherapy for metastatic colorectal cancer using a totally implantable infusion pump. *Am J Surg, 145:*285-290, 1983.

46. Cohen, AM, Kaufman, SD, Wood, WC: Treatment of colorectal cancer hepatic metastases by hepatic artery chemotherapy. *Dis Colon Rectum, 28:*389-393, 1985.

47. Schwartz, SI, Jones, LS, McCune, CS: Assessment of treatment of intrahepatic malignancies using chemotherapy via an implantable pump. *Ann Surg, 201:*560-567, 1985.

48. Kemeny, N, Daly, JM, Oderman, P, Shike, M: Hepatic infusion chemotherapy for metastatic colorectal carcinoma. Results and complications. (Abstr.) *Proc Am Soc Oncol, 123:*1983.

49. Kemeny, MM, Battifora, H, Blayney, DW, *et al.*: Sclerosing cholangitis after continuous hepatic artery infusion of FUDR. *Ann Surg, 202:*176–181, 1985.

50. Johnson, LP, Rivkin, SE: The implanted pump in metastatic colorectal cancer of the liver. Risk versus benefit. *Am J Surg, 149:*595–598, 1985.

W. JOHN B. HODGSON, M.D.

CHAPTER 10
Hepatic Resections

In keeping with the general philosophy of this book, this chapter will be concerned with simple hepatic resections in the beginning, and resections of increasing difficulty will be described as the chapter progresses.

HISTORICAL BACKGROUND

Much of the historical background of liver surgery has been covered in the previous chapters on Anatomy and Hepatic Artery Ligation. Suffice to say, Foster and Berman (1) note that Paulus Aeginata was said to have cauterized protruding portions of the liver after eviscerating injuries 1,300 years ago! Dagradi and Brearley (2) recorded that the first documented case of removal of a portion of human liver was in 1716 by Berta, who excised a protruding portion of the right lobe in a madman who had inflicted a knife wound in his own hypochondrium. In his "Report after Waterloo" John Thompson described 12 cases of wounds of the liver that were successfully treated (3). Removal of chunks of liver following trauma was a rare occurrence and survival thereafter was probably fortuitous (3, 4) but the first early steps had been taken.

In the mid 19th Century, Morton pioneered anesthesiology, Pasteur demonstrated that putrefaction was caused by bacteria and Lister transformed the practice of surgery by his successful use of antisepsis. These discoveries led to a great flowering of abdominal surgery. The liver, however, remained off limits because as Elliott pointed out it was so "friable, so full of gaping vessels, and so evidently incapable of being sutured that it had always seemed impossible to successfully manage large wounds of its substance" (5). On the other hand, in the laboratory, the principles of liver resection were being developed and liver regeneration was demonstrated (6-9).

The fable of Prometheus is relevant here. The secret of fire was given to man by Prometheus. As retribution the gods, there-

185

fore, bound him to the rocks and sent great birds to tear out his liver by day. But by night, according to this ancient Greek legend, the liver regenerated so that the punishment could be perpetuated.

The progress from laboratory to liver resection was rapid but more or less confined to removal of pedicled tumors. There was no anatomical understanding of the procedure in man at this time and the larger the pedicle, the more likely the patient would be to bleed to death. For example, Lius excised a solid tumor by ligating and cutting through a pedicled left lobe "adenoma" in 1886 but had difficulty controlling hemorrhage and the patient died 6 hours after the operation (10). In 1888 Langenbuch also resected a pedicled tumor of the left lobe and in this case, when the wound began bleeding on the evening of the operation, a re-operation did have a successful outcome although the postoperative course was long and stormy (11). As an aside, there was considerable controversy at that time as to whether the patient's tightly laced corset was responsible for the development of the tumor (12).

Although Tiffany is credited with the first American report of removal of a liver tumor, the tumor itself appeared to be the result of stone disease rather than neoplasia (13). W.W. Keen actually removed the first true neoplasm in the United States in 1892. He resected a 3½ inch cystic tumor from the edge of the right lobe in a 31–year–old female and found that he had problems using the hot cautery during the dissection but managed to complete the operation bluntly using his thumb nail (14). He also resected an angioma (15) in 1897 and a primary carcinoma of the left lobe of the liver (16) in 1899. He established some very useful principles of liver surgery. Perhaps the most important was the development of an artificial pedicle which was achieved by cutting through normal liver substance and attempting to ligate the vessels. In particular, his method during the removal of the angioma, was to place a rubber tube around the base of the developed pedicle and by tightening it up as much as possible he was able to exteriorize the tumor and then remove it 6 days later by transecting the pedicle without blood loss (15).

Much work was done in the animal laboratory to establish the technical aspects of liver resection. As in Keen's technique, most effort was put into devising methods for bringing tumors out on a stalk through the belly or using the approach of allowing delayed slough and peritoneal exclusion of the tumor and its stalk. Clamps were left in the wound and removed days later when thrombosis was secure and other devices such as hatpins, knitting needles, bulky removable ligatures and packs were also tried to allow delayed slough and peritoneal exclusion of the tumor and its stalk. The mainstay, of course, remained the heated cautery but most surgeons found that this was only suitable for smaller vessels. Kousnetzoff and Pensky (17) and also Auvray (18) established the value of blunt technique in that they passed large ligatures placed as through-and-through mattress sutures to control bleeding. Because ligatures tended to pull through soft liver tissue, Beck (19) used plates of decalcified bone or abdominal fascia to secure them. Cartilage of calf scapula, whale bone, and even plates of magnesium were all initially used (20). By means of using interlocking mattress sutures with blunt needles, reasonably good control was obtained and so by the beginning of the 20th Century most liver wounds were returned to the abdomen before closure of the abdominal wall.

The first significant anatomical advance was by Jay Hercath Pringle (21) who recommended digital compression of the hilar vessels to control bleeding from liver wounds in 1908 and this maneuver is used even today.

Sir Heneage Ogilvie (22) resected a metastasis from a rectal carcinoid tumor in 1951 and laid the ground work for the blunt technique used currently. In trying to apply a hemostat to a vessel divided by the knife, he was struck by the ease with which "the hemostat cut through liver tissue like butter, but met a resistance that could be appreciated when it reached the firmer tissue of Glisson's capsule in which the bleeding vessel lay." Thereafter, he used a fine pointed hemostat, closed for dividing the liver by very slow and gentle strokes, individually ligating the blood vessels and successfully completing the operation.

Anatomic principles were used by Wangenstein in 1951 who reported resection of all liver tissue to the right of the falciform ligament (23) but credit for the first lobectomy based on vascular anatomy with preliminary hilar ligation is usually given to Lortat-Jacob and Robert (24) in 1952. In 1953 Quattlebaum published a similar description (25).

Although Honjo and Araki (26) first reported their case in 1955 claiming no priority over Lortat-Jacob, it must be remembered that their case was first submitted in 1953 and contained more than one year's follow up so their operation may well have preceeded that of the French.

Clearly, the 1950s represented an explosion of clinical experience. Much knowledge was contributed by Quattlebaum (25) in

Georgia and by Pack (27), Brunschwig (28), and Bowden (29) of the Memorial Hospital in New York who performed most of the major hepatic resections from 1951-1954. Although their mortality rates were in the region of 30%, and this is a figure which still frightens many physicians even today, they did demonstrate that safe liver resection was a possibility. Healey (30, 31) demonstrated that the liver had a right and a left half and that each lobe was divided into subsections or segments. He advised segmental rather than lobar resection whenever possible but 30 years later surgical technique had not sufficiently advanced to bring this into general usage. Goldsmith and Woodburne (32) further clarified surgical anatomy and the work of Longmire, McDermott, Mersheimer and Clatworthy continues to be significant even now in America (33-37). The largest worldwide experience has been obtained in Asia and reported by Lin, Ong, Tung, Honjo and Balasegaram (38-42). Probably the greatest surgical anatomical influence on recent surgical· approaches has been provided by Starzl. His landmark series of right trisegmentectomies had only a 3% mortality (43). He later demonstrated in 1982 that the left trisegmentectomy was also a feasible possibility (44). Fortner has picked up the mantle at the Memorial Hospital and has continued to demonstrate excellent results with surgical resection of metastatic carcinoma of the liver (45). The work published from the Mayo Clinic by Adson (46) and from Duke University by Hank (47) has encouraged such surgery as possible in many major teaching centers (48-52), and indeed, even in community hospitals with well found cancer centers (53).

However, the actual technique of liver resection has remained a major problem due to the inability of the surgeon to have complete control during the procedure when using finger fracture. Laceration of a draining hepatic vein or the inferior vena cava is a major disaster with a high likelihood of fatality and the development of techniques to avoid such complications is a top priority.

TECHNICAL ADVANCES

The development of the Lin clamp (54) was a step forward and is used routinely in the Far East for non-anatomic liver resections. One problem is that multiple heavy mattress sutures are usually required to control bleeding before it is possible to remove the clamp. This leaves a 1-2 cm area of potentially necrotic liver ripe for abscess formation. Also, placement of the clamp may tear vessels during the manipulation required to set up the tumorous area for resection. If a branch of the inferior vena cava is hit, a major problem is at hand at the commencement of surgery. Ryan *et al.*, however, recently assessed the clamp and felt that they could half their blood loss during major hepatic resection using this approach (55).

Further technological advances have been applied to liver resections, and the only method receiving widespread support is the use of the CUSA system, pioneered by the author, who demonstrated even less blood loss and greater control (56, 57).

The CUSA System

Following animal work since 1979, the CUSA system (ultrasonic scalpel) was found to be useful in skeletonizing hepatic vessels by removing mesenchymal tissue from them in a controlled manner so they could be demonstrated intra–operatively and secured before division (58).

The ultrasonic scalpel itself has a free–standing control and power console (Figure 10.1) with a separate gas sterilizable lightweight hand piece (Figure 10.2). The power console uses regular operating room electricity and is self-contained. A 15–foot disposable cable is attached to the hand piece. This pencil grip hand piece contains a magneto strictive transducer placed in an electric coil. When an alternating current is passed through this coil, the transducer oscillates longitudinally at 23 kHz. These vibrations are then passed through the connecting body to a hollow conical titanium tip which acts as an amplifier. At maximum power of about 100 watts, the excursion of the tip is up to 300 microns. The hand piece itself is cooled by water run through a stainless steel jacket and sucked out by vacuum. There is a separate stream of saline solution irrigation which runs under a plastic flue surrounding the tip except at its very end. This protects the tissues from undue contact with the hand piece.

When the exposed tip contacts target tissue, cavitation occurs with resultant implosion and fragmentation. The greater the water content, the easier it is for this process to occur. When the power is reduced, the total stroke of the tip is also reduced and so the instrument can be used in various situations and organs which require different power ranges. After the tissue has been fragmented, the irrigating saline suspends the fragments and then they

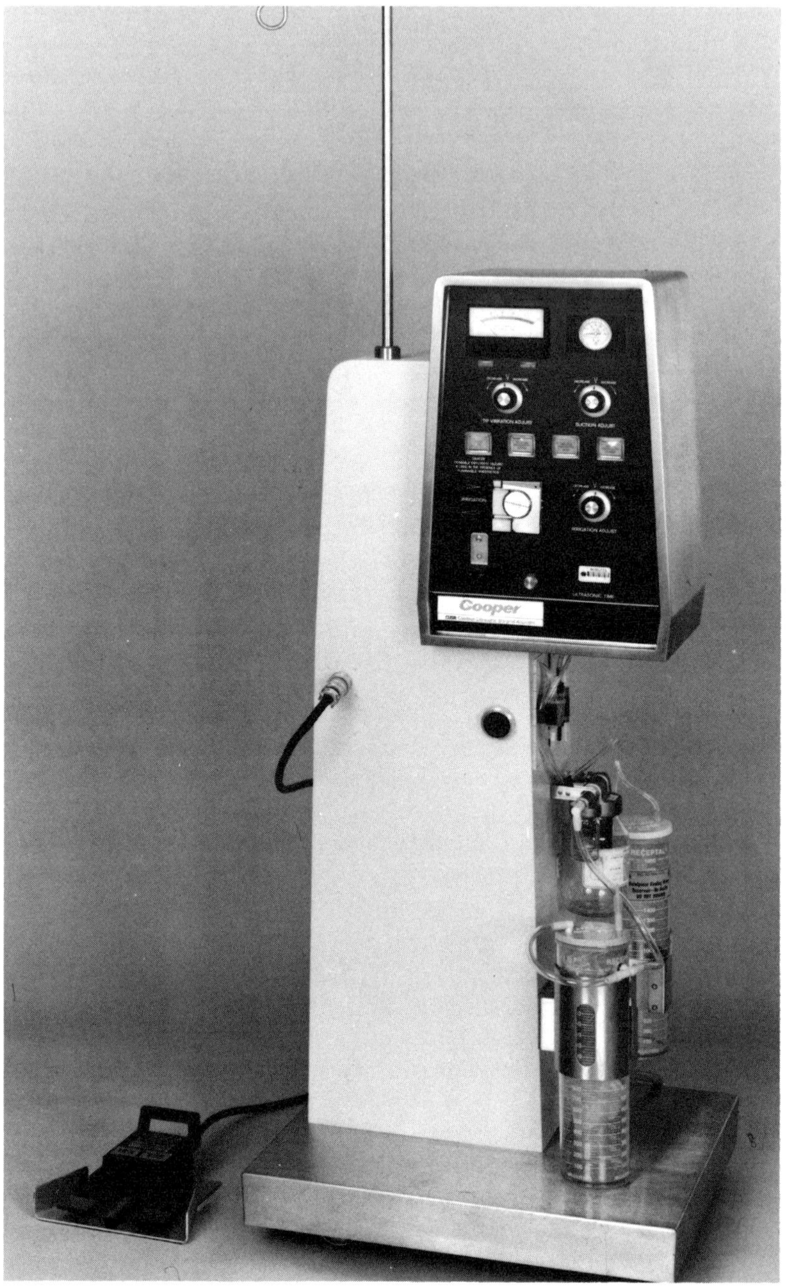

Figure 10.1. Control and power console of the CUSA System (ultrasonic scalpel).

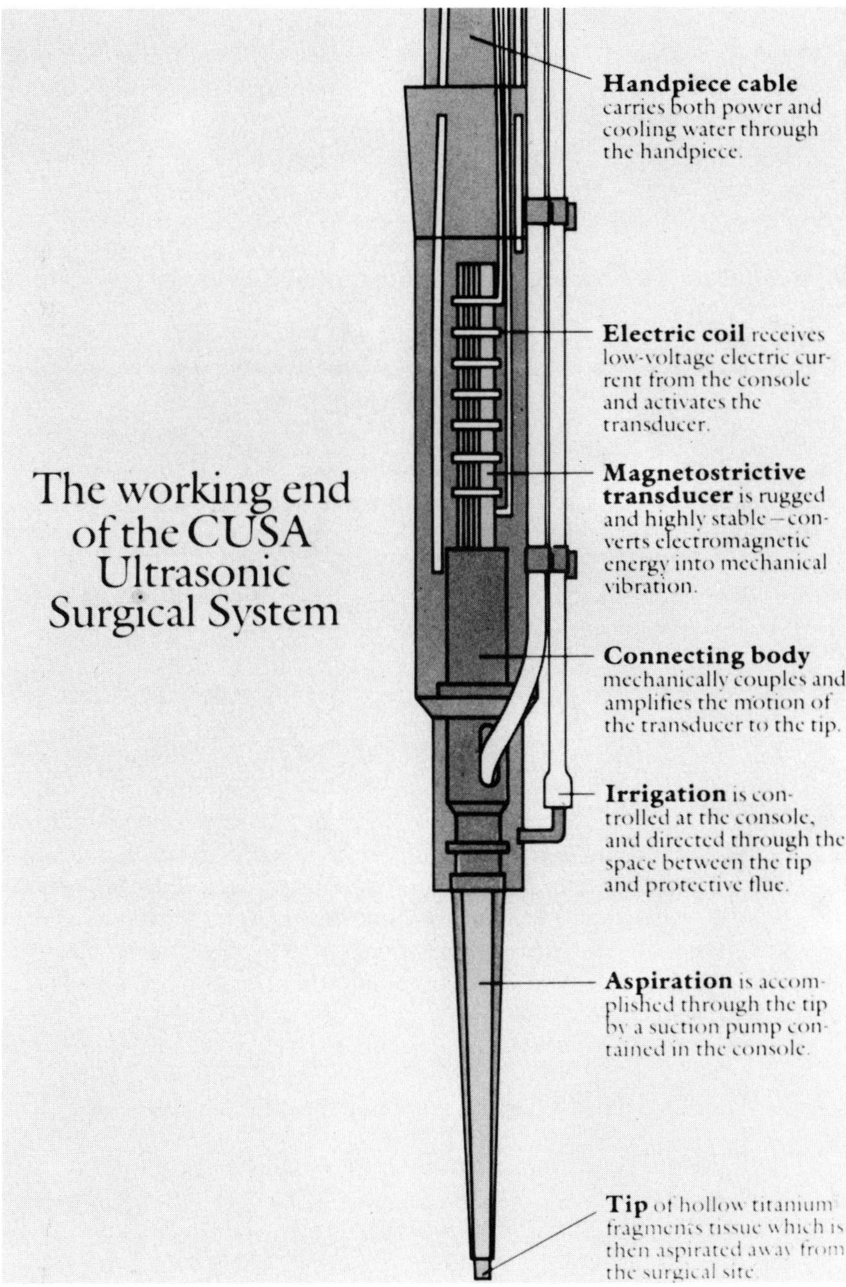

Figure 10.2. Diagram of CUSA handpiece.

can be aspirated from the operative field leaving a clear view. Because blood vessels have a high collagen and elastic tissue content, it is relatively easy to spare them and the surgeon can feel these vessels during the course of dissection and avoid them.

Histological studies indicate that the depth of cell damage using the ultrasonic scalpel is in the same range as that caused using an ordinary steel scalpel. Damage is, therefore, far less than that caused by the cautery or laser. The final appearance of the cut liver is of a smooth almost glossy surface, and histologically there appears to be a coating of adherent red cells on the surface (59).

WEDGE EXCISION

The technique of wedge excision can be used for any small tumor situated on the inferior border of the liver or a slightly more sophisticated version of this technique can be used for small tumors situated on the dome of the liver.

The only danger areas are those between the gall bladder and the falciform ligament. Occasionally the inferior branch of the left portal vein maintains a course close to the inferior border of the left lateral segment for 1-2 cm and it is important to watch out for this.

Any incision which allows adequate exposure of the involved tumor is used. Very small nodules can be removed with a knife after simple placement of a zero absorbable stitch on either side of the nodule. A third stitch is then placed behind the nodule as a through-and-through stitch. The needle is placed from above and passed through the liver before being re-introduced from below to exit on the superior surface of the liver. These sutures are tied firmly but not so tightly as to cut through the liver tissue and hemostasis is obtained.

WEDGE RESECTION (SUBSEGMENTECTOMY)

It should be noted that it has become fashionable to describe wedge resections as ·subsegmentectomy, based on the anatomical segments of the liver described by Couinaud (60) and as strongly advocated by Bismuth (61). This has the advantage of more accurately describing the extent of liver tissue removed but the disadvantage that it still does not take into account the variable venous drainage of the liver (62). This may trap the unwary surgeon who tries to follow such described segments too rigidly. On the other hand, preservation of the normal parenchyma is particularly important in primary carcinoma of the liver, and the intraoperative use of sonography (63–65) is allowing more and more accurate local wedge resections or subsegmentectomies to be done (66, 67).

With this in mind, the ultrasonic scalpel at a setting of 8–9 is used in a probing motion through Glisson's capsule to punch out a series of openings into the liver to delineate the area to be wedged out (Figure 10.3). A small amount of bleeding occurs when this is done and the ultrasonic scalpel is then used to enlarge the holes which have been made. As it does this, surgeons can see small blood vessels which can then be cauterized or clipped before division. The liver incision is rapidly opened up using this method and as vessels are seen, the movement of the tip is changed to a side-to-side movement to dissect parenchyma off them so that they can be very quickly controlled (Figure 10.4). Small tumors

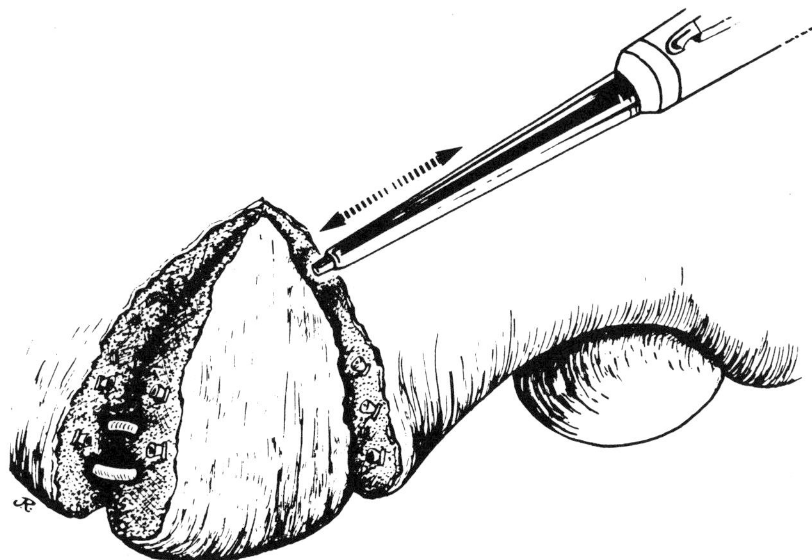

Figure 10.3. Probing motion of the ultrasonic scalpel in superficial dissection and small wedge resections of the liver. (Reproduced with kind permission from Hodgson, WJB, DelGuercio, LRM: Preliminary experience in liver surgery using the ultrasonic scalpel. *Surgery, 95:*230–234, 1984.)

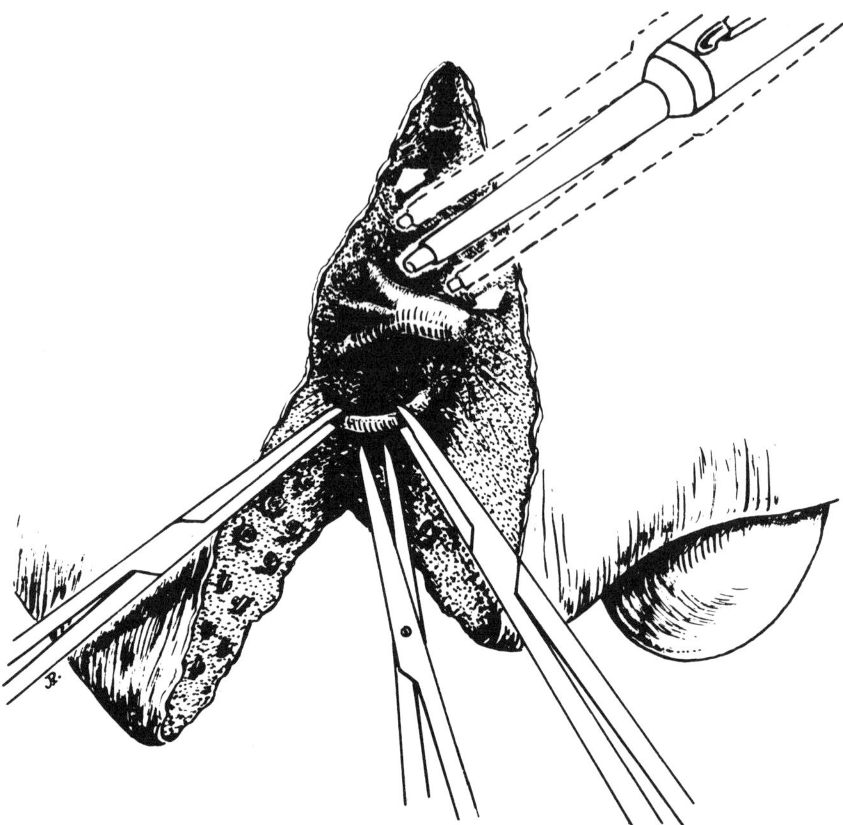

Figure 10.4. Lateral sweeping motion of the ultrasonic scalpel in deep dissection of the liver, which clears blood vessels and allows them to be clamped, cut, and sutured. (Reproduced with kind permission from Hodgson, WJB, DelGuercio, LRM: Preliminary experience in liver surgery using the ultrasonic scalpel. *Surgery*, *95*:230–234, 1984.)

can be removed in this way with dispatch. Where such a small peripherally situated lesion is due to a secondary deposit, it is recommended that it is removed at the same time as the primary cancer is excised.

Where the tumor may be on the dome of the liver, a circle is cut out using the ultrasonic scalpel by a probing motion so that an area is delineated around the tumor. This is then taken down carefully equidistantly from the tumor to a depth of about 1 cm and at that point some traction is used on the tumor itself to try and lift it out of the liver tissue. The vessels supplying the tumor are then put on the stretch and are more easily dissected out using the ultrasonic scalpel. At this point the side–to–side movement is used with a power setting of 7-8 and the stretched vessels quickly pop up into the field of vision and can then be clipped and cut or cauterized. The tumor is then undercut, so to speak, and the operation appears to be progressing rather slowly. Suddenly, however, it is apparent that the other side has been reached and the tumor can very quickly be removed after a clamp is placed across the remaining attachments. The resulting hole in the liver may occasionally need a #000 silk suture if a small vessel persists in bleeding. Multiple small tumors up to 3 cms in size can be removed in this manner. In fact, I have even removed tumors as large as 10 cms in this way but full mobilization of the liver is required before large tumors should be excised (Figure 10.5).

LEFT LATERAL SEGMENTECTOMY

The usual approach of a midline or left subcostal incision is used for this resection. The stomach is then retracted inferiorly and laterally and the liver is retracted medially. This exposes the

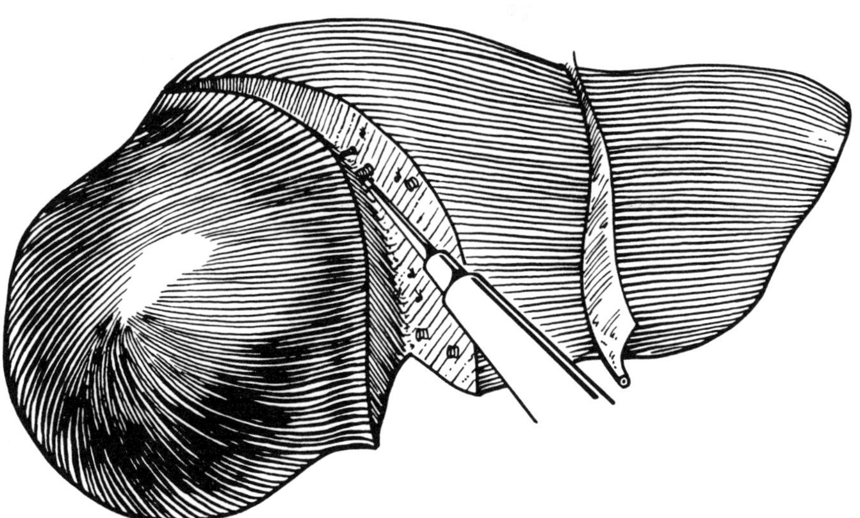

Figure 10.5. Wedge resection of large tumor from right lobe of liver. (Reproduced with kind permission from Putnam, CW: Technique of ultrasonic Dissection in resection of the liver. *Surg, Gynecol, Obstet, 157*:474-478, 1983.)

left triangular ligament which can be divided taking care not to injure the phrenic vessels themselves which run to the inferior vena cava near the attachment of the ligament to the diaphragm (Figure 10.6).

It is not usually necessary to dissect out the porta hepatis with this approach so I normally then proceed directly from the inferior border of the liver using the ultrasonic scalpel at a power setting of 8 or 9 to punch a series of holes just lateral to the falciform ligament. As soon as the first small blood vessels appear, these are cauterized and I then reduce power to 7–8 and change to a side–to–side transverse movement taking great care to search for an inferior branch of the portal vein. This is often found at this stage in the operation and can then be very quickly dissected out,

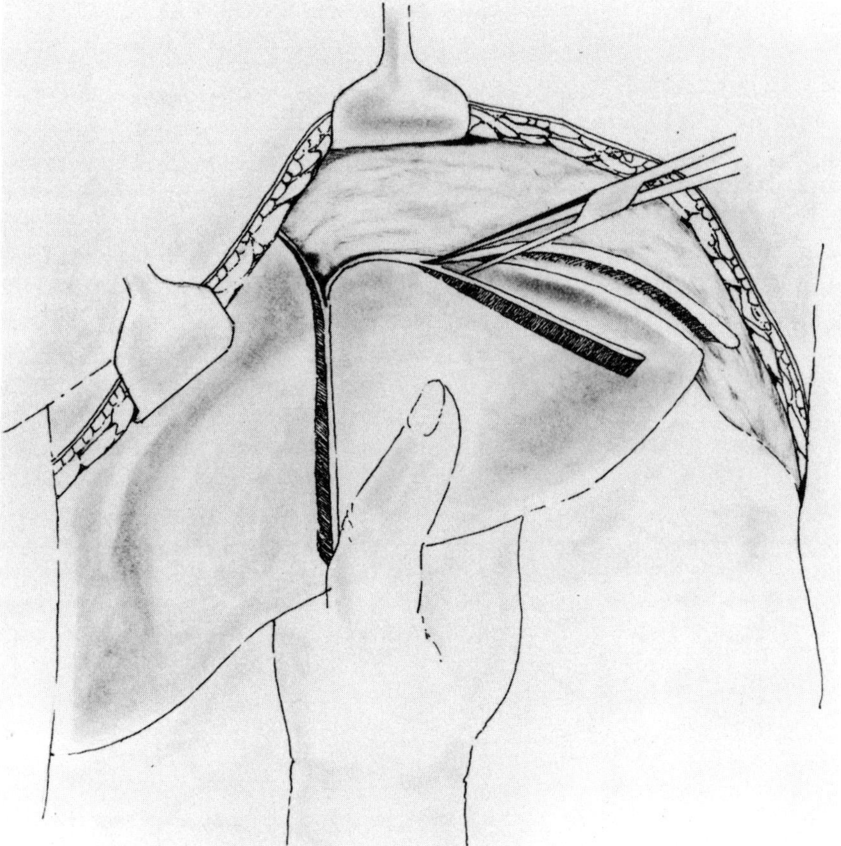

Figure 10.6. Division of left triangular ligament.

clamped off and suture ligated after division. More frequently, however, the vein is a little higher and some mesenchymal tissue must first be dissected away in order to identify it. In any event, the dissection is continued from below upwards and as the procedure is followed, it will be found that once the portal vein has been identified, there are no other major venous structures until the left hepatic vein is encountered up near the diaphragm.

The portal vein can sometimes literally run up in the fissure that would be used for dissection and gives branches to both medial and lateral segments of the left lobe of the liver. When this occurs, the ultrasonic scalpel is simply used to dissect out the lateral branches one by one which can then be clamped, divided and tied with #000 silk. The medial branches can be left intact and the dissection can be taken very close to the ascending branch of the portal vein itself.

When the left hepatic vein is approached, power is reduced to a setting of 6-7 and gentle traction of the diaphragm upwards, together with gentle traction of the liver away from the line of incision will help in visualizing this vessel. Sometimes it is useful to use a Satinski clamp to control it but usually I find that simple dissection of the mesenchymal tissue from the vein itself is sufficient. Because this vein is thinner-walled than the portal vein, it is easy to puncture a hole in it especially as it is usually near the end of the case and the surgeon is anxious to get finished. Care must, therefore, be taken until the vein is completely secured, divided and tied. At this point, the specimen is removed (Figure 10.7).

LEFT HEPATIC LOBECTOMY

This operation is an increase in magnitude over previously described resections in this chapter because it involves a dissection of the porta hepatis as a first step (Figure 10.8).

As with either right or left hemihepatectomy, dissection is facilitated by division of the falciform ligament as a first step back to the inferior vena cava. The left triangular ligament is divided so that the left lobe of the liver can be mobilized to the inferior vena cava and the inferior vena cava can be observed below the liver on the left. Then the hepatoduodenal ligament is explored for the hepatic artery. This will have been identified previously by angiography so that the surgeon will have some idea of where to look

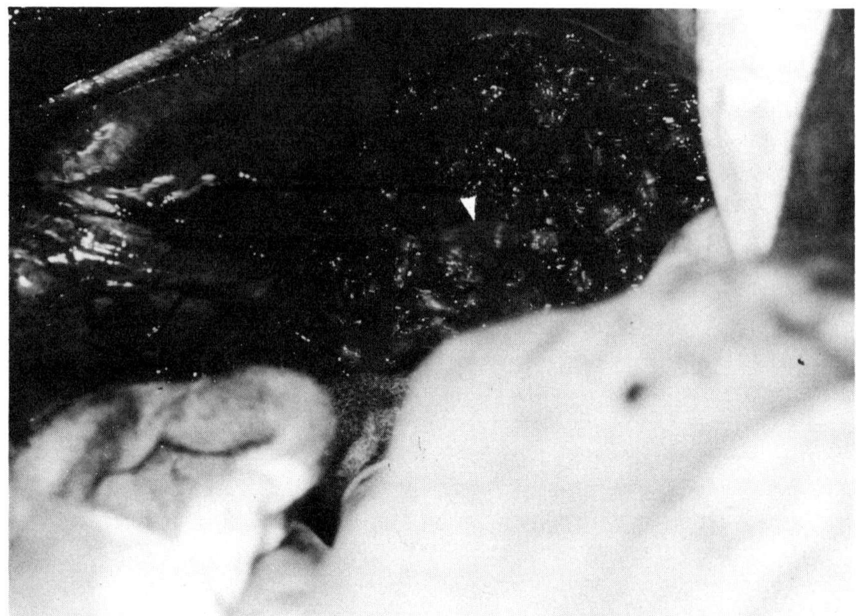

Figure 10.7. Photograph of completion of ultrasonic left lateral segmentectomy showing intact left main branch of the portal vein.

but it is an essential first step in the procedure. Once the artery has been identified and lifted by slings from the portal vein, I then find that a dissection of the common duct follows. This can also be carefully dissected off the portal vein and again protected by slings and the dissection can be taken up to the division of the bile ducts into right and left main hepatic ducts. Sometimes, however, the bifurcation of the common hepatic duct is frequently hidden by liver parenchyma. When this is the case, I leave it until later in the dissection. Traction is then applied to the common hepatic duct medially and the portal vein is identified. This can carefully be dissected away from the anterior structures of the artery and the bile duct and care must be taken to identify the edges of this vein correctly so that it is not accidentally entered during the dissection. I have usually found that it was possible to dissect out the bifurcation of the hepatic ducts at this point by simple blunt dissection with a clamp along the line of the duct into the hepatic tissue. Putnam, however, uses the ultrasonic scalpel to carry out this portion of the operation (56). It is important that if the

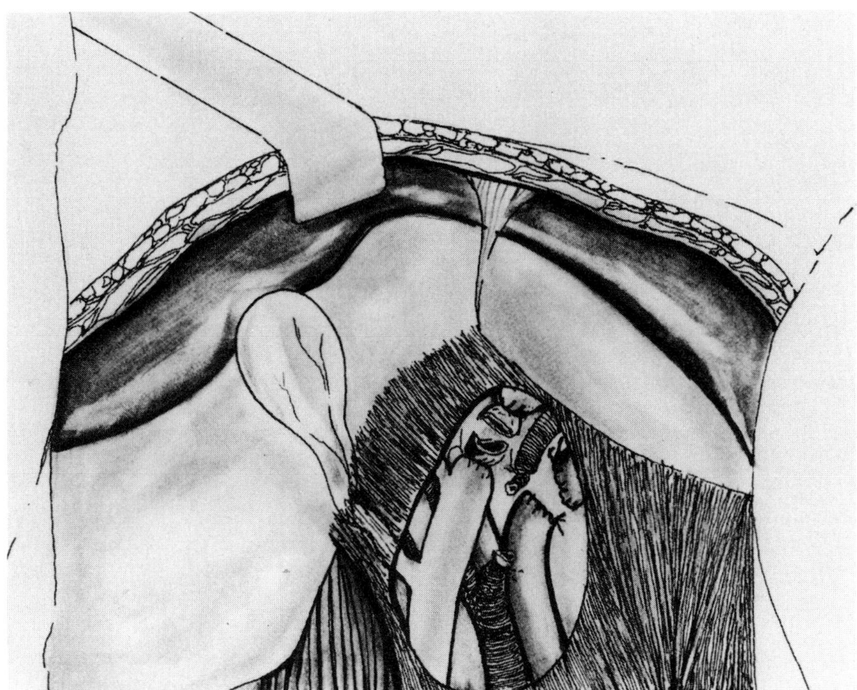

Figure 10.8. Dissection of porta hepatis with division of all left-sided structures (bile duct, hepatic artery and portal vein) prior to left hepatic lobectomy.

caudate lobe is to be preserved the dissection is taken up above the caudate bile duct on the left hepatic duct before this duct is divided.

At this point, the line of demarcation between the right and left side of the liver will clearly be seen. It is now a simple matter to divide the parenchyma of the liver back towards the inferior vena cava and the left hepatic vein to complete the procedure (Figure 10.9). However, some people prefer to place a Satinski clamp on the left hepatic vein before dividing the liver parenchyma itself but I have usually preferred to leave this until later because of the possibility of a branch of the vein coming off within the first centimeter which may be torn during clamping. Also, because of the high percentage of middle hepatic veins which run into the left hepatic vein and the anatomical disposition thereof, clamping with a Satinski in a blind fashion is a dangerous pro-

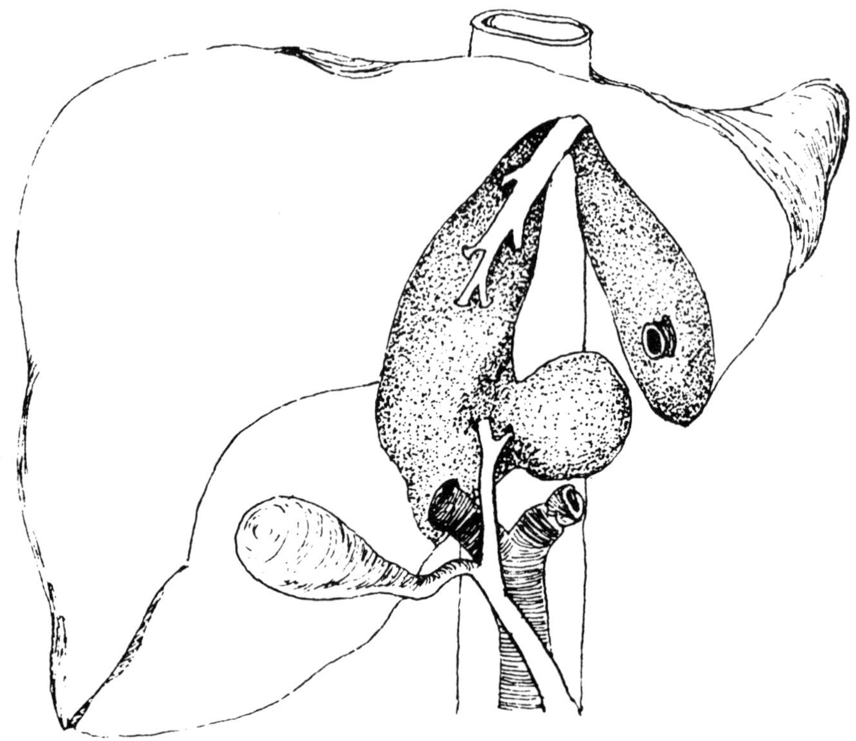

Figure 10.9. Completion of left hepatic lobectomy. Note the middle hepatic vein preserved in the plane of division between right and left lobes.

cedure. But, if a clear view can be obtained of this area, then at a setting of 6, the ultrasonic dissector can be used to take off the parenchyma from the left hepatic vein sufficiently far back for the vein and its branches to be identified so that it can be clamped under vision. The correct adjustment of the ultrasonic dissector is important so that it can be applied directly to the hepatic vein without damage and this can then be dissected safely even when there are unanticipated variations of anatomy.

In general, the surgeon should be aware of the position of the left hepatic vein whether or not it has been clamped before the next step is commenced. This step is division of the hepatic parenchyma itself. A simple way of doing this is to start on the superior surface of the liver at the gall bladder bed and for this reason, it may be safer to remove the gall bladder even with a left hemihepatectomy. The direct punching movement of the ultrasonic scalpel into the liver tissue is used initially with a power setting of 8-9. Small vessels and ductules are adequately exposed and readily secured by cautery and gradually the liver parenchyma is opened up as the surgeon works backwards into the tissue. As the trench deepens, power is reduced and the side–to–side movement of the ultrasonic scalpel is used. Care must be taken not to rush this stage as it is easy to tear out a major branch of the inferior vena cava. It is claimed in some centers that the transection of this portion of the liver can be completed in 10 minutes using finger fracture but unfortunately this is a highly dangerous procedure and the surgeon can easily spend the next 3-4 hours trying to stop the bleeding. However, with a careful dissection using the ultrasonic scalpel a transection should take no more than one hour and it would also be relatively blood–free since important vessels and ducts can be detected before damage. They could also be dissected out away from dangerous places so that hepatic veins running into the inferior vena cava in anomalous situations can be detected: the branches can be individually ligated leaving a safely controlled stump of a centimeter or two well away from the IVC. The only trouble I have ever had using the ultrasonic scalpel during hemihepatectomy has been when I have tried to rush. A patient progressive method is required for safe surgery. It should also be remembered that there are several small vessels situated low down in the posterior portion of the liver going directly to the inferior vena cava. Care must be taken to avoid tearing out these vessels as the cava is approached. The dissection can be accomplished with little risk and as the left hepatic vein is approached, it can be safely dissected out, its branches tied off, and blood loss can readily be kept to the minimum. If the hepatic vein has been previously successfully clamped with a vascular clamp, it can be tied off and divided at this stage.

After completing the transection, it is noteworthy that the cut surface of the liver is smooth and dry and that any residual bleeding points can be rapidly and easily controlled with #000 silk sutures. Bile leakage is unusual and can easily be seen and the leaking duct oversewn. The smooth dry feature of transection with the ultrasonic scalpel is not seen with other techniques. Consequently a closed drainage system is sufficient and it can be removed within 5-6 days when the drainage is down to about 50 cc per day and the length of hospitalization can consequently be shortened.

LEFT HEPATIC LOBECTOMY
INCLUDING CAUDATE LOBE

When it is necessary to also remove the caudate, the steps of left hemihepatectomy are repeated in the same way as have been discussed except that the caudate lobe is very carefully lifted off the inferior vena cava during the procedure and its directly draining hepatic veins are very carefully taken so as to avoid damage to this great vein (Figure 10.10). The ultrasonic scalpel is particularly useful here as caudate tissue can be literally dissected away to expose the veins for careful ligature.

VARIATIONS ON LEFT HEMIHEPATECTOMY

Because the ultrasonic scalpel so easily demonstrates all vessels during a dissection, it is no longer necessary to anatomically arrange for special subsegmental dissections. This makes particular sense as these areas have no relationship with venous drainage at all, but only with portal venous and hepatic arterial input. It is, therefore, possible to literally take out a segment in the middle portion of the liver by simply ensuring that it is possible to perform a Pringle maneuver beforehand and then starting from the outside superiorly and working around the area of the tumor to be resected by first using the probing motion of the ultrasonic scalpel and then the side–to–side movement when vessels are encountered. Gradually, if great care is taken, structures which are going to be included can be removed and structures which are going to be retained can be deliberately left behind. It is quite possible to run along a large vein for some distance using the ultrasonic scalpel and take only the branches to the side of the segment which is coming out and leave the remaining trunk or other branches. Indeed, one of the major advantages of this system is that this local resection can be carried out in a quick, efficient, safe manner.

CENTRAL HEPATIC LOBECTOMY

It is necessary to know the method for this type of resection in order to have the ability to radically treat Klatskin tumors (68-72). The approach is through a right subcostal incision and then the procedure is commenced by dissecting the gall bladder

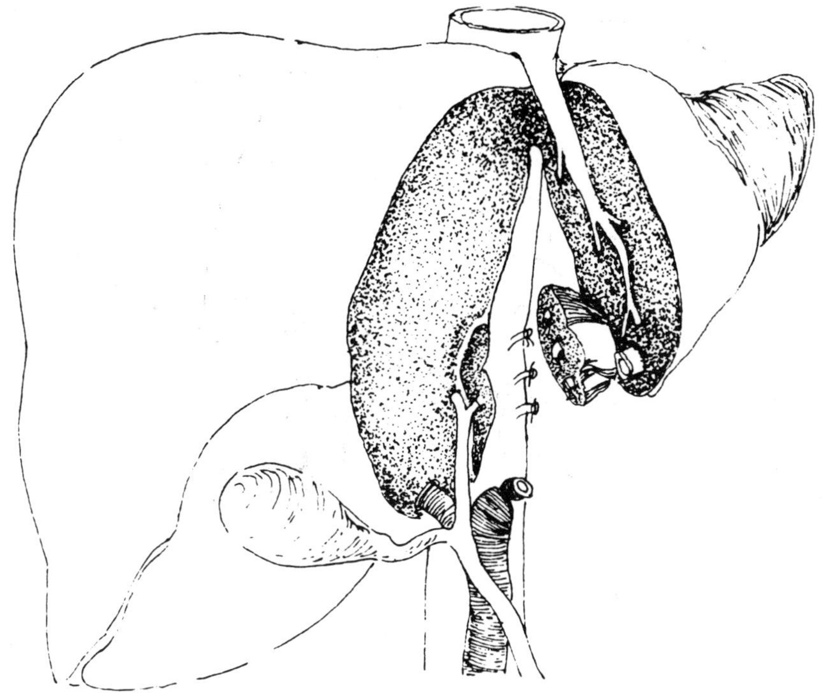

Figure 10.10. Completion of left hepatic lobectomy including caudate lobe. The middle hepatic vein is usually taken with the specimen.

off the gall bladder bed from the fundus downwards. When the cystic duct has been identified running into the common bile duct, the structures of the portal triad are dissected out.

The important points to remember are that it is possible to define a plane above the portal vein and below the hepatic arteries (Figure 10.11). Since the usual position of the bile ducts is above the hepatic arteries, then it should be possible to dissect into the liver beneath the duct and at the arteries in a bloodless plane. This is done with care using a probing motion with the finger in order to identify the division of the portal vein into right and left major branches. The left major branch is followed for about 2–3 cms into the liver taking great care to remain in the region of Glisson's capsule so that the mesenchymal tissue of the liver itself is not accidentally entered. The finger will be able to dissect out a small triangular area which will indicate to the surgeon whether or not the tumor is resectable as the tumor will lie anterior to the finger.

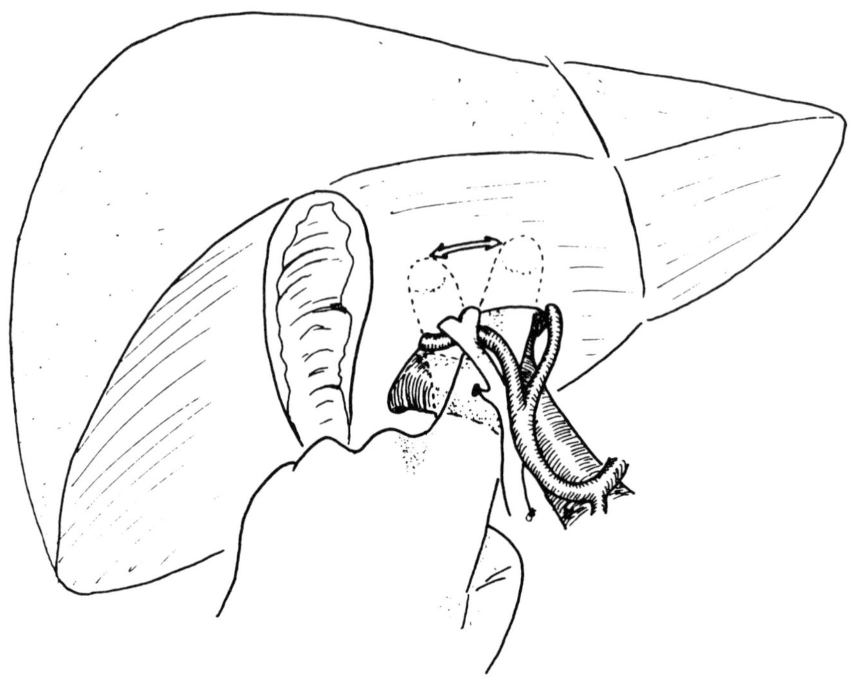

Figure 10.11. Plane of dissection anterior to the portal vein in central hepatic lobectomy.

If it is felt that the tip of the finger is beyond the tumor, then it is resectable.

The common bile duct is usually divided beyond the insertion of the cystic duct and these structures are reflected upwards, taking the lymphatics with them. It is then possible to dissect them off the hepatic artery but should the tumor involve these vessels, no hesitation should occur in taking them with the bile ducts. Arterial blood will find its way to the liver within two weeks (see Chapter 10).

The anterior surface of the liver can now be entered using the CUSA system in the usual way and a square or circle of hepatic parenchymal tissue can be dissected out in this manner in an antero-posterior direction. The finger lying above the left portal vein should act as a guide so that the dissection is not taken down too deeply. This will avoid injury to the cava and keep the dissection limited in extent so that the last structures to be divided will be the left and right hepatic ducts. In order to avoid retraction of these structures, it is suggested that a small stay stitch is placed before the ducts are divided for purposes of identification (Figure 10.12).

The reconstruction is carried out by hepaticojejunostomy (Figure 10.13) either using the Smith mucosal graft (73) or, perhaps more simply, by means of developing a cone around the duct of mesenchymal tissue. This can be very rapidly achieved with the ultrasonic scalpel. The cone will then project a small

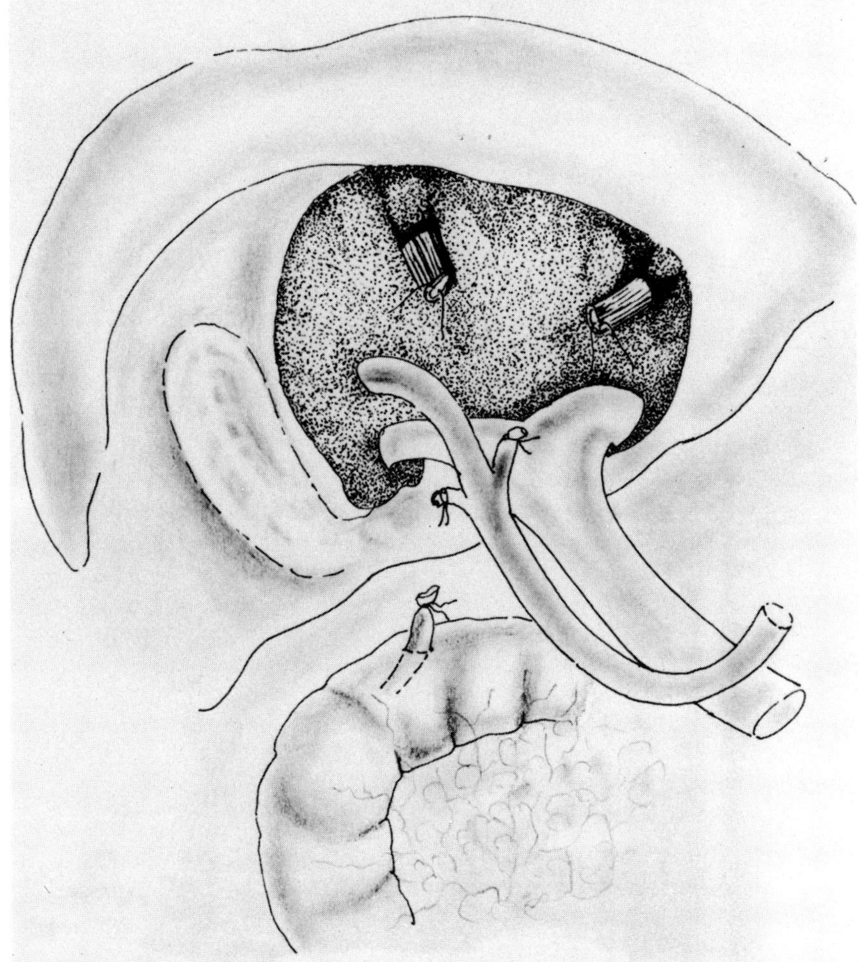

Figure 10.12. Completed central hepatic lobectomy.

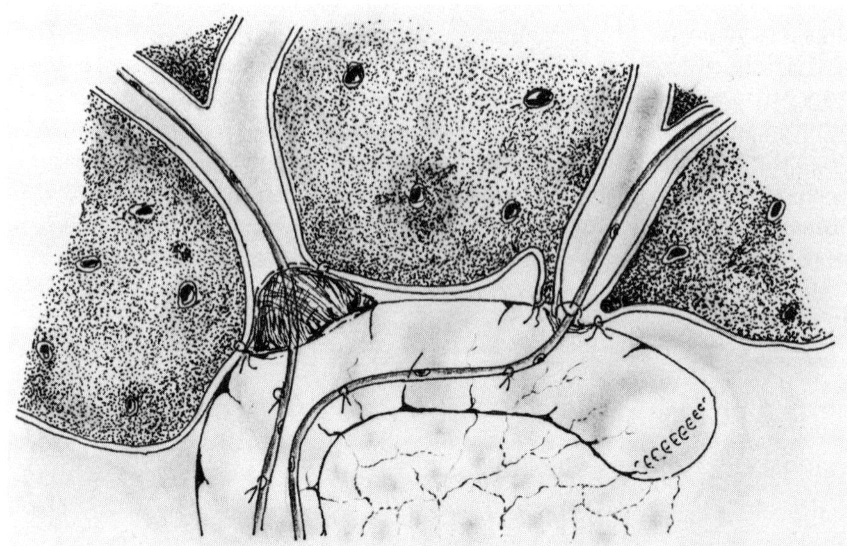

Figure 10.13. Reconstruction after central hepatic lobectomy with Smith mucosal graft to the right hepatic duct and a cone anastomosis to the left hepatic duct.

distance into the jejunum and will be rapidly covered by mucosa. Stents are usually placed in the transhepatic position with the tips brought out percutaneously so that postoperatively at intervals, cholangiograms can be performed to demonstrate that all is well. When this is demonstrated after two months or so, the tubes can be removed.

RIGHT HEPATIC LOBECTOMY

The right hemihepatectomy is carried out using a suitable incision such as the right subcostal or thoracoabdominal in a patient with a deep chest. It differs from the left hemihepatectomy only in that the right side of the liver represents somewhat more liver tissue than the left. Ong (74) says that the right side of the liver represents about 54% by weight of liver tissue. On scans, it seems that about 60% of the liver is represented in this way.

The right triangular ligament and superior and inferior coronary ligament must be divided. This division may need to be done somewhat blindly in the patient with a large tumor and great care must be exercised to avoid dividing a superior renal branch of the inferior vena cava during the course of this maneuver. Preferably, as the liver is lifted up and the inferior vena cava is approached from the lateral side, this portion of division of the coronary ligament inferiorly to expose the bare area should be done under direct vision. Similarly, ideally, division of the superior coronary ligament should also be done under direct vision so as to approach the hepatic vein safely and to avoid cutting an anomalous right phrenic vein which would lead to considerable blood loss from the vena cava.

The next step is to perform a cholecystectomy as the cystic duct will lead directly to the common bile duct. When the common bile duct has been identified, it can be dissected off the portal vein and isolated with slings. The next step is to identify and isolate the right hepatic artery and although its position is variable, it is usually to the left of the common duct. The right hepatic artery itself can then be traced and although it may be posterior to the right duct, the initial cholecystectomy and dissection of the common duct makes isolation of the right hepatic artery straightforward. I prefer to ligate the artery with #00 silk and then to ligate the right hepatic duct similarly before division. The right portal vein comes into view at this point and the main vein is clearly demonstrated by simple traction of the common duct and at the hepatic artery. The right branch is quite short and great care again must be exercised in its division so that it is not torn. Careful dissection is required to obtain clear delineation of the edges of the bifurcation and the right branch itself. Having carried this out, I normally place slings around the vein for identification before tying it off with #00 silk ligatures proximally and distally. Also, I then clamp it proximally, divide the vein and oversew its short cut edge with #000 silk (Figure 10.14).

Again controversy arises as to whether or not extrahepatic division of the hepatic veins should be undertaken. Because they may have a branch within 1 cm of the inferior vena cava, blind clamping of the vein can be dangerous (62).

Where I have seen the hepatic vein outside the hepatic parenchyma, I have then felt that it could be clamped. However, where the hepatic parenchyma has not given a view of the hepatic vein, I have not tried to clamp it at this point. On the other hand, Putnam advises dissection of this portion of hepatic parenchyma first with the ultrasonic scalpel in order to expose the vein (56).

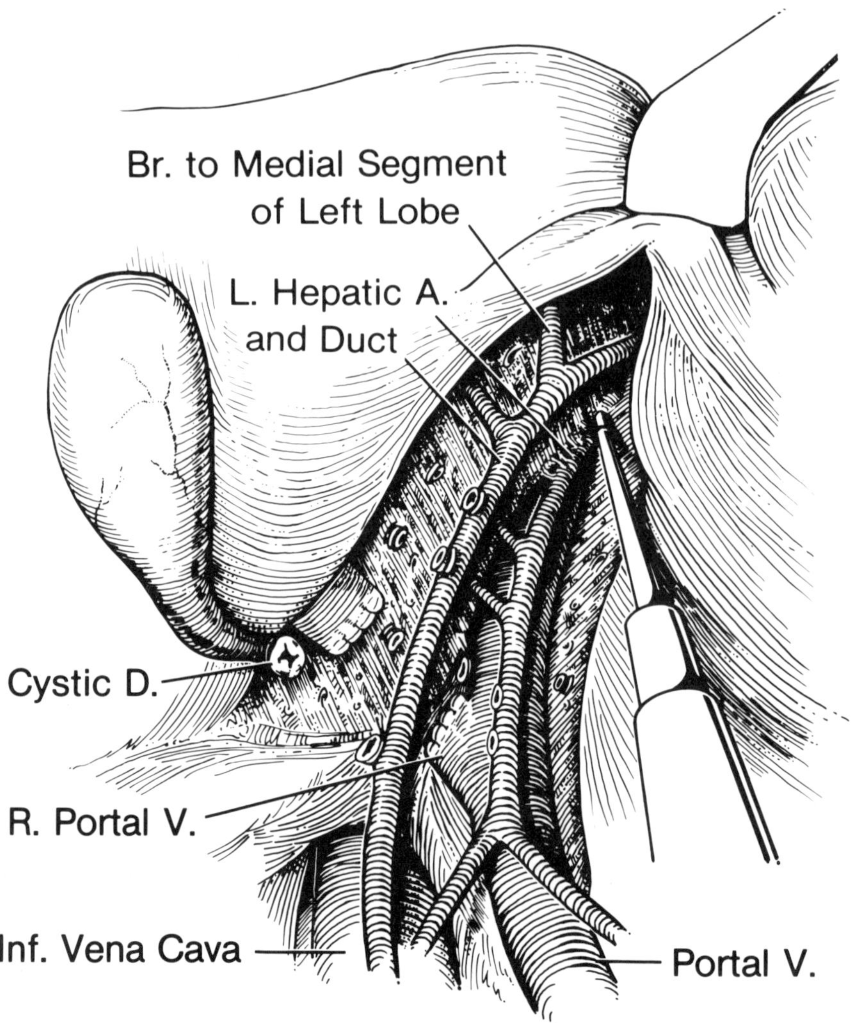

Figure 10.14. Dissection of the portal triad in right hepatic lobectomy. (Reproduced with kind permission from Putnam, CW: Technique of ultrasonic dissection in resection of the liver. *Surg, Gynecol, Obstet, 157:*474–478, 1983.)

If it is decided that the vein will be cleared and divided at this point, it is essential that it is oversewn rather than simply ligated.

Division of the liver is accomplished by starting at the gall bladder bed and progressing posteriorly from the dorsum of the

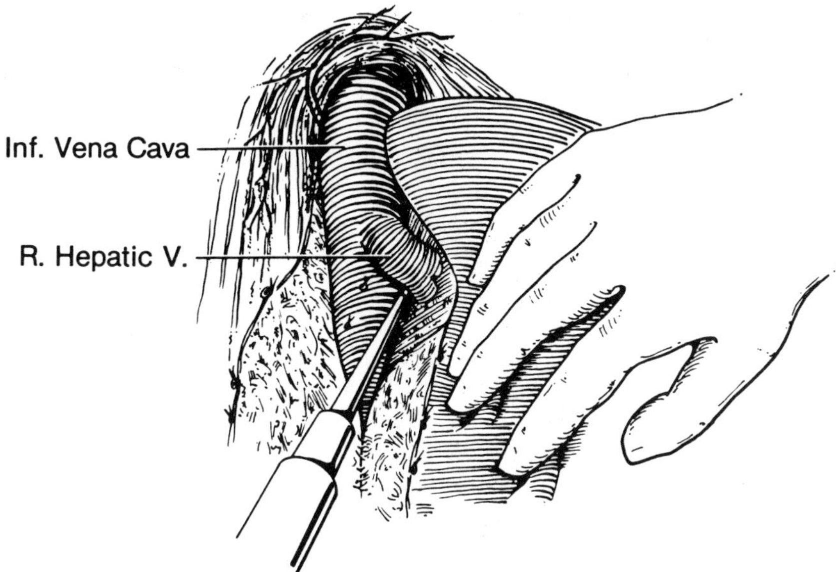

Figure 10.15. Dissection of right hepatic vein with the ultrasonic scalpel as a first step in right hepatic lobectomy. (Reproduced with kind permission from Putnam, CW: Technique of ultrasonic dissection in resection of the liver. *Surg, Gynecol, Obstet, 157:*474-478, 1983.)

liver using the ultrasonic scalpel in a probing motion initially over the first centimeter in depth and then switching to a side-to-side motion in order to preserve as many small vessels and ducts as possible. Normally the initial power setting is about 8 and is gradually reduced as the depths of the liver are opened. This is because larger vessels appear deeper within the liver tissue and the middle hepatic vein may be very big and run across the line of resection. Also, there may be a large dorsal hepatic vein which can be as large, if not larger, than the right hepatic vein and surprise the unwary surgeon (Figure 10.16). These major veins can be identified and parenchyma dissected off in order to place clamps and then divide and tie them. The branches themselves can also be dissected if necessary and ligated individually to keep the point of ligation away from the inferior vena cava and thus maintain the safety of the procedure.

Again, because the ultrasonic scalpel leaves the cut surface remarkably smooth and dry, it is quite simple to see small bleeding points and to oversew them and also to see any bile leakage

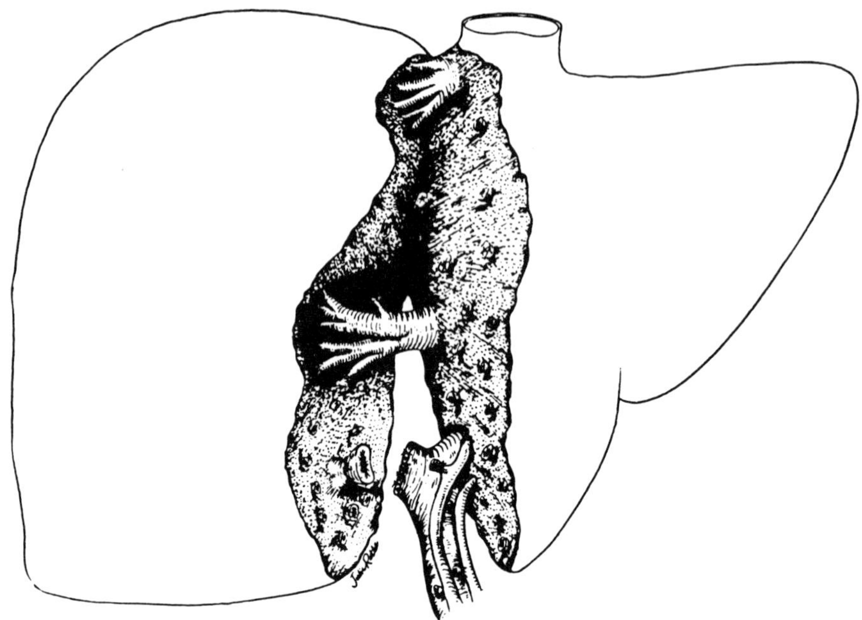

Figure 10.16. Illustration of the ability of the ultrasonic scalpel to dissect out the branches of the major hepatic vascular structures before clamping, which allows a highly controlled division of these vessels to take place without the chance of a caval or portal tear. (Reproduced with kind permission from Hodgson, WJB, DelGuercio, LRM: Preliminary experience in liver surgery using the ultrasonic scalpel. *Surgery, 95:*230-234, 1984.)

and oversew the source to stop this. Closed drainage systems are adequate and the patient will normally need to be watched closely only for about 24 hours and should be ready for discharge home in about one week to ten days.

VARIATIONS ON HEPATIC LOBECTOMY

Right Trisegmentectomy

The classical method of right trisegmentectomy was described by Starzl (43) in 1975. The operation consists of removal of the right lobe of the liver and also removal of the left medial lobe. The reason that it is called a trisegmentectomy is that the right lobe is, for practical purposes, divided into anterior

and posterior segments and these two plus the medial segment of
the left lobe make up the three. In a way, the term used by Pack
and his associates of extended right hepatic lobectomy (75) is
fairly accurate because the operation of trisegmentectomy is not
much different in magnitude from that of right hepatic lobectomy.
The reason for this is that the midline of the liver extends from
the gall bladder towards the inferior vena cava and actually slants
to the left posteriorly. The line of division between right and left
extends towards the falciform ligament and this is the structure
separating the left medial and lateral segments. In extending right
hemihepatectomy to trisegmentectomy all that is required is to
also remove the anterior portion of the liver on the right lateral
side of the falciform ligament and this will include the middle
hepatic vein; this vein is transected with right lobectomy (Figure
10.17).

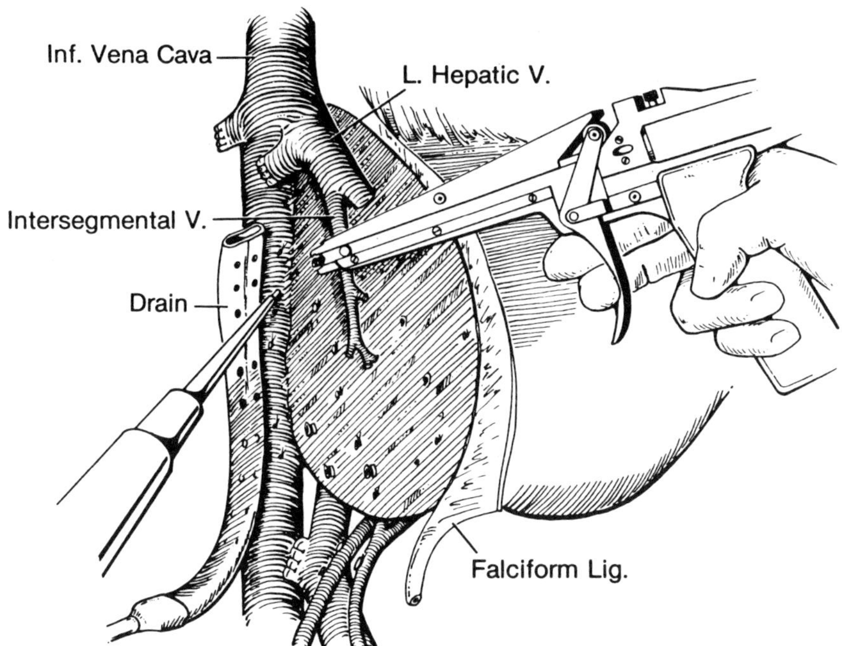

Figure 10.17. Completion of right trisegmentectomy showing stumps of right
portal vein, right hepatic vein and middle hepatic vein. (Reproduced with
kind permission from Putnam, CW: Technique of ultrasonic dissection in
resection of the liver. *Surg, Gynecol, Obstet, 157:*474-478, 1983.)

The technique used by Starzl is to begin with a right subcostal incision which is then extended into the chest across the costal margin or up to the sternum. Then, after exposing the liver and determining the extent of tumor and, therefore, the extent of resection, the right triangular and coronary ligaments are incised so that the bare area of the liver is broadly entered in order that the organ can be lifted into the wound and retracted to the left should this become necessary. It will give the surgeon the ability to view the right hepatic vein or the inferior vena cava. Starzl usually keeps the falciform ligament and the ligamentum teres intact for this operation.

The next step in trisegmentectomy as in right hepatic lobectomy is dissection of the hilus of the liver (Figure 10.18). It is not

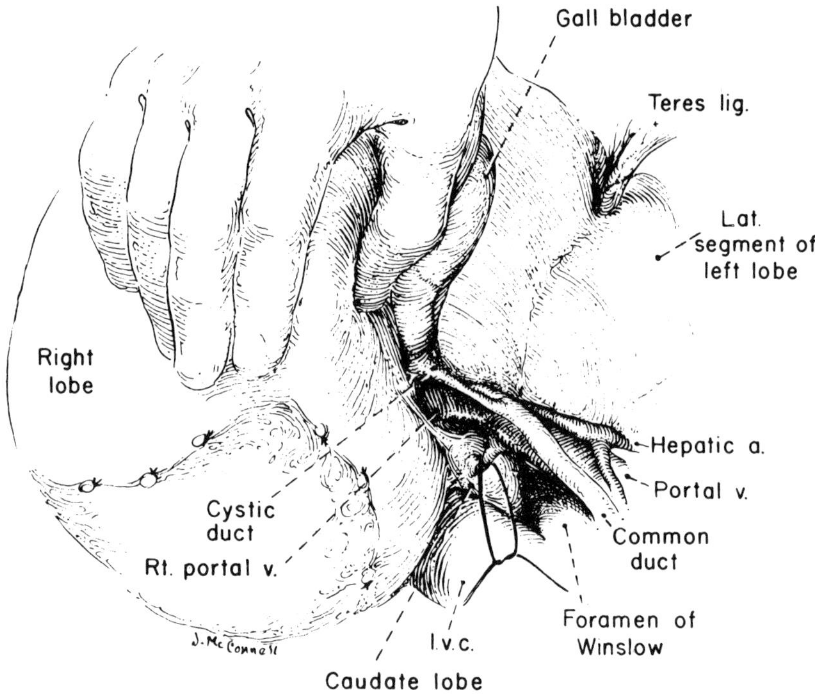

Figure 10.18. Posterior approach in dissecting the bifurcation of the portal vein. This maneuver is made possible by retracting the right lobe of the liver anteriorly and to the left. (Reproduced with kind permission from Starzl, TE, *et al.*: Hepatic trisegmentectomy and other liver resections. *Surg, Gynecol, Obstet, 155:*21–27, 1982.)

necessary to remove the gall bladder with this procedure but it is necessary to divide the cystic duct and cystic artery along with the right hepatic artery and right portal vein. This will provide a line of demarcation which will act as a guide between true right and left lobes.

At this point, the common bile duct is followed to its bifurcation which may be within the substance of the liver. The right duct is then ligated and divided so that all the structures for the left side can be retracted laterally.

There is a posterior tissue bridge concealing the umbilical fissure; this is often not as thick as the liver itself at the line of demarcation between right and left lobes. Starzl points out that there are no large structures passing through the umbilical fissure which, therefore, can easily be opened (Figure 10.19). Again, the most bloodless approach towards this is to use the ultrasonic scalpel at a power setting of 7 working back and forth so that minor vessels are identified and sealed before division. As this tissue bridge is opened, the left branches of the triad structures will be seen lying in the base of this area (Figure 10.20). The portal vein will divide and the branches to the left medial lobe will need to be individually ligated and divided. Sometimes, this vein runs in the umbilical fissure and can be a problem if ignored. It is best to try and keep this medial branch intact and simply divide its ramifications in order to ensure the best possible blood supply to the lateral segment. There is, of course, a danger of de–arterializing the lateral segment remnant and occasionally when the hepatic artery enters in a very lateral position, this is advantageous. However, if the artery is carefully followed into the left lateral segment, then it can be preserved.

Mobilization is not continued all the way posteriorly until a decision has been made about removal or retention of the caudate lobe. The last two major branches of the portal vein pass posteriorly to the left portion of the caudate lobe and if these are divided, the caudate lobe will be de–vascularized. If this is the case then this lobe is removed taking care to identify and ligate all the draining branches to the inferior vena cava. However, the procedure is simplified if the caudate lobe can be left intact.

At this point, the liver remains attached by the right hepatic vein and the middle hepatic vein (Figure 10.21). The dangers of clamping these before they are completely visualized have been previously discussed in this chapter (62). When they are seen, they are carefully ligated before division. The feedback structures

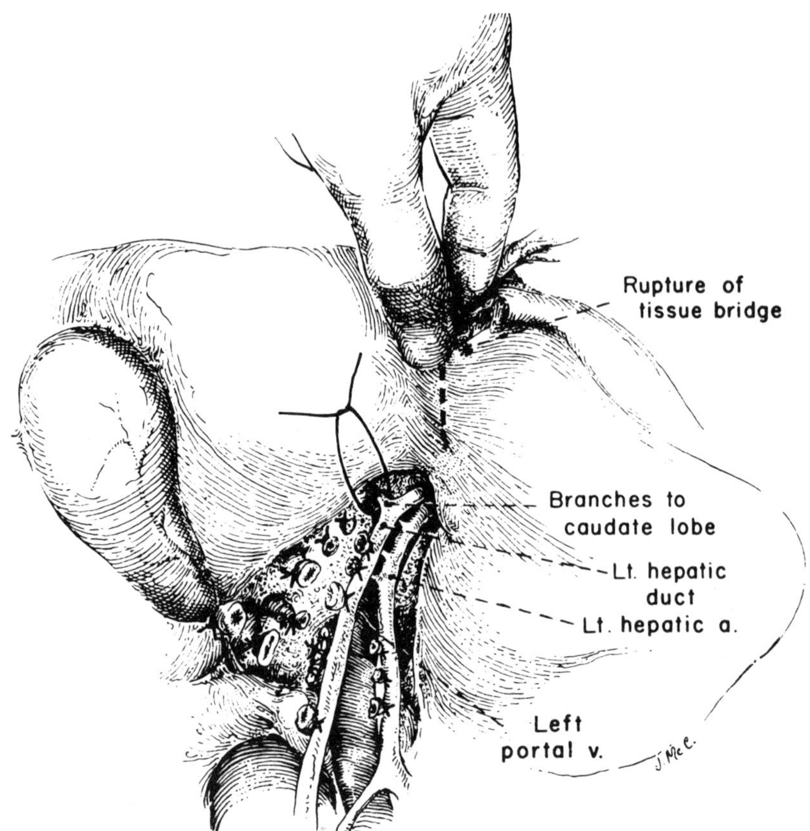

Figure 10.19. Nearly completed mobilization of the left branches of the portal triad. The tissue bridge is being broken down to permit access to the umbilical fissure. The final two branches before the main trunk reaches the umbilical fissure go to the left portion of the caudate lobe. These final branches or at least the last one should be preserved unless all of the caudate lobe is to be removed. Total caudate removal is not usually necessary. (Reproduced with kind permission from Starzl, TE, *et al.*: Hepatic trisegmentectomy and other liver resections. *Surg, Gynecol, Obstet, 155:* 21–27, 1982.)

found just to the right of the falciform ligament are then the final vessels to be secured. These are best attacked from the anterior surface and great care must be used to be sure that they are seen extending into the left lateral segment of the liver. They are left intact so that they do extend into this segment and only the branches to the left medial lobe are divided.

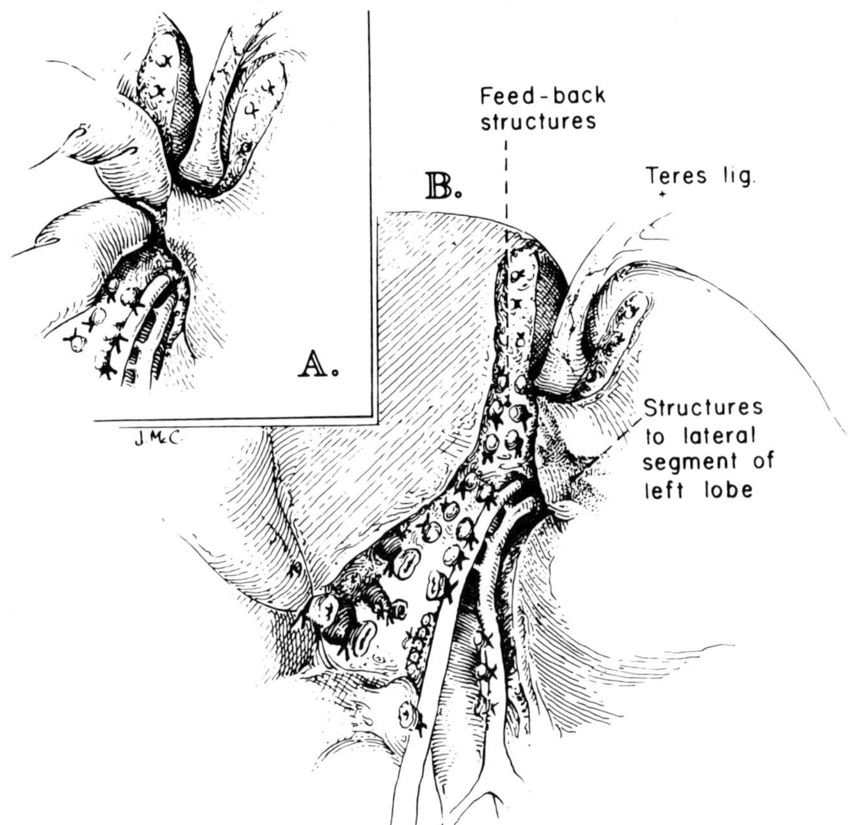

Figure 10.20. Structures feeding back from the umbilical fissure to the medial segment of the left lobe. A) These are encircled usually by blunt dissection within liver substance just to the right of the falciform ligament and umbilical fissure without entering the fissure. Note that the hepatic tissue bridge concealing the umbilical fissure has been broken down. B) The three segments of the specimen are not devascularized. (Reproduced with kind permission from Starzl, TE, *et al.*: Hepatic trisegmentectomy and other liver resections. *Surg, Gynecol, Obstet, 155:*21-27, 1982.)

A clean dry surface should remain and although there is a large subphrenic dead space, the space is rapidly filled by the colon, stomach and small bowel and again a closed drainage system is enough to be able to keep this space under control. A rapid increase in size of the left lateral segment of the liver occurs due to the entire portal venous blood running into the lobe initially

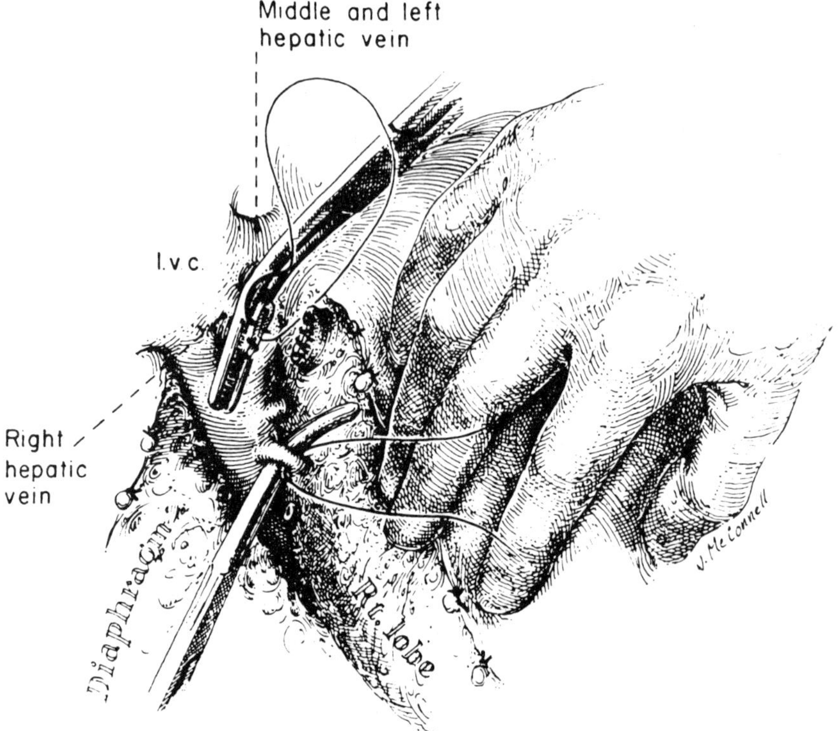

Figure 10.21. Division of the right hepatic vein. With the right lobe of the liver retracted anteriorly and to the left, the vein is divided between Pott's clamps and oversewn with vascular sutures. Several smaller hepatic veins must be ligated as they enter the retrohepatic vena cava more inferiorly. (Reproduced with kind permission from Starzl, TE, *et al.*: Hepatic trisegmentectomy and other liver resections. *Surg, Gynecol, Obstet, 155:*21-27, 1982.)

and later to true regeneration. This will also reduce the size of the cavity on the right.

Left Hepatic Trisegmentectomy

This is probably the most difficult liver operation of all and was described and published by Starzl (44) in 1982. A bilateral subcostal incision is used and after mobilization of the left lobe, a hilar dissection is carried out in the usual way but in particular the gall bladder is taken by dividing the cystic duct and cystic artery. The left portal vein is ligated and divided; the left hepatic artery is also dealt with in the same way and the left hepatic duct is divided as well. The liver is retracted medially and the caudate lobe is seen lying on the inferior vena cava. The caudate lobe is lifted and its draining veins are divided so that it can be lifted off the inferior vena cava. A standard left lobectomy could now be completed following the line of demarcation from the gall bladder bed to the inferior vena cava.

However, according to Starzl the additional requirement of a left hepatic trisegmentectomy is to scalp off the anterior segment of the right lobe of the liver. The main difficulty is to identify correctly the plane between the anterior and posterior right lobar segments (Figure 10.22). Starzl does this by beginning superiorly. He

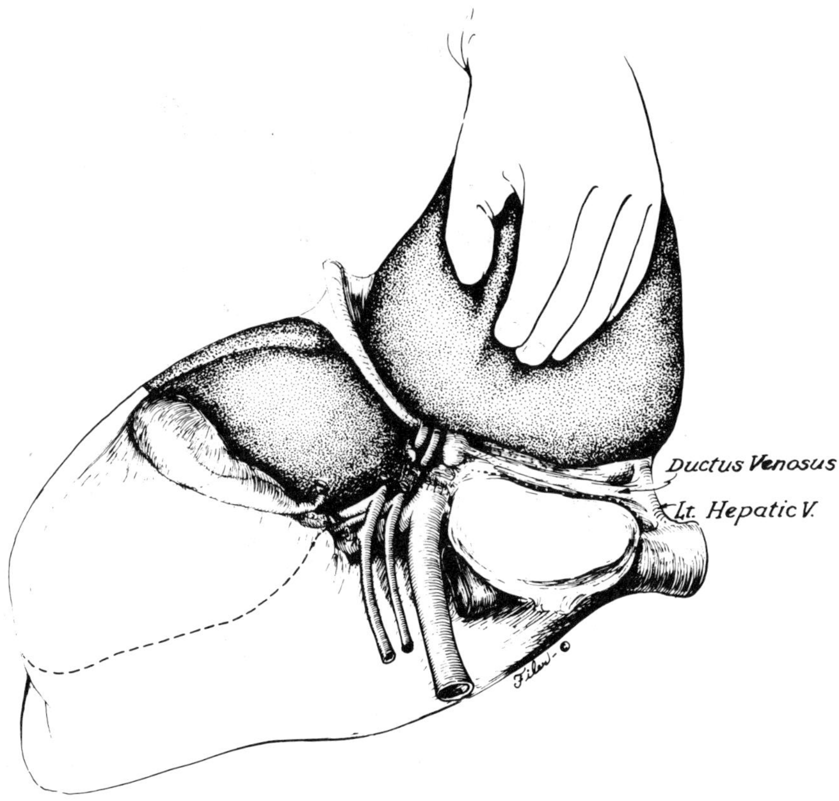

Figure 10.22. Demonstration of the plane between the anterior and posterior right lobar segments. (Reproduced with kind permission from Starzl, TE, et al.: Left hepatic trisegmentectomy. *Surg, Gynecol, Obstet, 155*:21-27, 1982.)

uses the point of transection of the left hepatic vein as a starting point. This line goes to the right and anterior to the right hepatic vein and if the middle hepatic vein is encountered it must be transected and ligated if this has not already been done. The specimen is retracted downwards whilst the superior to inferior scalping maneuver is continued looking for a resistance-free plane and clamping and ligating all resistant strands (Figure 10.23). The plane should emerge near the base of, and at right angles to, the gall bladder bed (Figure 10.24).

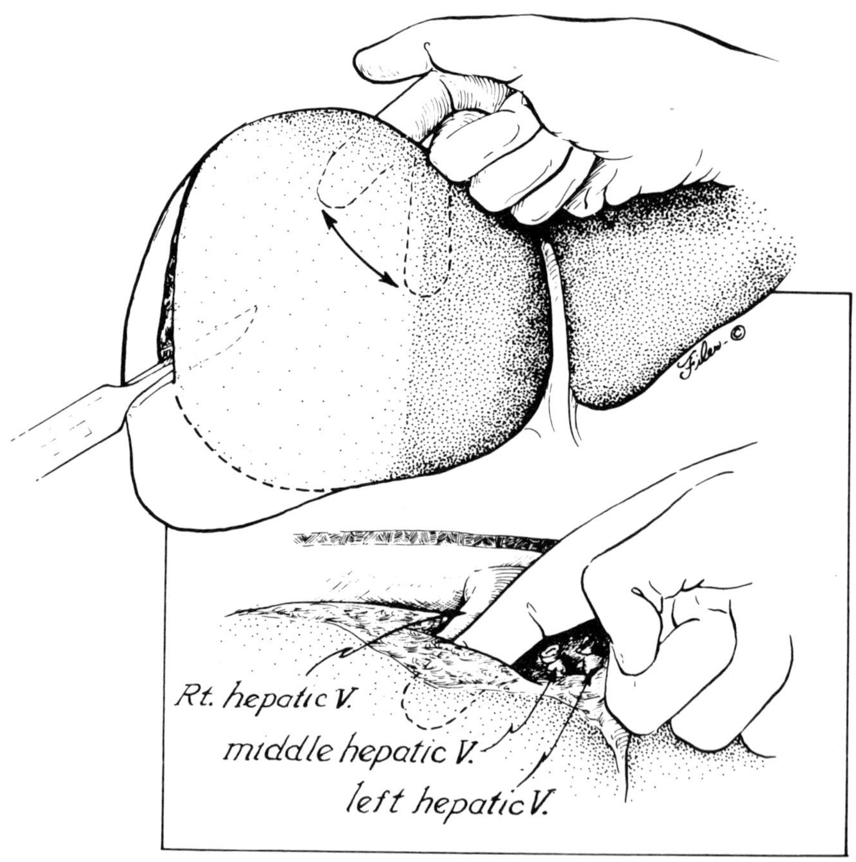

Figure 10.23. Superior to inferior scalping of the anterior segment of the right lobe. Inset - Note that the dissecting finger is kept anterior to the right hepatic vein, the left and middle hepatic vein having been ligated or sutured. (Reproduced with kind permission from Starzl, TE, *et al.*: Left hepatic trisegmentectomy. *Surg, Gynecol, Obstet, 155:* 21-27, 1982.)

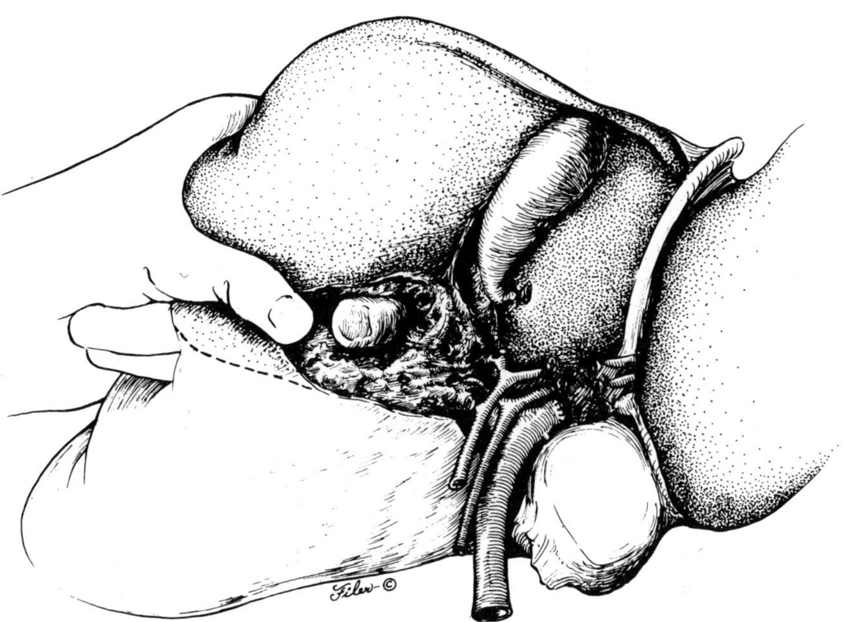

Figure 10.24. Further development of plane between the anterior and posterior segments of the right lobe of the liver. (Reproduced with kind permission from Starzl, TE, *et al.*: Left hepatic trisegmentectomy. *Surg, Gynecol, Obstet, 155:*21-27, 1982.)

Starzl uses the finger fracture technique and carries it out expeditiously in order to try and reduce blood loss. He finds it necessary occasionally to perform the Pringle maneuver since this anterior segment is supplied by the right hepatic artery and right portal vein which are not divided during this procedure. Only when the blood supply is finally interrupted does the anterior segment become cyanotic.

We have tried this procedure in a patient with a massive hemangioma that was sequestering platelets but found that the bleeding was excessive. However, we did not hesitate in abandoning the procedure with all the structures to the left lobe ligated. Indeed, the patient did very well with shrinkage of a football-sized hemangioma down to one the size of an apple and a rapid improvement in the platelet count postoperatively. This is an important point to be borne in mind with liver surgery as long as the draining veins are not themselves damaged. Division of the inflow may be enough to control the situation and it may be safer to stop when control is still apparent than to plunge ahead and try to be heroic and lose a patient.

RESULTS OF HEPATIC RESECTIONS

In our series of 46 patients, we have carried out 80 resections. There has only been one operative death and that was in a patient who had tumor invading the inferior vena cava and when the cava was clamped to remove this tumor, the patient arrested. Two other patients who had extensive liver disease with tumor involvement died two weeks after wedge resection to obtain a biopsy in one case of widespread pancreatic tumor and in the other case to stop bleeding from a ruptured hepatoma.

None of the other patients had significant postoperative problems and were able to leave the hospital in a short time. We have had a significant bile leak in one patient who returned three months after his right hemihepatectomy with a large biloma which required percutaneous drainage. It is interesting that in this patient, his tumor was massive and although we were able to carry out all the stages of hepatic resection for right hemihepatectomy previously described except for division of the right hepatic vein, we found that we were completely unable to lift the tumor out of the bed of the right lobe of the liver in order to visualize the inferior vena cava. I felt under these circumstances, that the risk of tearing the cava was unacceptable and, therefore, the procedure was halted at this point. We placed an Infusaid pump and went back three months later to complete the procedure.

Twenty-five of our patients had colon carcinoma metastatic to the liver. The longest survival time is 57 months, 12 patients have died and the median survival was 21 months.

Morrow and his group (51) operated on 64 patients with metastatic disease and had a cumulative survival rate of 45% at 2 years and 34% at 5 years. However, they had a significant operative mortality of 20%. Patients with metachronous metastases had almost double the survival rate of those with synchronous metastases at 2 years but at 5 years the rates were the same in both groups. It is noteworthy that more extensive resections were not associated with a higher long term survival rate but did have a higher operative mortality.

In Fortner's review of his experience over eight years of the management of 310 patients with liver metastases (76), he was able to report that in those patients having major hepatic resection that his operative mortality was 9% and claimed an 81% 3-year actuarial survival if the disease was limited to the liver. This is difficult to interpret as nobody else approaches these results. However, when he specifically published the results of resection on 65 of his patients operated on from March 1971 through May 1982, the results were somewhat clearer (77). The 3-year survival for stage I disease was 66%. These are patients defined as having tumor confined to the resected portion of the liver without invasion of major intrahepatic vessels or bile ducts. The 3-year survival for patients with stage II disease was 58%. These are defined as patients having regional spread. This presumably means tumors which are attached to omentum and in whom the omentum can also be removed along with the disease. Stage III disease is defined as those patients having metastases to lymph nodes or extra-regional sites. However, even in this group, survival after resection of two or more years was obtainable.

At Duke University 21 patients had hepatic resection between 1974 and 1981. A 5% mortality rate was noted. The overall survival for a 7-year period was 34% and in the patients with colorectal metastases to the liver this rate was 29% (78).

A recent publication from Kyushu University in Fukuoka, Japan evaluated the applicability of limited hepatic resection in cases of primary liver cancer in cirrhotic patients. The mortality rate in these patients with limited resection was only 10.8% which is a reduction in the usual mortality rate for lobectomy in these patients of 15.4%. The survival rates up to 5 years in the two groups was similar with 32.6% surviving after limited resection and 22.5% surviving after massive lobar resection. But in Hiroshima, Nagasue found that hepatocellular carcinomas were frequently resectable even in the presence of liver cirrhosis provided that they were discovered at a relatively early stage (80).

Since the discovery of the fibrolamella variant hepatocellular carcinomas, it has been pointed out that this young group of patients do particularly well, even after extensive and risky resections (81-84).

Longmire's work was summarized from Los Angeles by Thompson and Tomkins (85) and in 138 patients there was only one intraoperative death. There was no operative mortality and minimal morbidity in patients operated on for benign liver tumors. The 5-year survival in patients with hepatocellular carcinoma was 38% but there was a high 30-day mortality in this group of patients. If those who died earlier as a result of liver failure were excluded, a 5-year survival rate of 51% was obtainable. The 5-year cumulative survival of 22 patients who had colorectal metastases was 31%.

Starzl's results in 150 patients operated on over an 18-year period again show similar excellent results (86). His morbidity is minimal as is his mortality which is in the region of 6.5% for right lobectomy and right trisegmentectomy. His 3-year survival rate of patients with primary carcinoma of the liver was 56% and in those following treatment for metastatic disease to the liver it was 66%.

Adson (87) has recently pointed out that removal of small solitary hepatic metastases is a worthwhile procedure. He also says that patients who have large multiple lesions live longer after resection than we would expect. For metastases to the liver, his overall 5-year survival rate was 25%. He achieved an operative mortality of only 4%. On the other hand, in Logan's review (50), survival time was significantly better for solitary lesions (mean 33 months) than for multiple lesions (mean 16 months). Petrelli found in an analysis of 36 patients that survival after hepatic resection was not altered by the type of surgical resection nor the presence of solitary compared with multiple lesions in metastatic colon carcinoma (88).

The message that comes through time and time again is that in major centers hepatic resection for tumor is a worthwhile procedure as it significantly prolongs the patient's survival time. But, surgery need not be confined to such major centers. Nims demonstrated that liver resections done in a community hospital having an active cancer unit are worthwhile. He performed 20 resections on the liver in a 16-month period and at the end of two years 9 out of 10 patients who had metastatic tumor resected from the liver were alive (53).

Recently, doubts have been expressed that liver resection achieves anything at all, since the suggestion has been raised that patients do very well with simple observation, so that, for example, 67% of patients with solitary metastases survive one year, whilst 40% of patients with wide-spread disease also survived one year. Almost 20% of the patients with solitary liver metastases were alive at three years (89). Similar results were noted at the Society of University Surgeons (90) and also in Swedish reports (91). But I have problems with these figures when at the same time I read of median survival rates of only 10 months in trials of Vitamin C versus no treatment (92) which gave similar results to trials of

5-Fluorouracil (93). A more recent trial of combination chemotherapy of Methotrexate and 5-Fluorouracil achieved no improvement of survival compared with historical controls (94). We see many patients at the time their chemotherapy is "no longer controlling the tumor." Invariably, this occurs within a few months from the time of diagnosis and, of course, at that point it is too late to buy any more time.

All recent publications make the same point that hepatic resection is getting safer with an acceptably low operative mortality in the region of 5-10% and also an acceptably low postoperative morbidity. Survival rates in the region of 50-60% can be obtained for the first year and this high rate is maintained over 5 years with only a gradual drift downward to 25%. It is notable that no one survives 5 years without hepatic resection having sustained metastatic tumor deposits within the liver. However, no patient can be completely evaluated for inoperability unless a laparotomy has been performed and the liver examined carefully and mobilized. Sometimes it is surprising that the findings are in favor of the patient and surgeon and are not always grave as would be expected. A final plea, therefore, is that physicians should be aggressive in their management of patients with liver tumors since a nihilistic policy can only deprive the patients of the only realistic chance they have at the present time of extended survival.

REFERENCES

1. Foster, JH, Berman, MM: Solid liver tumors. *Maj Probl Clin Surg*, *22:*10, 1977.

2. Dagradi, A, Brearley, R: The surgery of hepatic tumors. *Postgrad Med J*, *38:*670, 1962.

3. Mikesky, WE, Howard, JM, DeBakey, ME: Injuries of the liver in 300 consecutive patients. *Int Abstra Surg*, *103:*323, 1956.

4. Longmire, WP, Jr.: Hepatic surgery: Trauma, tumors and cysts. *Ann Surg*, *161:*1, 1965.

5. Elliott, JW: Surgical treatment of tumors of the liver with the report of a case. *Ann Surg*, *26:*83, 1897.

6. Tillmans, H: Experimentelle und anatomische Untersuchugen über Wunden der Leber und Niere. *Virchows Arch*, *78:*437, 1897.

7. Glück, T: Ueber die Bedeutung physiologisch-chirurgischer Experimente an der Leber, *Arch Klin Chir*, *29:*139, (Berlin) 1883.

8. Ponfick, E: Ueber Leber Resektion und Leber Recreation. *Verh Dtsch Ges Chir*, *19:*28, 1890 (Congress).

9. von Meister, E: Recreation des Lebergeweber nach Abtragung ganzer Leberlappen. *Beitr Pathol Anat, 15:*1, 1894.

10. Lius, A: Di un adenoma del fegato. *Centralblatt fur Chir, 5:*99, 1887. Abstra. from Ganzy delle cliniche 1886, Vol. XXIII, No. 15.

11. Langenbuch, C: Ein Fall von Resection eines linksseitigen Schnurlappens der Leber. *Heilung Klin Wochenschr, 25:*37, 1888.

12. Resection Editorial: Resection of the left lobe of the liver. *Lancet, 1:*237, 1888.

13. Tiffany, LM: Surgery of the liver. *Bost Med Surg J CXXII, 23:*557, 1890.

14. Keen, WW: On resection of the liver, especially for hepatic tumors. *Bost Med Surg J, 126:*405, 1897.

15. Keen, WW: Removal of an angioma of the liver by elastic constriction external to the abdominal cavity, with a table of 59 cases of operations for hepatic tumors. *PA Med J, 1:*193, 1899.

16. Keen, WW: Report of a case of resection of the liver for the removal of a neoplasm with a table of 76 cases of resection of the liver for hepatic tumors. *Ann Surg, 30:*267, 1899.

17. Kousnetzoff, M, Pensky, J: Études cliniques et experimentales sur la chirurgie du foie sur la resection partielle du foie. *Rev Chir, 16:*954, 1896.

18. Auvray, M: Études experimentale sur la resection du foie chez l'homme et chez les animaux, *Rev Clin, 17:*318, 1897.

19. Beck, C: Surgery of the liver. *J Amer Med Assn, 38:*1063, 1902.

20. Moynihan, B. *Abdominal Operations,* Third Edition. London: W.B. Saunders, Co., 1914.

21. Pringle, JH: Notes on the arrest of hepatic hemorrhage due to trauma. *Ann Surg, 48:*541, 1908.

22. Ogilvie, H: Partial hepatectomy. *Brit Med J, 2:*1136, 1953.

23. Wangensteen, OH: *Cancer of the Esophagus and Stomach.* New York: American Cancer Society, 1951.

24. Lortat-Jacob, JL, Robert, HG: Hépatectomie droit réglée. *Princ Med, 60:*549, 1952.

25. Quattlebaum, JK: Massive resection of the liver. *Ann Surg, 137:*787, 1953.

26. Honjo, I, Araki, C: Total resection of the right lobe of the liver. *J Int Coll Surg, 23:*23, 1955.

27. Pack, GT, Baker, HW: Total right hepatic lobectomy. Report of a case. *Ann Surg, 138:*253, 1953.

28. Brunchwig, A: The surgery of hepatic neoplasms with special reference to secondary malignant neoplasms. *Cancer, 6:*725, 1953.

29. Foster, JH, Berman, MM: Solid liver tumors. *Maj Probl Clin Surg, 22:*22, 1977.

30. Healey, JE, Jr., Schroy, PC: Anatomy of the biliary ducts within human liver, analysis of prevailing patterns of branching and major variations of biliary ducts. *Arch Surg, 66:*599, 1953.

31. Healey, JE, Jr., Schroy, PC, Sorenson, RJ: The intrahepatic distribution of the hepatic artery in man. *J Int Coll Surg, 20:*133, 1953.

32. Goldsmith, NA, Woodburne, RT: The surgical anatomy pertaining to liver resection. *Surg, Gynecol, Obstet, 105:*310, 1957.

33. Longmire, WP, Jr., Marable, SA: Clinical experiences with major hepatic resections. *Ann Surg, 154:*460, 1961.

34. Longmire, WP, Jr.: Hepatic surgery: Trauma, tumors and cysts. *Ann Surg, 161:*1, 1965.

35. McDermott, WV, Greenberger, NS, Isselbacher, KJ, *et al.*: Major hepatic resection: Diagnostic techniques and metabolic problems. *Surgery, 54:*56, 1963.

36. Mersheimer, WL: Successful right hepato-lobectomy for primary neoplasm--preliminary observations. *Bulletin NY Med Coll, Flower and Fifth Ave Hosps, 16:*121, 1953.

37. Clatworthy, HW, Jr., Boles, ET, Jr., Newton WA: Primary tumor of the liver in infants and children. *Arch Dis Child, 35:*22, 1960.

38. Lin, TY: Resectional therapy for primary malignant hepatic tumors. *Int Adv Surg Oncol, 2:*25, 1979.

39. Ong, GB, Chan, PKW: Primary carcinoma of the liver. *Surg, Gynecol, Obstet, 143:*31, 1976.

40. Tung, TT: *Chirurgie d'exérèe due foie.* Hanoi, 1962.

41. Honjo, I, Mizumoto, R: Primary carcinoma of the liver. *Amer J Surg, 128:*31, 1974.

42. Balasegaram, M: Hepatic resection for malignant tumors. *Surgical Rounds, September:*14, 1979.

43. Starzl, TE, Bell, RH, Beart, RW, Putnam, CW: Hepatic trisegmentectomy and other liver resections. *Surg, Gynecol, Obstet, 141:*429, 1975.

44. Starzl, TE, Iwatsuki, S, Shaw, BW, *et al.*: Left hepatic trisegmentectomy. *Surg, Gynecol, Obstet, 155:*21, 1982.

45. Fortner, JG, Maclean, BJ, Kim, DK, *et al.*: The 70's evolution in liver surgery for cancer. *Cancer, 47:*2162, 1981.

46. Adson, MA, VanHeerden, JA: Major hepatic resections for metastatic colorectal cancer. *Ann Surg, 191:*576, 1980.

47. Hanks, JB, Meyers, WC, Filston, HC: Surgical resection for benign and malignant liver disease. *Ann Surg, 191:*584, 1980.

48. Foster, JH, Lundy, J: Liver metastases. *Curr Probl Surg, 18:*157, 1981.

49. Rajpal, S, Dasmahapatra, KS, Ledesma, EJ, Mittelman, A: Extensive resection of isolated metastases from carcinoma of the colon and rectum. *Surg, Gynecol, Obstet, 155:*813, 1982.

50. Logan, SE, Meier, SJ, Ramming, KP: Hepatic resection of metastatic colorectal carcinoma; a 10-year experience. *Arch Surg, 117:*25, 1982.

51. Morrow, CE, Grage, TB, Sutherland, DER, Najarian, JS: Hepatic resection for secondary neoplasms. *Surgery, 92:*610, 1982.

52. Tomas-de la Vega, JE, Donahue, EJ, Doolas, A, *et al.*: A 10-year experience with hepatic resection. *Surg, Gynecol, Obstet, 159:*223, 1984.

53. Nims, TA: Resection of the liver for metastatic cancer. *Surg, Gynecol, Obstet, 158:*46, 1984.

54. Lin TY: Results in 107 hepatic lobectomies with a preliminary report on the use of a clamp to reduce blood loss. *Ann Surg, 177:*413, 1973.

55. Ryan, WH, Hummel, BW, McClelland, RN: Reduction in the morbidity and the mortality of major hepatic resection. *Amer J Surg, 144:*740, 1982.

56. Putnam, CW: Techniques of ultrasonic dissection in resection of the liver. *Surg, Gynecol, Obstet, 157:*474, 1983.

57. Hodgson, WJB, DelGuercio, LRM: Preliminary experience in liver surgery using the ultrasonic scalpel. *Surgery, 95:*230, 1984.

58. Hodgson, WJB, Poddar, PK, Mencer, EJ, *et al.*: Evaluation of ultrasonically powered instruments in the laboratory and in the clinical setting. *Amer J Gastroent, 72:*133, 1979.

59. Williams, JW, Hodgson, WJB: Histologic evaluation of tissue sectioned by ultrasonically powered instruments (A preliminary report). *Mt Sinai J Med, 46:*105, 1979.

60. Couinaud, C: Le foie: Études anatomiques et chirurgicals. *Paris Masson and Cie:* 9-12, 1957.

61. Bismuth, H: Surgical anatomy and anatomical surgery of the liver. *World J Surg, 6:*3-9, 1982.

62. Nakamura, S, Tsuzuki, T: Surgical anatomy of the hepatic veins and the inferior vena cava. *Surg, Gynecol, Obstet, 152:*43-50, 1981.

63. Castaing, D, Kunstlinger, F, Habib, N, Bismuth, H: Intraoperative ultrasonographic study of the liver. Methods and anatomic results. *Amer J Surg, 149:*676-682, 1985.

64. Igawa, S, Sakai, K, Kinoshita, H, Hirohashi, K: Intraoperative sonography: Clinical usefulness in liver surgery. *Radiology, 156:*473-478, 1985.

65. Makuuchi, M, Hasegawa, H, Yamazaki, S: Ultrasonically guided subsegmentectomy. *Surg, Gynecol, Obstet, 161:*346-350, 1985.

66. Belli, L, Romani, F, Palmieri, B, Rondinara, G: Clinical experience with sublobar liver resection. *Ital J Surg Sci, 14:*295-299, 1984.

67. Nagasue, H, Yukaya, K, Ogawa, Y, *et al.*: Segmental and subsegmental resections of the cirrhotic liver under hepatic inflow and outflow occlusion. *Brit J Surg, 72:*565-568, 1985.

68. Klatskin, G: Adenocarcinoma of the hepatic duct at its bifurcation within the porta hepatis: An unusual tumor with distinctive clinical and pathological features. *Amer J Med, 38:*241, 1965.

69. Launois, B, Campion, JP, Brissot, P, Gosselin, M: Carcinoma of the hepatic hilus. Surgical management and the case for resection. *Ann Surg, 190:*151, 1979.

70. Todoroki, T, Okumura, T, Fukao, K, *et al.*: Gross appearance of carcinoma of the main hepatic duct and its prognosis. *Surg, Gynecol, Obstet, 150:*33, 1980.

71. Tsuzuki, T, Ogata, Y, Hosoda, Y, *et al.*: Hepatic resection upon patients with jaundice. *Surg, Gynecol, Obstet, 153:*387, 1981.

72. White, TT, Hart, MJ: Central resection for carcinoma of the hepatic bifurcation. *Contemp Surg, 20:*41, 1982.

73. Knight, M, Smith, R: Surgery of benign strictures of the extrahepatic bile ducts. In *Liver Surgery*, Calne, RY and Della Rovere, GQ (Eds). Italy: WB Saunders, 1982, pp. 91-121.

74. Ong, GB: Techniques and therapies for primary and metastatic liver cancer. *Curr Probl Cancer*, Vol II, No. 6. Chicago: Yearbook Medical Publishers, 1977.

75. Pack, GT, Miller, TR, Brasfield, RD: Total right hepatic lobectomy for cancer of the gall bladder. *Ann Surg, 142:*6, 1955.

76. Fortner, JG, Papachristou, DN: Surgery of liver tumors. *Int Adv Surg, Oncol, 2:*251, 1979.

77. Fortner, JG, Silva, JS, Golbey, RB, *et al.*: Multi-variate analysis of a personal series of 247 consecutive patients with liver metastases from colorectal cancer. I. Treatment by hepatic resections. *Ann Surg, 199:*306, 1984.

78. Kortz, WJ, Meyers, WC, Hanks, JB, *et al.*: Hepatic resection for metastatic cancer. *Ann Surg, 199:*182, 1984.

79. Kanematsu, T, Takenaka, K, Matsumata, T, *et al.*: Limited hepatic resection effective for selected cirrhotic patients with primary liver cancer. *Ann Surg, 199:*51, 1984.

80. Nagasue, N, Yukaya, K, Araki, G: Hepatic resection in the treatment of hepatocellular carcinoma: Report of 60 cases. *Brit J Surg, 72:*292-295, 1985.

81. Craig, JR, Peters, RL, Edmonson, HA, Omata, M: Fibrolamella carcinoma of the liver: A tumor of adolescence and young adults with distinct clinicopathologic features. *Cancer, 46:*372-379, 1980.

82. Berman, MM, Libbey, NP, Foster, JH: Hepatocellular carcinoma. Polygonal cell type with fibrous stroma - an atypical variant with favorable prognosis. *Cancer, 46:*1448-1455, 1980.

83. Nagorney, DM, Adson, MA, Weiland, LH, *et al.*: Fibrolamella hepatoma. *Amer J Surg, 149:*113-119, 1985.

84. Soreide, O, Czerniak, A, Blumgart, LH: Large hepatocellular cancers: Hepatic resection or liver transplantation? *Brit Med J, 291:*853-858, 1985.

85. Thompson, HH, Tompkins, RK, Longmire, WP, Jr.: Major hepatic resection: A 25-year experience. *Ann Surg, 197:*375, 1983.

86. Iwatsuki, S, Shaw, BW, Starzl, TE: Experience with 150 liver resections. *Ann Surg, 197:*247, 1983.

87. Adson, MA, VanHeerden, JA, Adson, MH, *et al.*: Resection of hepatic metastases from colorectal cancer. *Arch Surg, 119:*647, 1984.

88. Petrelli, NJ, Nambisan, RN, Nerrera, L, Mittelman, A: Hepatic resection for isolated metastases from colorectal carcinoma. *Amer J Surg, 149:*205-209, 1985.

89. Wagner, JS, Adson, MA, VanHeerden, JA, *et al.*: The natural history of hepatic metastases from colorectal cancer. *Ann Surg, 199:*502-507, 1984.

90. Finley, IG, McArdle, CS: Role of occult hepatic metastases in colo-

rectal carcinoma. Presented at the 46th Annual Meeting and 6th Tripartite Meeting of the Society of University Surgeons. Boston, Massachusetts, Feb., 1985.

91. Bengtsson, G, Carlsson, G, Hafstrom, L, Johnsson, PE: Natural history of patients with untreated liver metastases from colorectal cancer. *Amer J Surg, 141:*586-589, 1984.

92. Moertel, CG, Fleming, TR, Creagan, ET, *et al.*: High dose Vitamin C versus placebo in the treatment of patients with advanced cancer who have had no prior chemotherapy. *N Engl J Med, 312:*137-141, 1985.

93. Lavin, P, Mittelman, A, Douglass, H, Jr., *et al.*: Survival and response to chemotherapy for advanced colorectal adenocarcinoma. *Cancer, 46:*1536-1543, 1980.

94. Herrman, R, Spehn, J, Berger, JH, *et al.*: Sequential Methotrexate and 5-Fluorauracil. *Clin Oncol, 2:*591-594, 1984.

JOHN SAVINO, M.D.

CHAPTER 11
Pre and Postoperative Management

INTRODUCTION

The liver is the metabolic center of the body where nutrients are assimilated, modified, and then stored until needed; waste products and foreign substances are detoxified, catabolized, and/or excreted; and finally, components of certain critical systems, such as the blood coagulation mechanisms, are maintained almost in their entirety. There are certain basic functions which can be measured with respect to the level of present capacity and which can be supported by the administration of specific nutrients and/or exogenously produced active components.

EVALUATION

Biochemistry and Laboratory Evaluation

A minimal biochemical examination to evaluate liver disease includes a serum glutamic oxalacetic transaminase (SGOT), serum glutamic pyruvic transaminase (SGPT), gammaglutamyl transpeptidase (GGTP), total bilirubin, alkaline phosphatase, total serum protein, serum albumin, prothrombin time and partial thromboplastin time.

These liver chemistries do not accurately reflect the overall function of the liver; rather they provide only an estimate of any dysfunction. An adequate evaluation requires an understanding of the natural history of the liver disease, a careful physical examination, determinations of liver chemistries, and frequently a percutaneous needle biopsy of the liver. Liver and spleen size should be established and signs of retained fluid, encephalopathy, and malnutrition noted. Jaundice, fluid retention, and hepatic encephalopathy are signs of marked functional impairment and increased surgical morbidity and mortality. If the liver chemistries are abnormal, they should be repeated on one or more occasions at least 7 to 10 days apart, since some fluctuation is expected. A prolonged prothrombin time which does not respond to Vitamin K therapy carries a poor prognosis, particularly in alcoholic liver disease, and is a strong contraindication to elective surgery.

There are, however, four laboratory tests that have proven to be of considerable value and do reflect with moderate accuracy the overall state of liver function at any given point in time (1, 2). These are the blood glucose, the blood ammonia, the serum bilirubin, and serum albumin. Elevations in ammonia and bilirubin indicate significant impairments in catabolism and subsequent excretion of two specific waste products, while hypoglycemia and hypoalbuminemia demonstrate an inability to maintain, assimilate, and/or manufacture certain critical substances from the diet taken.

Tolerance of major surgery and actual clinical course, irrespective of the operation performed appears to correlate quite well with these four tests of liver function (1). Liver histology as noted through biopsy, on the other hand, is seldom reliable (3). Granted active hepatitis (whether alcoholic or viral) is uniformly associated with a poor prognosis and has, therefore, become an almost absolute contraindication to surgery. Exclusive of this single microscopic finding, predictability of outcome and guidance in supportive therapy must always be based upon the four stated laboratory tests and the patient's clinical course to date, i.e., presence and intractability of ascites, neurologic disorders of ammonia intoxication, and state of nutrition.

Clinical Evaluation

Based upon these few laboratory and clinical features, Child has proposed a classification for patients who potentially have sustained some compromise in functional liver reserve (Table 1) (1). Although originally designed to select out those cirrhotic patients who would not be good candidates for surgical decompression of the portal venous system, the method can be applied with equal usefulness to all subjects considered for any major operation as well as for those specific individuals for whom liver resection is planned (1, 4).

In Class A, patients have no detectable stigmata of significant liver disease, have normal hepatic reserve, require no special preoperative measures, and can tolerate all forms of major surgery. Regardless of prior disease states, these individuals are normal for all intents and purposes.

TABLE 1
CLASSIFICATION OF HEPATIC FUNCTION

Class	A:	B:	C:
Functional impairment	Minimal	Moderate	Severe
Serum bilirubin (mg percent)	< 2.0	2.0 to 3.0	> 3.0
Serum albumin (gm percent)	> 3.5	3.0 to 3.5	< 3.0
Ascites	None	Easily controlled	Poorly controlled
Neurologic disorders	None	Minimal	Moderate to severe
Nutrition	Excellent	Good	Poor, wasted
Operative mortality	$< 1\%$	10%	$> 50\%$

In Class B, there are definite limitations to the functional reserve of the liver. Only emergency, life-saving operations, should be performed without prior preparation by dietary supplements, ascites control, and occasionally even infusions of salt-poor albumin and fresh frozen plasma. Portosystemic shunting should be considered only if there is splanchnic decompression without diversion of portal flow away from the liver (the Warren distal splenorenal shunt) (5). Hepatic resections of greater than 10 to 15% of liver substance are always contraindicated.

In Class C, there is minimal to almost no liver reserve. Such patients are continually in and out of liver failure, although an occasional patient may appear to move up from a "Class C" to a "Class B" with intensive medical management. Nevertheless, functional liver capacity is so severely restricted that essentially all operations are contraindicated, that is, except for emergency procedures demanded by acute life-threatening disease or injury.

As a general rule, Class A patients can be compared to individuals who have been deprived of 30% or less of their hepatic parenchyma. Class B patients emulate liver resections of 50 to 70%, while Class C patients are similar to subjects who have just undergone a 90 to 95% resection. The major difference, however, is if liver function has been limited by disease preoperatively, regenerative processes have already been maximally stimulated, and thus little improvement in liver function can be expected at any time during the postoperative phase. By contrast, patients who have had hepatic resection and whose livers are otherwise normal almost uniformly regain their preoperative liver reserve within a few weeks following even a relatively massive ablation.

The crux is whether parenchymal regenerative mechanisms are essentially spent or are still basically intact.

In synthesis, Class A patients really have no limitations and should respond normally to all operations with a normal ability of the liver to regenerate. Class B patients have some limitation to liver function and will have an altered response to all operations, but if prepared well preoperatively usually tolerate most procedures. Class C patients obviously demonstrate severe limitations in liver function with a poor response to all operations regardless of preparatory efforts and liver resection should usually be contraindicated in this group.

PRE-OP PREPARATION

Nutrition

Normal patients and those with known liver disease, yet with a Class A status, require no special diet or medications prior to operation (1). Class C patients, as a general rule, are never operative candidates, although they should receive supportive measures in an effort to improve their functional status and thereby to make them eventually operable. Thus, it is the Class B patient who warrants energetic and detailed preparations for surgery.

Patients with compromised liver function should be placed on a diet as high in protein as ammonia tolerance will permit (5). This nitrogen load can additionally be increased by the oral administration of some nonabsorbable antimicrobial agent (neomycin) in order to suppress the bacterial population of the colon and thereby to limit the intestinal absorption of free ammonia and/or ammonium compounds released by these microbes.

Many patients with primary or secondary liver involvement are undernourished; there may also be a history of alcoholism and the combination may result in extensive fatty infiltration. This state imposes increased surgical risk in terms of normal metabolic response to surgical stress and increases mortality. McDermott and Ackroyd (6) have stressed the importance of delaying surgery if possible until some degree of nutritional repletion can be accomplished in malnourished patients. The mode of nutritional rehabilitation may involve p.o., tube, or parenteral feedings, with the route and the nutrient composition depending upon the clinical situation.

The indications for TPN depend on an evaluation of many variables. Weight loss is a known prognostic indicator (7, 8, 9) and a common component of various performance scales that are widely used to stratify patients entering antineoplastic therapeutic trials. Epidemiologic studies have described a large proportion of hospitalized patients as malnourished. Within these patient groups, the prevalence of hypoalbuminemia has been 26 to 50% (10, 11). Abnormalities of anthropometric indexes, diminution in acute-phase reactants, decreases in transferrin levels, plasma vitamin and mineral deficiencies, decreases in the creatinine–height ratio, and demonstrations of immunoincompetence have all been used as screening tests to identify malnourished patients (12, 13, 14). Unfortunately, such data are imprecise in individual patients and are altered by hydration, stress, and prior starvation. Although these determinations may be of value in epidemiologic studies, their value in individual patients has been questioned (15, 16), however, combinations of these indexes of malnutrition can predict outcome (17). We arbitrarily consider patients who are hospitalized without intake for more than 10 days or who have lost 10 to 15% of their pre–illness body weight as candidates for some form of nutritional support.

Once a decision about the need for nutritional support has been made and the gastrointestinal tract is not functioning, the techniques and requirements can be examined.

Of obvious concern is the possibility that nutritional support would stimulate tumor growth without benefit to the host. Data on this problem in human beings are lacking. In a recent conference on nutritional support in cancer, no stimulation of tumors was detected (18). The group with the greatest experience with TPN in cancer patients has not reported identifiable tumor stimulation (19). In one randomized study of the effects of TPN in patients given chemotherapy for metastatic colon cancer, the TPN group fared worse than the controls. Tumor progression was not identified as a possible cause of this outcome. All other studies have been conducted in animal models and have examined the relative benefits to tumor and host of various short–term intravenous nutritional regimens. It seems clear that incomplete intravenous dietary regimens, such as those using amino acids only, impair the host and either stimulate tumor growth or have no effect on it (20, 21, 22). In studies of more prolonged TPN, the host has been preserved, but with a larger tumor than that of the anorexic control (the ratio of tumor weight to host weight remaining the same) a situation that presumably could occur in human beings in the absence of specific, effective antineoplastic therapy.

Ascites

Efforts should always be made to totally eliminate, or at least to control effectively, ascites (1, 2, 5). A sodium–poor diet and diuretics specifically preventing obligatory sodium reabsorption (spironolactone with or without hydrochlorothiazide) are usually successful if the regimen is adhered to diligently. However, persisting ascites in the face of an otherwise Class B liver function may indicate the need for a more aggressive approach, such as the insertion of a LeVeen peritoneal–jugular shunt (23). Repeated paracenteses as independent procedures, even though the fluid is filtered and then reinfused intravenously, should be avoided.

Because of the humerally influenced positive sodium balance at the expense of excessive potassium excretion, body depletion of potassium and its consequent alkalosis are common. Renal retention of protons and thus a return of the acid–base balance toward normal can be accomplished only if sufficient potassium ions are available for exchange at the renal tubular level. Accordingly, large quantities of potassium must be given to both replete potassium losses as well as to correct the attendant alkalosis (1, 5).

Hypoxia

Discounting the physical trauma inflicted by retractors or purposeful cutting into liver substance itself, hepatic injury associated with operation is almost always caused by local tissue hypoxia or the anesthetic agent used (21). Hypotension secondary to blood loss or to the administration of some vasodilator and derangements in pulmonary ventilation and/or perfusion account for a majority of the cases of parenchymal hypoxia (24). Although greater stress is usually placed upon the effects of ischemia on other organs (kidney, brain, etc.), the liver is extremely susceptible to injury caused by oxygen lack. It is, however, the tremendous reserve capacity of the normal liver which masks this relatively common cellular injury. Should the patient have prior significant liver disease, the damage caused by hypoxia is much more overt and may of itself cause irreversible changes, even death. Thus shock, whether due to hemorrhage or pharmacologic agents, must always be minimized.

Cardiac Risk

Based on this concept we feel strongly that preoperative risk assessment and optimization of hemodynamic function is mandatory. Continued monitoring during the operative procedure and in the immediate postoperative period avoids the extrahepatic and hepatic complications related to poor perfusion and oxygen delivery.

The ability of cancer patients requiring surgery of the liver to meet the stresses of surgery and anesthesia should be assessed in the preoperative period in order to quantitate the cardiovascular, respiratory and metabolic functional deficits. The high risk patient who must undergo surgery presents a judgment decision for the internist, surgeon, and patient. Unfortunately, preoperative risk assessment without optimization of the patient does little to diminish intraoperative and postoperative morbidity and mortality.

Methods of predicting cardiac risk in preoperative patients rely heavily on history and clinical estimate of cardiac status. Goldman *et al.* (25) developed a scoring system for cardiac risk factors based on 1,001 patients over 40 years of age. The study attempted to determine which preoperative factors might affect the development of cardiac complications after major non–cardiac surgery. Nine independent significant correlates of serious cardiac complications were identified: 1) preoperative third heart sound or jugular venous distention, 2) myocardial infarction in the pre-ceeding six months, 3) more than five premature ventricular con-tractions per minute documented at any time before operation, 4) rhythm other than sinus or presence of premature atrial con-tractions on preoperative electrocardiogram, 5) age over 70 years, 6) intraperitoneal, intrathoracic or aortic operation, 7) emergency operation, 8) important valvular aortic stenosis, and 9) poor general medical condition.

More important than just the assessment of operative risk is the knowledge that this risk can be reduced with judicious pre-operative therapeutic interventions. A cardiopulmonary physiolog-ical assessment enables the clinician to determine the myocardial performance and oxygen delivery preoperatively, thereby, reduc-ing surgical morbidity in high risk surgical patients by correcting abnormal parameters.

Oxygen delivery, the final goal of the cardiorespiratory sys-tem is a direct function of the cardiac output and the arterial oxygen content. The cardiac output, the amount of blood ejected from the heart into the systemic circulation each minute, is a reflection of preload, afterload, myocardial contractility, and heart rate (26).

The preload is the degree of muscle fiber stretch imposed by filling of the ventricles during diastole. According to Starling's law of the heart this varies directly with the cardiac output and can be approximated by the pulmonary capillary wedge pressure (PCWP). This pressure can be obtained with the use of a pulmonary artery catheter when the balloon is inflated and the catheter tip progresses into a more distal branch of the pulmonary artery. This pressure measurement reflects the pressures of the left ventricle in cases where there is no mechanical obstruction between the balloon tip and the left ventricle (normal 1–15 mm Hg). Problems arise with mitral stenosis, left atrial venous, or pulmonary vein obstruction.

Also obtained from the use of this catheter are the pulmonary artery systolic and diastolic pressures. The systolic pressure (PAS) is obtained during the systolic phase of the cardiac cycle and reflects the pressure generated by the contraction of the right ventricle (normal: 15–25 mm Hg). The pulmonary artery diastolic pressure (PAD) is obtained when the cardiac cycle is in diastole and reflects diastolic filling pressure of the left ventricle (normal: 8–10 mm Hg). The right ventricle preload is reflected by the central venous pressure (CVP) (normal: 2–6 mm Hg or 2.7–12 cm H_2O).

The afterload is the impedance to cardiac ejection during systole imposed by vascular resistance, blood pressure and blood viscosity and is represented by the peripheral vascular resistance or total peripheral resistance (TPR). The pulmonary vascular resistance is a measure of the impedance applied by the pulmonary circuitry to the systolic effort of the right ventricle (PVR). The contractility refers to the state of health of the heart muscle and the rate at which the muscle fibers can shorten circumferentially around the bolus of blood within the ventricles. Any monitoring system designed to access the state of the myocardium must include these factors.

With the use of the Swan Ganz pulmonary artery catheter myocardial performance and reserve can be evaluated and extrapolations from the data to determine risk can be made. In order to measure the amount of blood ejected from the left ventricle each minute the thermodilution method is utilized. This method of calculating the output utilizes the theory of temperature change as an indicator of circulating volume.

We have previously described the use of right–sided heart balloon flotation catheters, and arterial sampling in the preoperative pressure measurements within the right atrium, right ventricle, and pulmonary artery were recorded and simultaneously mixed venous and arterial blood samples were obtained. Physiological variables representing left and right ventricle function, oxygen transport, metabolic parameters and ventricular function curves herein described were calculated from the information obtained utilizing a computerized hemodynamic profile, and the patients were divided into four groups according to the data.

Group I patients were without functional deficits and could be managed during and after surgery in a routine manner. Their derived and measured variables were all within normal range. Group II were patients with mild functional deficits for whom surgery did not need to be delayed but who required advanced intraoperative and postoperative monitoring utilizing arterial and mixed venous blood samples, as well as, measurements of cardiac output and pulmonary wedge pressures. Group III were patients with mild to moderate deficit in ventricular, pulmonary and oxygen transport function. The main difference between Group II and III patients was that the physiologic profiles of the latter group showed that they might benefit from physiologic optimizing of abnormal parameters. Surgery in this group was delayed for blood volume expansion, inotropic therapy, pulmonary therapy, or even a period of total parenteral nutrition. Optimization of protein–calorie nutrition by a period of parenteral or enteral supplementation improved cardiac and pulmonary function in some of these Group III patients. Reassessment of their physiologic status then determined whether they underwent the surgical procedure with careful invasive monitoring as in Group II; if they did not improve, they were placed in the Group IV category. Group IV were patients with moderate to advanced functional deficits that could not be corrected. These patients were offered either an alternative mode of therapy or a lesser operation under local anesthesia.

Of the original 148 patients, 19 were denied surgery, 16 died postoperatively and 113 were successfully operated upon. None of the 20 Group I (13.5%) patients died postoperatively. Eight of the 94 patients eventually assigned to Group II and III (63.5%) died postoperatively. Of the 34 patients assigned to Group IV (23%) seven underwent lesser anesthesia and surgery without mortality, 19 did not receive surgery, and 8 underwent surgery as originally planned only to die postoperatively.

Clearly, the risk factors that led to assignment to Group IV were strongly associated with perioperative mortality, e.g., an arterial oxygen tension below 50 mm Hg or a pulmonary venoatrial admixture above 20%. Elevated pulmonary artery pressure, high pulmonary vascular resistance, poor left ventricular contractility as determined from ventricular function plots, high arteriovenous oxygen differences and incorrigible ventricular failure were risk factors leading to assignment to Group III or IV.

The American Society of Anesthesiologists developed a classification of physical status as a method of assessment. This classification involved assigning a number from I to V to a preoperative patient depending on his physical status at the time of surgery. Status I normally healthy patient, status II mild systemic disease, status III severe system disease, status IV severe systemic disease that is a constant threat to life, status V moribund patient who is not expected to survive for 24 hours with or without operation. This number is a powerful prognosticator of postoperative outcome. In a study of 68,388 surgical cases collected from 11 U.S. Naval Hospitals mortality rates at 48 hours were 0.08, 0.27, 1.8, 7.8 and 9.4% respectively for status I through V (28).

In this latter study, the incidence of death rose progressively from age 31 on and was highest after age 81 years. However, correlation of physical status rather than age seemed to be the more important factor in determining death rates.

Physiologic staging of the patients in our study was compared with the anesthesia physical status, and postoperative deaths categorized as due to errors in diagnosis, errors in technique, errors in judgment, or the patient's disease. Classification of physical status by anesthesiologists correlated well with many of the variables in the study. The significant difference was the lack of specificity regarding the functional deficit and that stage III and IV patients were not distinguishable from a mortality standpoint. This unfortunate shortcoming relates to the subjectivity of the various anesthesiologists' opinions compared to a more objective, specific physiologic assessment.

Physiologic Assessment Unit

The data from our original study clearly indicated that invasive preoperative assessment of elderly patients disclosed a high percentage of serious physiologic abnormalities requiring a delay in surgery in some and cancellation in others. This frequent observation of subtle underlying defects in cardiac reserve in patients who otherwise appeared healthy to the clinician precipitated the opening of the preoperative assessment unit at the Westchester Medical Center in January 1983.

This special unit is comprised of 4 beds and is equipped for continuous EKG and hemodynamic pressure monitoring. However, it is used exclusively for preoperative hemodynamic assessment and optimization.

Thus, all our high risk preoperative patients are routinely admitted to this unit 24–48 hours prior to the intended operation. The clinical history and physical examination including measurements of height and weight are then completed. After obtaining informed consent, a Swan Ganz catheter is then inserted under local anesthesia via either a right internal jugular or subclavian approach. Serial pressure measurements within the right atrium, right ventricle, and pulmonary artery are recorded. Then mixed venous and arterial blood samples are obtained after x–ray confirmation of catheter-tip placement. Cardiac outputs are then measured by thermodilution technique with automated calibration accomplished by a programmable calculator. Blood samples are analyzed for pH, gas tensions, carboxy hemoglobin saturation, hemoglobin, hematocrit and lactate values.

Primary and derived data of ventricular function include cardiac index, pulse rate, stroke index, left ventricular stroke work, pulmonary vascular resistance, and a Sarnoff ventricular function curve. Arteriovenous oxygen difference, oxygen consumption, and venoarterial admixture are calculated as measures of oxygen transport and respiratory function. Simultaneous measurements of venous oxygen saturation and oxygen tension with correction factors for carboxyhemoglobin concentration, temperature and pH allowed computation in vivo and standard p50 values reflecting acute and chronic displacements of the oxyhemoglobin dissociation curve exclusive of the Bohr effect. The adequacy of oxygen transport in meeting metabolic requirements is reflected by the blood lactate level and calculated base deficits. All of these derived variables are analog plotted on a preprinted logical format previously described as the Automated Physiologic Profile. The normal values for the Automated Physiologic Profile represented one standard deviation from the mean for healthy young male adults in the resting state (29).

The profile is evaluated and appropriate therapeutic interventions are initiated to optimize oxygen transport and myocardial function. More importantly in this preoperative controlled setting myocardial reserve is assessed by hemodynamically stressing the patients with fluid augmentation (preload) to a predetermined pulmonary capillary wedge pressure in the range of 12 to 14 mm Hg. Cardiac outputs are then repeated to assess the Starling Curves as being normal to subnormal. In the case of diminished myocardial performance inotropic agents and/or afterload relaxants are utilized in an attempt to normalize the parameters and ventricular function curves (Figure 11.1).

Included is the preoperative hemodynamic profile of a 58-year-old woman with metastatic colon carcinoma of the liver, status post four years coronary artery bypass surgery (Figure 11.2). Her medications included digoxin and lasix daily. The profile clearly demonstrated an elevated wedge pressure (20 mm Hg) and evidence of diminished contractility on the Sarnoff curve. Left ventricular hemodynamic assessment revealed a diminished cardiac index, stroke index and left ventricular stroke work with a total peripheral resistance increased. The oxygen transport parameter of arterial venous oxygen content difference demonstrated increased extraction of oxygen to compensate for the diminished left ventricular function.

This patient was started on dobutamine at a dose of 5 micrograms per kilogram per minute to treat persistent congestive heart failure. After approximately twelve hours the effect of the therapeutic intervention was assessed with a repeat profile (Figure 11.3). Clearly at this point, the patient was optimized and was allowed to undergo a left lateral segmentectomy of the liver.

This patient had an uneventful recovery. Her Swan Ganz catheter was removed on the second postoperative day and she was discharged from the surgical intensive care unit to the hospital floor level.

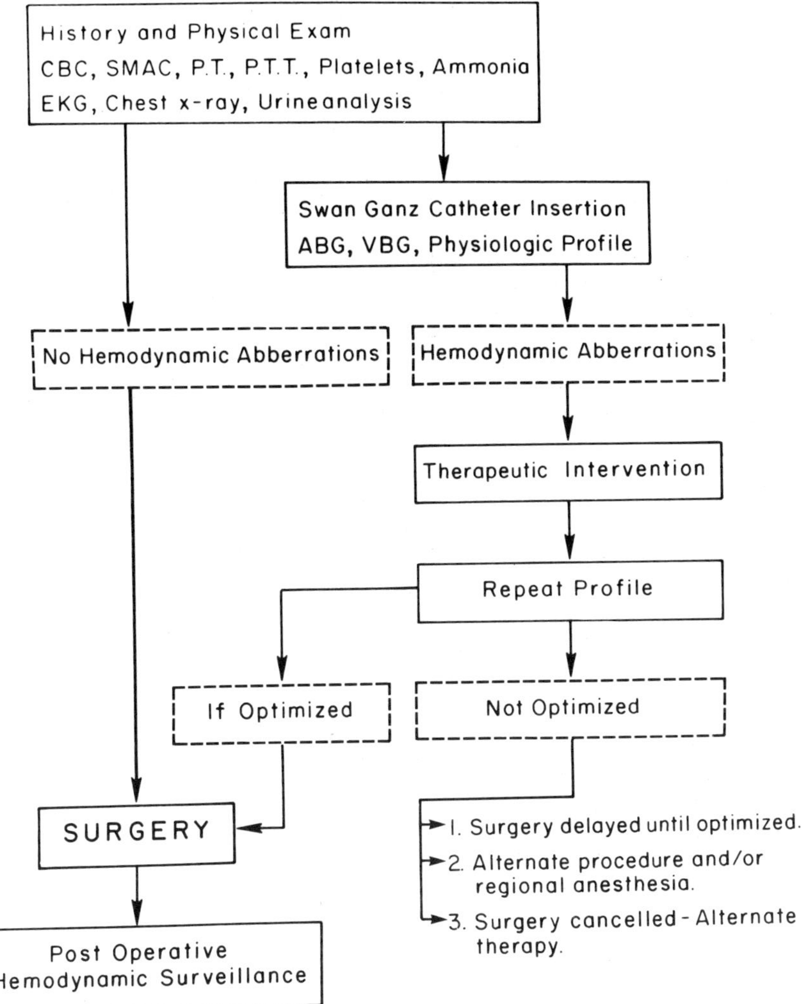

Figure 11.1. Flow chart for hemodynamic management of pateints admitted to the Preoperative Unit.

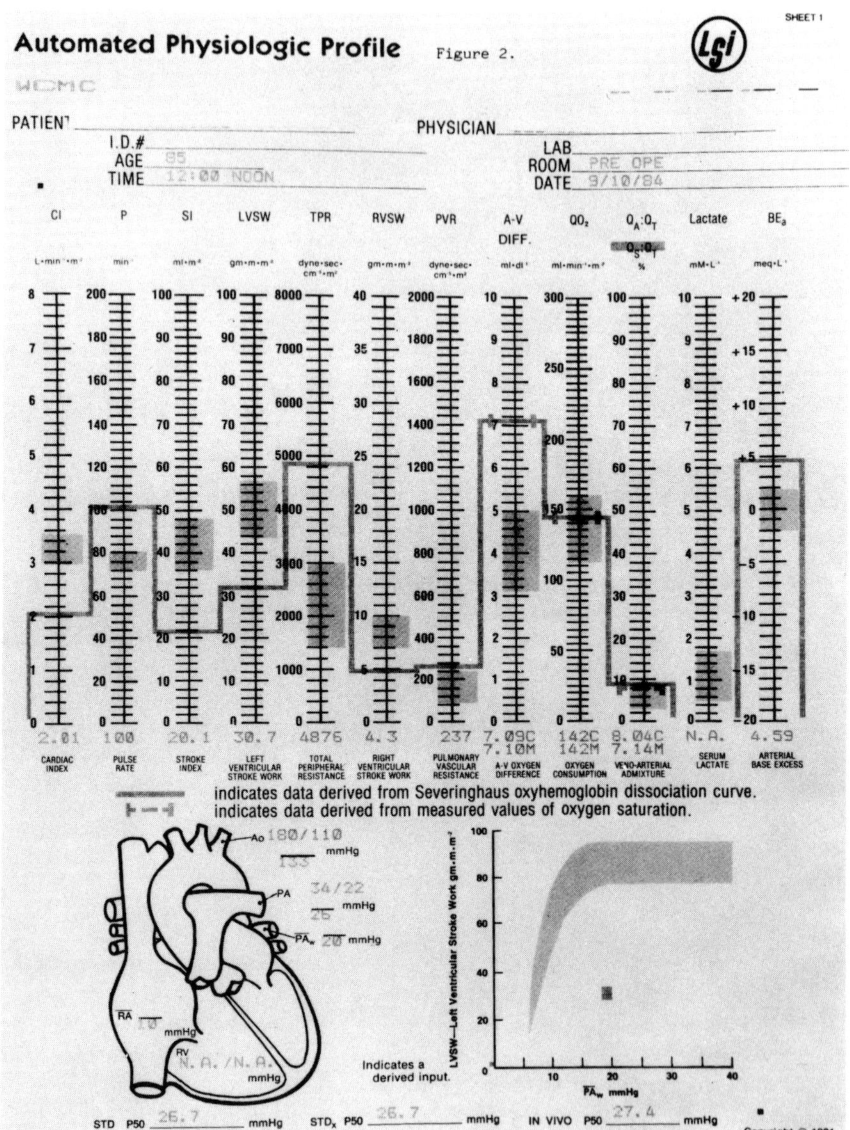

Figure 11.2. Physiological profile in a preoperative patient demonstrating myocardial insufficiency which could lead to significant surgical complications if left uncorrected.

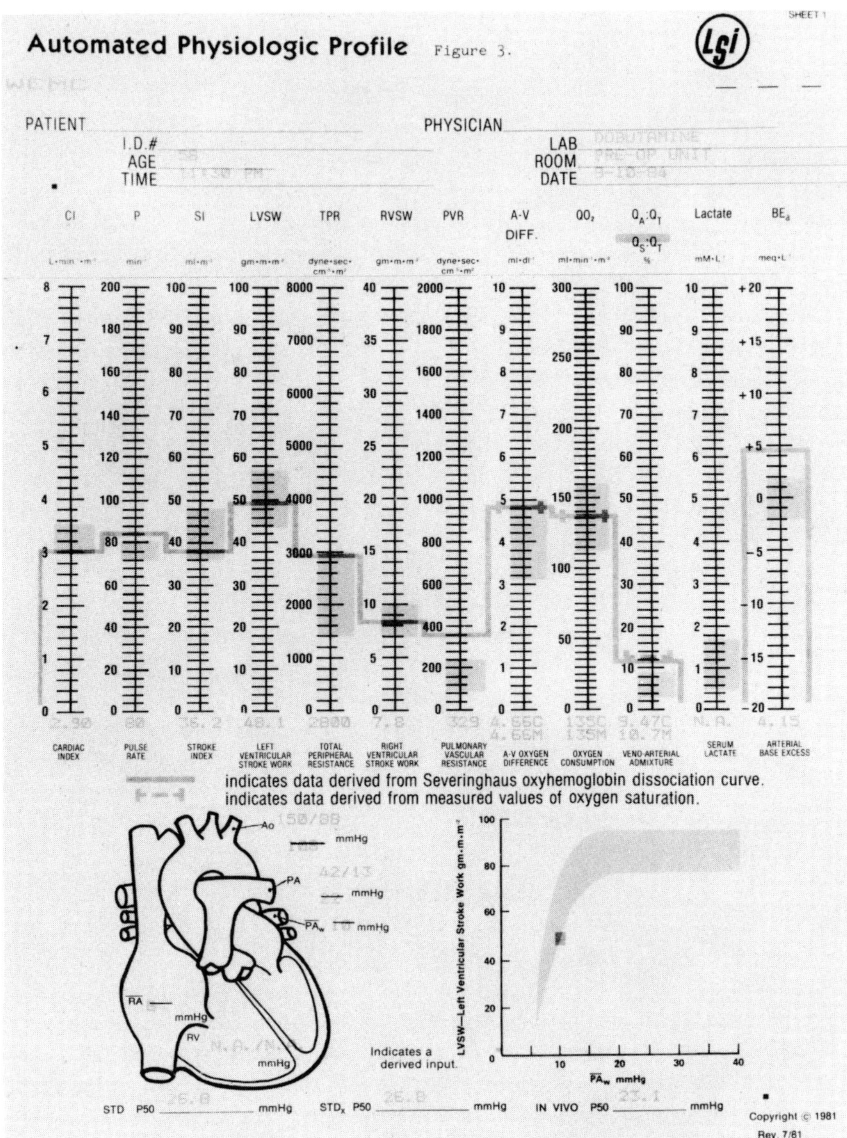

Figure 11.3. Physiological profile showing same patient as in Figure 11.2 after correction of persistent congestive heart failure.

POST-OP MANAGEMENT

Monitoring

Continued hemodynamic monitoring is continued in the recovery room and immediate postoperative period until patients have stable parameters, usually 24 to 48 hours. Previously reported hypovolemia secondary to splenchnic sequestration (24) of blood is thus avoided by continuous hemodynamic monitoring and support.

After operation — regardless as to whether on the liver, portal venous system, or elsewhere in the body — care of the patient with comprised liver function (Class Bor C) is based upon those same measures applied during the phase of preoperative preparation. Such include: close attention to nitrogen balance, evidence of ammonia intoxication, and level of serum albumin; sodium and water restriction, spironolactone diuretics, and extra aliquots of potassium, always keeping in mind the potential for development of a secondary hypovolemia; the occasional addition of more energetic measures for ascites control; and the generous administration of fresh frozen plasma to treat or prevent the occurrence of any bleeding disorder. Otherwise, care becomes routine for the individual operative procedure performed.

Regeneration

Normal liver tissue is endowed with a tremendous capacity for regeneration. Nevertheless, after major hepatic resection the early biochemical and metabolic changes that can occur can be serious and life-threatening. Appropriate steps are necessary to manage these changes to permit recovery and rapid regeneration. A significant drop in blood sugar following resection of 70% or more, and severe hypoglycemia has been noted in patients following total hepatectomy and liver transplantation (30). Other groups have not observed such marked blood sugar changes following resection, perhaps because of routine use of glucose postoperatively (31). In any case, it seems wise to obviate this danger by monitoring blood sugar and infusing 10% glucose solution i.v. continuously for at least the first several days or until adequate p.o. intake of carbohydrates is assured. Often following p.o. carbohydrate, blood sugar may be elevated for several weeks. Since the liver is the site of albumin synthesis, it is not surprising that hypoalbuminemia will occur to a significant degree unless replaced by parenteral administration. Failure to do so can lead to a progressive fall in osmotic pressure in the vascular compartment and accumulation of marked interstitial fluid with increased vascular load and the danger of pulmonary edema. The need for supplementary albumin persists for approximately one week. The amounts of albumin given have usually averaged 26 g/day for the first five days or so (30). According to Coppa *et al.* (31), these albumin requirements can be as high as 200–300 grams per day. By the end of the third postoperative week, nearly normal albumin levels are usually found. However, with the utilization of the techniques advocated in this text albumin levels are frequently maintained in the postoperative period without the need of excessive replacement.

Preoperatively, some patients may have elevated serum prothrombin time, which is corrected by preoperative administration of Vitamin K. Oxide i.m. Fibrinogen, prothrombin, and other coagulation factors (V, VII, IX, X) that are synthesized by the liver will fall following major resection (30). Despite the postoperative administration of Vitamin K, prothrombin levels remain depressed in the postoperative phase; such depression is not reflected in any clinical disorder. These factors gradually return to normal as hepatic regeneration progresses (31). Probably, the most reliable approach has been to give fresh frozen plasma, both during the operation as well as in the immediate postoperative period. By this means, almost the entire complement of noncorpuscular clotting elements can be replenished (24).

After subtotal hepatectomy there is a rapid fall in serum triglycerides. This is expected since the liver is the major source of serum triglycerides and since peripheral tissues are continuously removing circulating fat. As serum triglycerides fall there is a rapid rise in levels of nonesterified fatty acids, that reflects an increased mobilization of fatty acids from adipose tissue (30). As hepatic regeneration proceeds there is progressive rise of the triglycerides and a fall in nonesterified fatty acids over the first several weeks. Decreased total serum calcium reflects a fall in serum albumin. Transient low serum sodium and potassium have been reported in some patients after liver resection (32), while others have reported low levels of serum inorganic phosphates following clinical hepatic resection and hepatic transplantation. Hypophosphatemia in dogs following partial hepatectomy is associated with increased hepatic uptake and diminished urinary excretion of phosphate (30).

Decompensation

Evidence of liver decompensation has been observed in cases of extended right hepatic lobectomy (30). In such instances reduction of protein intake and initiation of a medical regimen for hepatic precoma are indicated. These disturbances disappear in a short period. At this time it is important to provide sufficient intake of protein and other nutrients to permit optimum liver regeneration. When hepatic dysfunction persists following resection or liver transplantation, and especially when this is associated with portal vein shunting, the i.v. amino acid regimen developed by Fischer *et al.* (33) may be useful. The rationale for this therapy has been reviewed by Soeters and Fischer (34). They postulate that, in catabolic states such as liver failure and associated conditions such as sepsis, catecholamine discharge is associated with marked increases in glucagon secretion and a decreased insulin: glucagon ratio. The result is a release of a large amount of amino acids from protein sources; the aromatic amino acids cannot be catabolized by the failing liver and accumulate in the circulation. Decreased plasma branch-chain amino acids together with the increased aromatic amino acids allow toxic aromatic amino acids to penetrate the blood-brain barrier in increased amounts and encephalopathy develops. The nutrient formulation is designed to reverse the catabolic state by providing sufficient calories and other nutrients and to reverse encephalopathy by increasing branch-chain amino acid concentration while decreasing aromatic amino acid concentraiton in order to restore the normal plasma molar ratio of branch-chain amino acids to aromatic amino acids and to reverse the amino acid losses from muscle and liver. The administration of the keto analogs of five essential amino acids (valine, leucine, isoleucine, methionine, and phenylalnine) and five amino acids (histidine, threonine, tryptophan, lysine, and arginine) i.v. or p.o. has been reported to improve portal-systemic encephalopathy in 8 of 11 patients.

Hepatic decompensation, pulmonary insufficiency, postoperative bleeding and hospital death were significantly higher in patients whose operative blood loss exceeded 5,000 ml according to Nagao and colleagues (35). To determine this, they measured hepatic functional reserve by the removal rate of indocyanin green (ICG.R max); they measured prothrombin time; they measured the lineality index of the oral glucose tolerance test (OGTT.Li). When the ICG.R max was above 0.8, the prothrombin time above

60% of normal and the OGTT.Li above 1, the patient had sufficient hepatic reserve. By noting changes in these values, they could determine postoperative prognosis.

Regeneration of a normally functioning liver can uniformly be expected, regardless of how massive the resection (i.e., 90 to 95%), provided that the retained liver parenchyma is viable, has an unobstructed duct and blood supply, and was not diseased itself. Thus, supportive care is indeed worthwhile until the residual piece of liver can alone take over two of its most important tasks — maintenance of both glucose and serum albumin.

Jaundice is usually low–grade and lasts for only 5 to 10 days. If more profound or if persisting into the third week, obstruction of the duct system should be suspected. Other parameters of liver function have seemed to be of little importance and of absolutely no use whatsoever. Nevertheless, monthly liver scans will document an actual increase in liver size which begins as passive congestion, progresses to hypertrophy, and then finally reflects a true cellular hyperplasia (24).

Nutrition

Worth elaborating upon is the hepatic dysfunction associated with total parenteral nutrition, which becomes significant if utilized in the postoperative period along with chemotherapy in these patients.

Hepatic dysfunction induced by TPN in the adult patient is usually more benign and reversible when compared to that in the pediatric patient. This complication is characterized by gradual elevations in alkaline phosphatase, SGOT, and occasionally bilirubin. Concurrent liver biopsies in patients who have developed liver function elevations while on TPN have revealed hepatic steatosis (36-40). These liver biopsies were characterized by both increases in glycogen stores and fatty infiltration within the hepatocyte. In most cases, hepatic architecture was well preserved.

Proposed etiologies for this phenomenon in the adult patient included excessive glucose administration (36, 37, 41), essential fatty acid deficiency (37, 38), tryptophan breakdown products (40), and carnitine deficiency.

Many of the adult patients who develop increases in liver function tests while receiving TPN will not require treatment because these elevations are only transient. The initial elevations of alkaline phosphatase and SGOT are generally seen after 7 to 10 days of TPN (37). Follow up liver function tests are mandatory to identify which patients have a persistent abnormality. If a patient has received a fat-free TPN regimen, administration of intravenous fat emulsions will correct the essential fatty acid deficiency and liver function tests may improve. Two to three 50 ml administrations of 10% lipid have reversed clinical and biochemical signs of EFAD (38, 39). This supplies 2-4% of the nonprotein kcal as linoleic acid in most TPN regimens. If the patient is fluid-restricted, 1-2 500 ml administrations of 20% lipid may be used. Patients who demonstrate a persistent rise in liver function tests while being administered TPN may be treated with cyclic TPN or protein sparing. Protein sparing will decrease the administered dextrose load to the patient and decrease serum insulin levels. This may allow resumption of lipolysis and clearance of trapped hepatic lipid. Cyclic TPN will shorten the infusion time for dextrose administration and allow an 8-12 hour dextrose-free period each day. It is presumed that insulin levels will decrease, allowing lipolysis to resume.

Recent work done by Buzby *et al.* (42) demonstrated massive hepatomegaly and fat deposition when protein-depleted rats were administered TPN with all of their nonprotein calories as either lipid or dextrose. The livers of the rats receiving only dextrose as a calorie source showed deposition of endogenously synthesized fat while those rate receiving only lipid as a calorie source had fatty livers secondary to lysosomal deposition of fat pigment within hepatocytes and Kupffer cells. The fatty livers in the rats receiving only lipid may represent sequestered exogenous lipid rather than endogenously synthesized lipid (42). A group of rats receiving 75% of their nonprotein calories as dextrose and 25% as lipid did not demonstrate the fatty liver seen in the other two groups. Although these data need to be studied in adult humans, they suggest a TPN regimen of balanced caloric composition may be an alternative to decreasing the carbohydrate load to prevent hepatic dysfunction. This would allow for optimal caloric and protein administration when nutritional repletion is critical (42).

Wagman *et al.* (43) have reported on liver function test elevation in a group of 143 cancer patients receiving 199 cycles of TPN. TPN induced a rise in alkaline phosphatase, SGOT and SGPT similar to that reported by others. No correlation with age, parenteral fat administration, tumor burden or caloric administration could be made with these liver function test evaluations (43).

REFERENCES

1. Child, CG, III: *The Liver and Portal Hypertension.* Philadelphia: W.B. Saunders Co., 1967, pp. 48-77.

2. Wirthlin, LS, Urk, HV, Malt, RB, Malt, RA: Predicators of Surgical Mortality in Patients with Cirrhosis and Nonvariceal Gastroduodenal Bleeding. *Surg, Gynecol, Obstet, 139:*65, 1974.

3. Sunderman, FW, Sunderman, FW, Jr.: *Laboratory Diagnosis of Liver Disease.* St. Louis: W.H. Green, Inc., 1968, p. 327.

4. Stone, HH: Major Hepatic Resections in Children. *J Pediatr Surg, 10:*127, 1975.

5. Galambos, JT, Warren, WD, Rudman, D: Selective and Total Shunts in the Treatment of Bleeding Varices. *N Eng J Med, 295:*1089, 1976.

6. McDermott, WV, Jr., Ackroyd, FW: Nutrient Demands Imposed by Surgery of the Liver. *Am J Clin Nutr, 23:*652-656, 1970.

7. DeWys, WD, Begg, C, Lavin, PT: Prognostic Effect of Weight Loss to Chemotherapy in Cancer Patients. *Am J Med, 69:*491-497, 1980.

8. Studley, HO: Percentage of Weight Loss: A basic indicator of surgical risk in patients with chronic peptic ulcer. *JAMA, 106:*458-460, 1936.

9. Hickman, DM, Miller, RA, Rombeau, JL, Twomey, PL, Frey, CF: Serum Albumin and Body Weight as Predicators of Postoperative Course in Colorectal Cancer. *J Per, 4:*314-316, 1977.

10. Hill, GL, Blackett, RL, Pickford, I: Malnutrition in Surgical Patients: An unrecognized problem. *Lancet, 1:*689-692, 1977.

11. Bistrian, BR, Blackburn, GL, Hallowell, E, Heddle, R: Protein Status of General Surgical Patients. *JAMA 230:*858-860, 1974.

12. Copeland, EM, MacFadyen, BV, Jr., Dudrick, SJ: Effect of Intravenous Hyperalimentation on Established Delayed Hypersensitivity in the Cancer Patient. *Ann Surg, 184:*60-64, 1976.

13. Copeland, EM, III, MacFadyen, BV, Jr., Lanzotti, VJ, Dudrick, SJ: Intravenous Hyperalimentation as an Adjunct to Cancer Chemotherapy. *Am J Surg, 129:*167-173, 1975.

14. Harvey, KG, Bothe, A, Jr., Blackburn, GL: Nutritional Assessment and Patient Outcome During Oncological Therapy. *Cancer 43:*2065-2069, 1979.

15. Forse, RA, Shizgol, HM: The Assessment of Malnutrition. *Surgery, 88:*17-24, 1980.

16. Ryan, JA, Jr., Taft, DA: Preoperative Nutritional Assessment Does Not Predict Morbidity and Mortality in Abdominal Operations. *Surg Forum, 31:*96-98, 1980.

17. Mullen, JL, Buzby, GP, Mathews, DC, Smole, BF, Rosato, EF: Reduction of Operative Morbidity and Mortality by Combined Preoperative and Postoperative Nutritional Support. *Ann Surg, 192:*604-613, 1980.

18. Brennan, MF, Copeland, EM: Panel Report on Nutritional Support of the Cancer Patient: Proceedings of an NIH sponsored conference. *Am J Clin Nutr, 34 (Suppl):*1199-1205, 1981.

19. Copeland, EM, III, Daly, JM, Ota, DM, Dudrick, SJ: Nutrition, Cancer and Intravenous Hyperalimentation. *Cancer, 43:*2108-2116, 1979.

20. Buzby, GP, Mullen, JL, Stein, TP, Miller, EE, Hobbs, CL, Rosato, EF: Host-Tumor Interaction and Nutrient Supply. *Cancer, 45:*2940-2948, 1980.

21. Steiger, E, Oram-Smith, J, Miller, E, Juo, L, Vars, HM: Effects of Nutrition on Tumor Growth and Tolerance to Chemotherapy. *J Surg Res, 18:* 455-461, 1975.

22. Goodgame, JT, Jr., Lowry, SF, Brennan, MF: Nutritional Manipulations and Tumor Growth. II. The Effects of Intravenous Feeding. *Am J Clin Nutr, 32:*2285-2294, 1979.

23. LeVeen, HH, Wapnick, S, Grosberg, S, Kinney, MJ: Farther Experience with Peritoneo-Venous Shunt for Ascites. *Am Surg, 184:*574, 1976.

24. Stone, HH: Preoperative and Postoperative Care. *Surg Clin N Am, 57:*409-419, 1977.

25. Goldman, L, Calderea, DL, Nussbaum, SB, *et al.*: Multifactional Index of Cardiac Risk in Noncardiac Surgical Procedures. *N Eng J Med, 297:* 845, 1977.

26. Del Guercio, LRM: Physiologic monitoring of the surgical patient. In: *Principles of Surgery,* Schwartz (Ed.), 1979 pp. 525-545.

27. Del Guercio, LRM, Cohn, JD: Monitoring Operative Risk in the Elderly. *JAMA, 243:*1350-1355, 1980.

28. Vaconti, CJ, Van Houten, RJ, Hill, RC: A Statistical Analysis of the Relationship of Physical Status to Postoperative Mortality in 68,388 Cases. *Anesth Analg Curr Res, 49:*564-566, 1970.

29. Cohn, JD, Engler, PE, Del Guercio, LRM: The Automated Physiologic Profile. *Crit Care Med, 3:*51-58, 1975.

30. Shils, ME: Effect on Nutrition of Surgery of the Liver, Pancreas and Genitourinary Tract. *Cancer Res, 37:*2387-2394, 1978.

31. Coppa, GF, Eng, K, Ranson, JH, *et al.*: Hepatic resection for metastatic colon and rectal cancer. An evaluation of preoperative and postoperative factors. *Ann Surg, 202:*203-208, 1985.

32. Aronsen, KF, Ericsson, B, Pihl, B: Metabolic Changes Following Major Hepatic Resection. *Ann Surg, 169:*102-110, 1969.

33. Fischer, JE, Rosen, HM, Ebeid, AM, James, JH, Keane, JM, Soeters, PB: The Effect of Normalization of Plasma Amino Acids on Hepatic Encephalopathy in Man. *Surgery, 80:*77-91, 1976.

34. Soeters, PB, Fischer, JE: Insulin, Glucogen, Amino Acid Imbalance and Hepatic Encephalopathy. *Lancet,* 880-882, 1976.

35. Nagao, T, Inoue, S, Mitzuta, T, *et al.*: 100 hepatic resections. Indications and operative results. *Ann Surg, 202:*42-49, 1985.

36. Kaminski, DL, Adams, A, Jellinek, M: The Effect of Hyperalimentation on Hepatic Lipid Content and Lipogenic Enzyme Activity in Rats and Man. *Surgery, 88:*93-100, 1980.

37. Sheldon, GF, Petersen, SR, Sanders, R: Hepatic Dysfunction During Hyperalimentation. *Arch Surg, 113:*504-508, 1978.

38. Jeejeebhoy, KN, Zohrab, EJ, Langer, B, *et al.*: Total Parenteral Nutrition at Home for 23 Months without Complication and with Good Rehabilitation. *Gastroenterol, 65:*811-820, 1973.

39. Langer, B, McHattie, JD, Zohrab, EJ, *et al.*: Prolonged Survival After Complete Small Bowel Resection Using Intravenous Alimentation at Home. *J Surg Res, 15:*226-233, 1973.

40. Grant, JP, Cox, CE, Kleinman, LM, *et al.*: Serum Hepatic Enzyme and Bilirubin Elevations During Parenteral Nutrition. *Surg, Gynecol, Obstet, 145:* 573-580, 1977.

41. MacFadyen, BV, Dudrick, SJ, Baquero, G, *et al.*: Clinical and Biological Changes in Liver Function During Intravenous Hyperalimentation. *JPEN, 3:*438-443, 1979.

42. Buzby, GP, Mullen, JL, Stein, TP, *et al.*: Manipulation of TPN Caloric Substrate and Fatty Infiltration of the Liver. *J Surg Res, 31:*46-54, 1981.

43. Wagman, LD, Burt, ME, Brennan, MF: The Impact of Total Parenteral Nutrition on Liver Function Tests in Patients with Cancer. *Cancer, 49:*1249-1257, 1982.

TAUSEEF AHMED, M.D.
MICHAEL L. FRIEDLAND, M.D.

CHAPTER 12

Chemotherapy of Primary and Metastatic Hepatic Neoplasms

INTRODUCTION

Malignant neoplasms involve the liver in up to 39% of all solid tumors (1), and cause 20-25% of all cancer deaths (2). Commonly, liver cancer represents the tip of the iceberg; however, destruction of hepatic function due to metastatic liver tumor often affects survival more significantly than metastases to other sites, e.g., lymph node or omentum.

Certain tumors may demonstrate a proclivity toward hepatic metastasis. A study from the Roswell Park Memorial Institute (1) examined 8,455 autopsies of patients with adult solid tumors and noted that metastasis confined to the liver occurred seven times more frequently when the lesion was drained by the portal vein, compared to lesions which arose outside the portal bed, where pulmonary metastases were more common. Other factors, including a selectivity by the liver for certain tumor cell sub-populations may be important. This was elegantly demonstrated by the work of Fidler, *et al.* (3), who described differences in the propensity of various sub-populations of B16 melanoma cells to metastasize to various organs. Host immunologic factors, hypercoagulability or trauma may also be important factors.

PHARMACOLOGY AND PHARMACODYNAMICS

The effect of drug dosages and schedules is readily apparent in animal tumor systems, but their importance is not so clear in human tumors. While intermittent boluses of chemotherapy are convenient, they necessitate substantial period of non-treatment. The half life (T ½) of several chemotherapy drugs such as anti-metabolites, e.g., fluorouracil (5-FU), is extremely short, i.e., to the order of 6-20 minutes (Chabner). Even with drugs with long half lives such as methotrexate (MTX) and cyclophosphamide (CYC) the T ½ is no longer than a few hours. The fraction of tumor cells undergoing DNA synthesis usually represents the subpopulation of cells that are responsive to cycle specific drugs. Among solid tumors, like colon cancer, only 2-3% of the entire cell population is in the phase of DNA synthesis. Thus, the theoretic probability of enhancing the effect of an agent by prolonging the duration of exposure is high.

Among the drugs often used to treat hepatic metastasis, especially from colorectal carcinoma, 5-Fluorouracil (5-FU) and fluoro-2'-deoxyuridine (FUDR) are the most important. These drugs are schedule dependent and cytotoxic effects are generally a function of the duration of exposure above a given drug concentration. Continuous infusions of fluoropyrimidines may be less myelotoxic than bolus injections (4). On the other hand, alkylators like Mitomycin-C or carmustine (BCNU) which work best when administered as a bolus, at higher peak exposure may produce more DNA damage while lower levels may allow repair processes to proceed (6).

Administering chemotherapy directly into a target organ, using appropriate infusion systems, affords one the opportunity to influence the time integrals of drug levels (i.e., the concentration times time or CXT) within the region being profused (7). Moreover, if the clearance of the drug by the target organ is high, one can obtain significant target watershed levels while maintaining low systemic concentrations and thus possibly obviate systemic toxicity (8). The blood levels in the hepatic artery of these drugs are 8-10-fold higher for 5-FU and 100-400-fold higher for FUDR (9) when these drugs are administered into the hepatic artery instead of systemically. Moreover, 50% of 5-FU and greater than 90% of FUDR is extracted by the liver at first pass (4). Thus, the fluoropyrimidines can be used advantageously to treat liver tumors. Since the concentration of drug in the hepatic artery is dependent on the rate of blood flow, a decrease in hepatic artery flow by 90% may increase the arterial blood concentration of a drug 10-fold (8). Infusing drugs after ligating the hepatic artery may be only marginally better than infusion with patent vessels, as collateralization around the ligated vessel often occurs (10). Moreover, ligation has the disadvantage of being irreversible. Temporary obstruction using balloon catheters (11) or vasoconstrictors (12) may be more useful for bolus injections. Although several innovative methods of decreasing hepatic arterial blood flow exist, their precise effect on tumor response still requires definition.

Modern totally implantable pumps not only allow one to deliver drug by a controlled continuous infusion, but also permit bolus injections through a side port (13). These pumps are expensive and cannot be reused, however. They are best utilized in patients who are good surgical candidates with a long-term potential. External pumps are cheaper and reusable, however, they are awkward for patients to carry around and have an increased risk of infection and possible arterial thrombosis. Patients who have far advanced disease and are poor surgical candidates may benefit from external pumps. Although reportedly better survivorship exists among patients with surgically placed catheters (14, 15), they might represent a better risk and thus enjoy better survival compared to those with percutaneously placed catheters who presumably represent worse surgical candidates.

DEFINITIONS OF RESPONSE

While several solid tumors lend themselves to accurate assessment by means of physical examination and/or imaging techniques, lesions in the liver are notoriously hard to evaluate. In fact, the very vagaries in the techniques used to evaluate these tumors and the definitions of response that are employed, lead in large part to major differences in response rates. For example, measurement of hepatomegaly by means of physical examination and its use as the primary method of evaluating the response presupposes that the entire liver is replaced by tumor, has large inter-observer variability and often fails to take into account the extent of disease sequestered behind the rib cage. Also variations in hepatic measurements due to ascites, weight loss, degree of inspiratory effort, posture and drug related hepatitis have to be considered.

Standard radionuclide scans often show lesions with hazy margins and do not allow precise measurements of tumor size. Radionuclide scanning is sub-optimal in most instances to quantitate a response. Often a decrease in hepatomegaly or symptoms or CEA may precede improvement in liver scan by 6-10 weeks. Computerized transaxial tomography, while often used for following indicator lesions, also suffers from innate problems. For example, tomographic cuts cannot be repeatedly obtained at the same precise spot, making follow up assessment patently inaccurate.

These problems have led to some observers using carcinoembryonic antigens and lactic dehydrogenase levels (LDH) for follow up and attempting to correlate them with survival data. Unfortunately these, and other tests of liver function, do not bear a quantitative relationship with tumor burden and liver. With these provisos, we use the following criteria for "objective response."

Complete Response: A complete response is defined as disappearance of all clinical, biochemical and radiologic evidence of tumor for at least one month.

Partial Response: A greater than 50% decrease in the summed products of the bidimensionally measurable diameters of all measurable lesions for at least one month. No new lesions may appear and no lesions may grow larger. Tumor response is based on shrinkage of hepatic size if there is independent evidence, either by pathologic means or by imaging techniques of involvement by a malignant process. The liver must be palpable 5 cm below the costal margin when the patient is supine and breathing quietly. Measurements from the costal margin to the liver edge are taken at 5 cm intervals from the mid–sternal line. A minimum of 50% decrease in the sum of the measurements for a minimum of one month is required to obtain a tumor response. Some cooperative groups and cancer centers accept a 30% decrement in hepatic measurements as evidence of response.

Minor response predicates a 25-49% decrease in tumor size for less than 1 month, *stabilization* denotes a less than 25% change in tumor size for more than 3 months, and *progression* is defined as a greater than 25% increase in tumor size.

CHEMOTHERAPY TRIALS

This review will summarize systemic and regional chemotherapy trials for both primary and metastatic liver tumors.

Primary Hepatic Carcinomas

The most common primary hepatic cancers include hepatocellular carcinomas and cholangiocarcinomas. They are rare in the United States and most of the western world, accounting for no more than 1% of all cancers. In parts of Africa, hepatomas may account for 30–40% of all cancer deaths (17), while cholangiocarcinoma is probably more common in the Orient (18), possibly due to clonorchis sinesis infestations. Hepatocellular carcinomas outnumber cholangiocarcinomas by a factor of 10 to 30. Hepatic cirrhosis (19), aflatoxin (20), nutritional deficiencies, exposure to hepatitis B (20) and alcohol (19) have all been implicated as etiologic factors. The following discussion will summarize the experience with hepatomas.

Systemic Chemotherapy for Hepatoma

The drugs most commonly employed to treat primary hepatomas systemically include fluorouracil and doxorubicin. Doxorubicin appears to be marginally more effective. In a recent review (21) of 100 selected cases reported in the literature, treated with doxorubicin alone, a 25% response rate was noted. This was in contrast to fluorouracil where the response rate was no better than 9% in 105 selected cases. The median duration of survival of 7-9 months with responders compared to 2-4 months for non-responders. Other chemotherapeutic agents such as the nitrosureas (22-25), mitomycin (26, 27), cytarabine (28), vinca alkaloids (29), and anti-folates (30) have all been used in combination with 5-FU and doxorubicin without any striking improvement in remission rates.

With the recent identification of hormone receptors in the tumors, trials employing hormonal agents are underway.

Given the overall dismal results using systemic chemotherapy with currently available agents, the authors feel that these tumors are probably best treated by investigational agents and/or approaches.

Regional Chemotherapy for Hepatoma

Regional chemotherapy is an attractive concept in that high levels of these agents can be directed to the target organ. Improvements in angiographic techniques, catheters and infusion pump technology have made it possible to administer continuous infusions via the hepatic artery. However, no randomized trials have been reported comparing the relative advantages of systemic chemotherapy to continuous intrahepatic infusions of chemotherapeutic agents in the treatment of hepatoma. Nevertheless, regional perfusion chemotherapy may be useful in highly selected instances. A review of the literature (29, 31-40) (Table 1) on fluoropyrimidines administered via hepatic artery infusion finds 44 responses in 101 evaluable cases with hepatoma, an overall response rate of 43%, apparently superior to the use of 5-FU as a

<table>
<tr><td colspan="4" align="center">TABLE 1
THERAPY OF PRIMARY HEPATOCELLULAR CARCINOMA
WITH INTRA-ARTERIAL FLUOROPYRIMIDINES</td></tr>
<tr><td>Ref.</td><td>No. Treated</td><td>No. Responding</td><td>Drug</td></tr>
<tr><td>29</td><td>17</td><td>9</td><td>FUDR</td></tr>
<tr><td>31</td><td>3</td><td>0</td><td>FU</td></tr>
<tr><td>32, 33</td><td>9</td><td>6</td><td>FU</td></tr>
<tr><td>34</td><td>19</td><td>0</td><td>FU</td></tr>
<tr><td>35</td><td>7</td><td>1</td><td>FU</td></tr>
<tr><td>36</td><td>1</td><td>1</td><td>FU</td></tr>
<tr><td>37</td><td>18</td><td>10</td><td>FU/FUDR</td></tr>
<tr><td>38</td><td>6</td><td>2</td><td>FUDR</td></tr>
<tr><td>39</td><td>8</td><td>6</td><td>FUDR</td></tr>
<tr><td>40</td><td>13</td><td>9</td><td>FUDR</td></tr>
</table>

single agent systemically. One must be cautious in interpreting these results since response criteria vary.

Catheters may be inserted percutaneously using the Seldinger technique. However, while this requires relatively less technical skill, long term infusions are rarely possible with this method. These catheters often become dislodged, infected, or clotted. The occasional excellent results noted with regional perfusion for hepatoma may justify its use in highly selected patients.

Chemotherapy of Metastatic Neoplasms to the Liver

The treatment of metastatic neoplasms to the liver is, in general, dictated with regard to the primary site. Neoplasia from gastrointestinal primaries frequently metastasize to the liver. Tumors that affect primary sites not drained by the portal venous system which commonly spread to the liver include lung cancer, breast carcinoma and malignant melanoma.

While 39% of solid tumors involve the liver, in only 2.5% are the metastases confined to the liver (1). Thus a systemic mode of therapy is often desirable. This section will deal with trials of chemotherapeutic agents administered systemically to patients with intra–abdominal primary tumors.

Colorectal Neoplasia

Seventy percent of patients with metastatic colorectal carcinoma develop metastasis (41). 5-Fluorouracil is the drug most commonly employed. The popularity that this drug has enjoyed over the past few decades probably stems from the fact that the alternative therapeutic modalities are even less desirable than this drug. It is generally agreed that the five-day loading schedule utilizing 15 mg/kg of 5-FU is superior to weekly bolus of 5-FU. In studies (42-45) where a response was defined as less than 50% reduction in tumor size the average response rate in 226 patients with metastatic colon cancer given 5-FU was 20% (Table 2). In two studies (42, 43) where patients with evaluable hepatic metastasis were identified, and a partial remission was defined as a greater than 50% decrease in tumor size, administration of 5-FU resulted in 21% objective remission rate in 42 cases. Interestingly, a high response rate was noted in one study (42) where 15 of 34 patients responded to a continuous infusion of 5-FU. Forty-eight hour infusions of 5-FU at a high dose (30 mg/kg/day) recycled weekly were noted to be similarly efficacious, where using strict criteria a 30% response rate was noted in 36 patients (46). Preliminary data from a prospective study (47) comparing systemic to intrahepatic therapy have recently become available. Of 34 patients with metastatic colorectal carcinoma involving only the liver, 15 were randomized to receive FUDR, infused continuously by means of an Infusaid® pump into the hepatic artery, and 19 received continuous systemic infusion of FUDR again using an Infusaid® pump. Forty-one percent of patients receiving intrahepatic chemotherapy responded as did 40% of patients receiving systemic infusions. In this trial it appears that the use of a systemic chemotherapeutic agent is at least as active as an intrahepatic infusion in treating metastatic tumor to the liver. Of note, however, in this trial the appearance of extrahepatic metastasis was markedly decreased in the group that received systemic infusions.

TABLE 2

EFFICACY OF FLUOROURACIL IN COLORECTAL CARCINOMA
SELECTED SERIES

Ref.	No. Treated	No. Responding
42	70	21
43	31	7
44	80	15
45	45	3
Total	226	46 (20.4%)

Acid peptic disease was the commonest form of toxicity in the hepatic artery infusion group while diarrhea was the least frequent toxicity in the systemic chemotherapy area. Another study (48) that is also presently ongoing has noted similar results.

Other attempts to improve upon the response rates observed with 5-FU include combinations of 5-FU with other agents. The combination of methyl-CCNU, vincristine and 5-FU (MOF) was originally reported by Moertel, *et al.* (49) to yield a response rate of 43%. However, subsequent studies (50-54) have failed to support these initial findings (Table 3). Randomized studies comparing 5-FU to MOF have failed to demonstrate superiority for the combination regimen. In fact, in a prospective study a response rate of 6% for MOF was noted (54). MOF-Strep similarly was initially reported to yield a 36% response rate (41). Subsequent trials (55) by other investigators have failed to confirm the superiority of MOF-Strep over MOF and, in fact, the response rates in a recent trial of MOF-Strep was only 16%.

Early results with sequential methotrexate (MTX and 5-FU) have been interesting. Methotrexate leads to an increase in the level of phosphoribosyl pyrophosphate which helps convert 5-FU to its active metabolite FUMP leading to an apparent increase in the biologic activity of 5-FU. This effect is schedule dependent (57) and it appears that a period of time must elapse between the administration of MTX and 5-FU. In a review of the literature (Table 4) (58-71) the response rate was lower (14%) in trials where MTX and FU were administered within one hour of each other compared to trials in which at least a 3-hour time difference existed between these drugs, where a 37% overall response rate was observed. In one recent study (72) where sequential MTX and 5-FU were compared to a combination of MOF + Streptozotocin,

TABLE 3
RESULTS WITH METHYL CCNU, VINCRISTINE AND 5-FU

Ref.	*No. Treated*	*No. Responding*
50	25	10
51	46	17
52	127	34
53	81	10
54	69	7
Total	348	78 (22.4%)

TABLE 4

RESULTS WITH METHOTREXATE AND 5-FLUOROURACIL IN COLORECTAL CARCINOMA

Ref.	MTX mg/m^2	Leucovorin	5-FU mg/m^2	Interval hrs.	No. Rx	No. Resp.
Simultaneous MTX and FU						
58	60	no	1500	0	30	1
Percent responding						3%, 1/30
One hour interval between MTX and FU						
59	250	yes	600	1	5	3
60	1500	yes	1500	1	7	2
61	250	yes	600	1	16	1
62	200	yes	600	1	7	0
63	200	yes	1000	1	9	2
63	200	yes	600	1	5	0
64	100	yes	600	1	20	5
65	250	yes	600	1	18	1
Percent responding						16%, 14/87
More than 3 hours between MTX and FU						
66	200-600	yes	300-4000	7	43	15
67	20 mg/kg	yes	600	4	29	10
68	40	no	600	4	8	3
68	200	yes	600	4	6	2
69	100	yes	600	4	10	8
70	200-300	yes	900	3	8	5
71	40	no	600	24	43	14
Percent responding						37%, 57/147

only one response was noted in 17 patients with metastatic colorectal cancer given MTX + 5-FU. Other methods of biochemical
modulation, including the use of hydroxyurea, allopurinol,
leucovorin, PALA and thymidine all appear to alter the usual
effects of 5-FU but rarely have these combinations been superior
to 5-FU alone.

In summary, 5-FU leads to an average response rate of 20%
in trials utilizing strict response criteria. Liver metastases appear to
respond as frequently as other metastases. MOF and MOF-Strep,
while reportedly statistically superior to 5-FU in controlled studies
have only a marginal edge. Biochemical modulation with various
chemicals in combination with fluorouracil is an interesting exercise
in tumor biology, but as yet its use has not resulted in markedly

superior response rates compared to 5-FU alone. The use of continuous infusions of 5-FU alone may have some merit, especially in patients with tumors confined to the liver. However, the numbers of patients treated with this modality is still small and its use requires further investigation. For patients with widely metastatic disease due to colorectal carcinoma involving the liver and other organs, therapy remains poor. In this situation, newer investigational agents have to be explored. Investigational agents are probably best used in the patient who has had no prior chemotherapy, since this allows one to detect activity with greater precision and at an earlier point in a disease oriented drug trial. Patients who develop progressive disease on an investigational agent have responded to 5-FU containing regimens with the expected frequency (73). Moreover, survival in patients given investigational drugs is equivalent to that noted in patients given 5-FU (74).

Gastro-intestinal Neoplasia

The gastro-intestinal neoplasia that frequently metastasize to the liver include gastric and pancreatic carcinoma. The drugs commonly used for these tumors include 5-FU, mitomycin C, doxorubicin and the nitrosoureas. Responses have also been noted with etoposide (VP-16) and cisplatin in selected patients with gastric carcinoma. A combination frequently used to treat gastric and pancreatic neoplasms is that of doxorubicin, mitomycin, and fluorouracil (FAM). In 5 trials involving 186 patients with gastric cancer, 57 responses were noted. The addition of a nitrosourea did not improve the response rate. The overall response rate with FAM in patients with gastric cancer with hepatic metastases is similar to that noted in patients without hepatic metastases.

Despite its prevalence, pancreatic cancer does not lend itself well to objective evaluation, and the life expectancy of patients with advanced disease is very poor. With 5-FU based combinations an overall response rate of 20% for advanced pancreatic cancer (22% for patients with a pancreatic carcinoma with liver metastases) can be achieved.

Malignant tumors involving the liver are, in general, associated with a poor prognosis. Nevertheless, using aggressive measures surivival may be improved in selected patients.

Hepatic Artery Infusions

Klopp and co-workers (75) reported on the successful delivery of a drug directly into the hepatic artery in 1950, but it was not until the early 1960s that this approach gained recognition (76-78). In 1965, Sullivan and Zurch (78) reported a 60% response rate in patients with hepatic metastases given hepatic arterial infusions of chemotherapy. Infusions using catheters attached to external pumps have been reported to result in response rates of 32-83% (14, 40, 43, 78-80).

Hepatic artery infusions in patients with metastatic colorectal carcinoma who have not received prior chemotherapy, reportedly result in response rates ranging from 39-75%. The differences in reported response rates depend in large part on the response criteria employed. In fact, in some series, the response rates observed could be increased by as much as 25-33% by applying differing response criteria, and changing definitions of patient eligibility and adequacy. Oberfield reported that responders lived longer, 8.5 months, compared to non-responders who lived a median of 2 months. No dose response relationship was observed in this trial, and prior therapy with 5-FU did not adversely effect the response rate.

Of late, there has been considerable interest in the use of a totally implantable pump to treat hepatic metastases. Neiderhuber *et al.* (81) recently reported an 83% response rate by infusing a fluoropyrimidine into the hepatic artery. Whether this response rate translates into an improved survival for responders is unclear, since in this study survival was measured from the time of diagnosis of metastases and not from the time of therapy, thus making the impact of therapy uncertain. Other investigators (83, 84) have failed to confirm this rate of tumor response. Table 5 (81-94) summarizes the results of trials utilizing hepatic arterial infusions of fluoropyrimidines. Differing response criteria, variations of drugs, drug schedules, and drug delivery techniques may all be important factors which influence the response rate and survival. One important prognostic factor appears to be the extent of hepatic involvement by tumor. In our experience at the New York Medical College (85), we find that prolonged survival can be achieved only if all visible tumor in the liver is surgically resected before infusional chemotherapy. Kemeny *et al.* (83) have also noted that survival is directly related to the extent of hepatic involvement by tumor: patients with less than 20% of the liver involved by tumor survived longer than patients with more than 60% liver involvement, 13.5 months vs. 6 months, p = 0.001. Thus, it is clear that patient selection is critical. Maximum benefit is observed when metastases are confined to the liver. Systemic

TABLE 5
HEPATIC ARTERIAL INFUSIONS OF FLUOROPYRIMIDINES
IN METASTATIC COLORECTAL CARCINOMA

Ref.	*No. Treated*	*% Responding*
43	31	34%
47	10	40%
48	17	41%
81	93	78%
82	51	71%
83	41	36%
84	17	35%
86	48	58%
87	27	33%
88	15	20%
89	8	75%
90	50	83%
91	31	30%
92	18	56%
93	17	29%
94	17	41%
95	26	53%
Total	517	54%

metastases are responsible for mortality if this principle is not observed. In recent studies it has become apparent that using higher doses of intra-hepatic boluses does result in increased toxicity, (95, 96) specifically acid peptic disease and chemical hepatitis. The development of acid-peptic disease and upper GI bleeding may also be related to surgical technique or the presence of portal hypertension. The various side effects noted with hepatic arterial infusions are listed in Table 6.

Whether hepatic arterial infusions are truly superior to systemic infusions is unclear (97). In a prospective multicenter trial (43) 61 patients were randomly assigned to receive either hepatic artery infusions of 5-FU or systemic 5-FU. No patients had received prior chemotherapy and all had disease confined to the liver. The response rate was higher (34%) for the hepatic artery infusion group compared to the systemic group (23%), but this difference did not achieve statistical significance. However, the group receiving systemic infusions was staged non-invasively as opposed to that receiving intra-hepatic therapy, and thus may

---

TABLE 6

COMPLICATIONS OF INTRA-ARTERIAL CHEMOTHERAPY

1. Acid peptic disease
2. Chemical hepatitis/biliary sclerosis.
3. Catheter occlusion, migration, dislodgment.
4. Hemorrhage.
5. Arterial thrombosis.
6. Stenosis of hepatic artery.
7. Pseudoaneurysm of hepatic artery.
8. Localized infection.
9. Pump pocket seroma.
10. Hepatic abscess.
11. Pulmonary atelectasis.
12. Ileus.
13. Acute pancreatitis.
14. Incorrect catheter placement.
15. Stomatitis, diarrhea.
16. Myelosuppression.
17. Nausea and vomiting.

---

have had more patients with advanced disease. Also this trial was biased in that the dose of 5–FU for the hepatic infusion arm was higher in the initial 3 weeks (350 mg/kg over 21 days) compared to the systemic arm (102 mg/kg over 21 days). Despite this apparent bias, myelosuppression and stomatitis were equally frequent in both arms. Nausea, vomiting and diarrhea were three times more frequent in the intra-hepatic arm, and arterial thrombosis occurred in 6% of the arterial infusion cases. Kemeny *et al.* (47) also compared the use of systemic infusion of a fluoropyrimidine to intra-hepatic infusion of the same drug in patients with surgically staged hepatic metastases. The response rate in both the systemic and intra-hepatic infusion arms was equal, but extrahepatic metastases occurred far more frequently in patients receiving an intra-hepatic infusion. Moreover, the incidence of gastrointestinal toxicity, including chemical hepatitis and upper GI bleeding, was significantly higher in the intra-hepatic group. Another similar randomized study (48) is presently in progress, but preliminary data show response rates to be marginally greater in patients given hepatic infusions.

Thus, although response rates may be high in patients given intra-hepatic infusions of fluoropyrimidines, there appears to be no clear cut survival advantage for this group. Systemic toxicity may be lower in patients given hepatic artery infusions, there is substantial morbidity with surgical implantation of catheters and pumps, and gastrointestinal and hepatic toxicity is also greater. Extra-hepatic metastases occur more frequently in patients receiving intra-hepatic therapy. Substantial palliation can be achieved in carefully selected patients given infusions of chemotherapy.

REFERENCES

1. Pikren, JW, Tsukada, Y, Lane, WW: Liver metastases: Analysis of autopsy data. In: *Liver Metastases*, Weiss, L, and Gilbert, HA (Ed.). Chicago: Year Book Medical Publishing, 5:2-18, 1982.

2. Cady, B: Natural history of primary and secondary tumors of the liver. *Semin Oncol, 10:*127-134, 1983.

3. Fidler, J, *et al.*: The biology of cancer invasion and metastases. *Adv Cancer Res, 28:*149-250, 1978.

4. Chabner, B: *Pharmacologic Principles of Cancer Treatment.* Philadelphia: W.B. Saunders Co., 1982.

5. Lokich, JJ: Infusion chemotherapy for cancer. *Curr Conc Oncol, 6:* 3-8, 1984.

6. Skipper, HE, Schakel, IM: Quantitative and cytokinetic studies in experimental tumor models. In: *Cancer Medicine*, Holland, JF, and Frei, E, III (Eds.). Philadelphia: Lea and Febiger, 1973, pp. 629-650.

7. Eckman, WW, Patlack, CS, Fenstermacher, JD: A critical evaluation of principles governing the advantages of intra-arterial infusions. *J Pharmakinet Biopharm, 2:*257-285, 1984.

8. Ensminger, WD, Gyves, JW: Clinical pharmacology of hepatic arterial chemotherapy. *Semin Oncol, 10:*176-182, 1983.

9. Ensminger, WD, Rosowsky, A, Raso, V, *et al.*: A clinical pharmacological evaluation of hepatic arterial infusions of 5-Fluoro-2'-deoxyuridine and 5-Fluorouracil. *Cancer Res, 38:*3784-3792, 1978.

10. Bengmark, S, Rosengren, K: Angiographic study of the collateral circulation to the liver after ligation of the hepatic artery in man. *Am J Surg, 119:*620-624, 1970.

11. Watkins, E, Jr., Hering, AC, Luna, R, *et al.*: The use of intravascular balloon catheters for isolation of the pelvic oxygenator perfusion of cancer chemotherapeutic agents. *Surg, Gynecol, Obstet, 3:*464, 1960.

12. Abrams, HL: The response of neoplastic renal vessels to epinephrine in man. *Radiology, 82:*217, 1964.

13. Blackshear, PJ, Dorman, FD, Blackshear, PL, *et al.*: The design and initial testing of an implantable infusion pump. *Surg, Gynecol, Obstet, 143:* 51-56, 1972.

14. Cady, B, Oberfield, RA: Regional infusion chemotherapy of hepatic metastases from carcinoma of the colon. *Am J Surg, 127:*220-227, 1974.

15. Oberfield, RA, McCraffey, JA, Polio, J, *et al.*: Prolonged and continuous percutaneous intra-arterial hepatic infusion chemotherapy in advanced metastatic liver adenocarcinoma from a colorectal primary. *Cancer, 44:*414-423, 1979.

16. Kemeny, N, Braun, D: Advanced colorectal carcinoma: Clinical and laboratory parameters as indicators of response and survival. *Proc ASCO and AACR, 22:*336, 1981.

17. Sumithran, E, Prathap, K: Hepatocellular carcinoma in the Malaysian Orang Asli. *Cancer, 37:*2263-2266, 1976.

18. Okuda, *et al.*: Primary liver cancers in Japan. *Cancer, 45:*2663-2669, 1980.

19. Purtilo, DT, Gottlieg, LS: Cirrhosis and hepatoma occurring at Boston City Hospital (1917-1968). *Cancer, 32:*458-462, 1973.

20. Blumberg, BS, Larouze, B, London, WT, *et al.*: The relation of infection with the Hepatitis B agent to primary hepatic carcinoma. *Amer J Pathol, 81:*669-682, 1975.

21. Remming, KP: The effectiveness of hepatic artery infusion in treatment of primary hepatobiliary tumors. *Semin Oncol, 10:*199-205, 1983.

22. Cheblewski, R, *et al.*: Clinical and pharmacokinetic aspects of adriamycin (ADR; Adria Laboratories, Dublin, Ohio) and Methyl-CCNU (MCCNU) therapy for biopsy proven hepatoma. *Proc ASCO and AACR, 19:*386, 1978.

23. Moertel, CG: Clinical management of advanced gastric cancer. *Cancer, 36:*675-682, 1975.

24. McIntire, K, *et al.*: Effect of surgical and chemotherapeutic treatment on alpha-feto-protein levels in patients with hepatocellular carcinoma. *Cancer, 37:*677, 1976.

25. Falkson, G, *et al.*: Chemotherapy of primary liver carcinoma. A parallel study in American and African Bantu patients. *Proc ASCO and AACR, 17:*21, 1976.

26. Umsawadi, T, Chainuva, T, Veronuva, T, *et al.*: Combination chemotherapy of hepatocellular carcinoma with 5-FU and Mitomycin C. *Proc ASCO and AACR, 19:*193, 1978.

27. Buroker, TR, *et al.*: Mitomycin C alone and in combination with fluorouracil to the treatment of disseminated gastrointestinal carcinomas. *Med Pediatr Oncol, 4:*35, 1978.

28. Gailani, S, Holland, JF, Falkson, G, *et al.*: Comparison of treatment of metastatic gastrointestinal cancer with 5-FU to a combination of 5-FU with cytosine arabinoside. *Cancer, 29:*1308-1313, 1972.

29. Al-Sarraf, M, *et al.*: Primary liver cancer. *Cancer, 33:*574, 1974.

30. Umsawadi, T, *et al.*: FAP protocol for hepatoma. *Cancer Chemotherap Rep, 59:*1167-1169, 1975.

31. Massey, WH, Fletcher, WS, Judkin, MP, *et al.*: Hepatic artery infu-

sion for metastatic malignancy using percutaneously placed catheters. *Am J Surg, 121:*160-167, 1977.

32. Ansfield, FJ, Ramirez, G, Skibba, JL, *et al.*: Intrahepatic arterial infusion with 5-FU. *Cancer, 28:*1147-1160, 1971.

33. Davis, HL, Ramirez, CS, Ansfield, FJ: Adenocarcinoma of stomach, pancreas, liver, and biliary tracts: Survival of 328 patients treated with fluoropyrimidine therapy. *Cancer, 33:*193-202, 1974.

34. Ong, GB, Chan, PKW: Primary carcinoma of the liver. *Surg, Gynecol, Obstet, 143:*31-38, 1974.

35. Ramming, KP, Sparks, FC, Eilber, FR, Morton, DL: Management of hepatic metastases. *Semin Oncol, 4:*71-80, 1977.

36. Anderson, JM, Patrick, RS, Short, DW, *et al.*: Disappearance of hepatic cancer after intra-arterial fluorouracil. *Br Med J, 3:*454-461, 1972.

37. Cady, B, Oberfield, RA: Regional infusion chemotherapy of hepatic metastases of carcinoma of the colon. *Surg, Gynecol, Obstet, 138:*220-227, 1974.

38. Watkins, E, Khazei, AM, Nebra, KS: Surgical basis for arterial infusion chemotherapy of disseminated carcinoma of the liver. *Surg, Gynecol, Obstet, 130:*581-586, 1970.

39. Ryan, R, Metman, EH, Oberfield, R, Clause, M: Percutaneous infusion of the liver with fluorinated pyrimidine for primary and metastatic cancern. *Bull Cancer (Paris), 64:*409-420, 1970.

40. Reed, M, Vaitkevicius, V, Al Sarraf, M, *et al.*: The practicality of chronic hepatic artery infusion therapy of primary and metastatic hepatic malignancies: Ten year results of 124 patients on a prospective protocol. *Cancer, 47:*402-409, 1981.

41. Kemeny, N, Yagoda, A, Braun, D, *et al.*: Therapy of metastatic colorectal carcinoma with a combination of methyl CCNU, 5-Fluorouracil, vincristine, and streptozotocin (MOF-Strep). *Cancer, 45:*876-881, 1980.

42. Seifert, P, Baker, LH, Reed, MD, *et al.*: Comparison of continuously infused 5-Fluorouracil with bolus injections in patients with colorectal adenocarcinoma. *Cancer, 36:*123, 1975.

43. Grage, TB, Vassilopoulos, P, Shingleton, WW, *et al.*: Results of a prospectively randomized study of hepatic artery infusion with 5-Fluorouracil vs. intravenous 5-Fluorouracil in patients with hepatic metastases from colorectal cancer: A Central Oncology Group Study. *Surg, 86:*550-555, 1979.

44. Moore, G, Bross, I, Ausman, R, *et al.*: Effects of 5-Fluorouracil (NSC 19893) in 389 patients with cancer. *Cancer Chem Rep, 52:*641, 1968.

45. Brennan, MJ, Talley, RW, San Diego, EL, *et al.*: Critical analysis of 594 cancer patients treated with 5-Fluorouracil. In: *Proceedings of the International Symposium on Chemotherapy of Cancer*, Plattner, PA (Ed.). New York: Elsevier, 1964, pp. 118-150.

46. Shah, A, MacDonald, WC, Gudanskas, GA, Sullivan, B: Weekly 48 hour 5-Fluorouracil (5-FU) intravenous infusions in advanced colorectal cancer. *Proc ASCO, 2:*116, 1983.

47. Kemeny, N, Daly, J, Oderman, P, *et al.*: Randomized study of intra-hepatic vs. systemic infusion of fluorodeoxyuridine in patients with liver metastases from colorectal carcinoma. *Proc ASCO, 3:*14, 1984.

48. Stagg, RJ, Friedman, M, Lewis, B, *et al.*: Current status of the NCOG randomized trial of continuous intra-arterial (IA) vs. intra-venous (IV) floxuridine in patients with colorectal carcinoma metastatic to the liver. *Proc ASCO, 3:*148, 1984.

49. Moertel, CG, Schutt, AL, Hahn, GR, *et al.*: Therapy of advanced colorectal cancer with a combination of 5-Fluorouracil, methyl-1-2-ciw (2 chloroethyl)-1-nitrosourea, and vincrisitine, brief communication. *J Natl Cancer Inst, 54:*69, 1975.

50. MacDonald, JS, Kisner, DF, Smythe, T, *et al.*: 5-Fluorouracil (5-FU), methyl CCNU, and vincristine in the treatment of advanced colorectal cancer. Phase II study utilizing weekly 5-FU. *Canc Treat Rep, 60:*1597, 1976.

51. Falkson, G, Falkson, H: Fluorouracil, methyl CCNU, and vincristine in cancer of the colon. *Cancer, 38:*468, 1976.

52. Moertel, CG: Chemotherapy of gastro-intestinal cancer. *NEJM, 229:* 1049, 1978.

53. Engstrom, P, MacIntyre, J, Douglass, H, Jr., *et al.*: Combination chemotherapy of advanced bowel cancer. *Proc ASCO and AACR, 19:*384, 1978.

54. Kemeny, N, Yagoda, A, Golbey, RB: A randomized study of two different schedules of methyl CCNU, 5-FU, and vincristine for metastatic colorectal cancer. *Cancer, 43:*78, 1978.

55. Kemeny, N, Yagoda, A, Braun, D: Metastatic colorectal carcinoma: A prospective randomized trail of methyl CCNU, 5-Fluorouracil (5-FU), and vincristine (MOF) vs. MOF plus streptozotocin (MOF-Strep). *Cancer, 51:* 20-25, 1983.

56. GITSG: Phase II study of Methyl CCNU, vincristine, 5-Fluorouracil and streptozotocin in advanced colorectal cancer. *J Clin Oncol, 2:*770, 1984.

57. Bertino, JR, Sawiki, WL, Lindquist, CA, Gupta, VS: Schedule dependent anti-tumor effects of methotrexate and fluorouracil. *Cancer Res, 37:*327-328, 1977.

58. Rajagopal, RR, Jaffer, A, Bedikian, AY, McKelvey, EM, Bodey, GP: Sequential conventional dose methotrexate (MTX) and fluorouracil (5-FU) in the primary treatment of metastatic colorectal carcinoma. *Proc ASCO, 2:* 125, 1983.

59. Alan, M, Coat, S, Hedley, D, Fox, RM, Rhagavan, RM, Tattersall, MHN: Randomized trial of sequential methotrexate (M) following 5-Fluorouracil (F) vs. F following M. *Proc AACR, 24:*140, 1983.

60. Tisman, G, Wu, SJG: Effectiveness of intermediate dose methotrexate and high dose 5-Fluorouracil as sequential chemotherapy in refractory breast cancer and as primary therapy in metastatic adenocarcinoma of the colon. *Cancer Treat Rep, 64:*829-835, 1980.

61. Cantrell, JE, Brunet, R, Largarde, C: Phase II study of sequential methotrexate–5–FU therapy in advanced measurable colorectal cancer. *Cancer Treat Rep, 66:*1563-1565, 1982.

62. Blumenreich, MS, Woodcock, T, Allegra, M, *et al.*: Sequential therapy with methotrexate (MTX) and fluorouracil (5-FU) for adenocarcinoma of the colon. *Proc ASCO, 1:*102, 1982.

63. Panasci, D, Margolise, R: Sequential methotrexate (MTX) and fluorouracil (FU) in breast and colorectal cancer. Results of increasing the dose of FU. *Proc ASCO, 1:*101, 1982.

64. Hansen, R, Ritch, R, Anderson, T: Sequential methotrexate (MTX), 5-Fluorouracil (5-FU), and leucovorin (LCV) in colorectal cancer. *Proc ASCO, 2:*117, 1983.

65. Burnet, R. Smith, TP, Hoerni, B, Lagarsch, C, Schein, P: Sequential methotexate–5–Fluorouracil in advanced measurable colorectal cancer. Lack of appreciable synergism. *Proc AACR/ASCO, 22:*370, 1981.

66. Drapkin, R, McAloon, E, Lyman, G: Sequential methotrexate (MTX) and 5-Fluorouracil in advanced measurable colorectal cancer. *Proc ASCO, 2:*118, 1982.

67. Weinermann, B, Schipper, H, Bowman, D, Levitt, M: 5-Fluorouracil (F), methotrexate (M), and leucovorin (LR) in the treatment of metastatic colorectal cancer (CRC). *Proc AACR/ASCO, 22:*450, 1981.

68. Solon, A, Vogl, SE, Kaplan, BH, *et al.*: Sequential chemotherapy of advanced colorectal cancer with standard or high dose methotrexate followed by fluorouracil. *Med Ped Oncol, 10:*145-149, 1980.

69. Mehrotra, S, Rosenthal, CJ, Gardner, B: Biochemical modulation of antineoplastic response in colorectal carcinoma: 5-Fluorouracil (F), high dose methotrexate (M) with calcium leucovorin (FML) in two sequences of administration. *Proc ASCO, 1:*100, 1982.

70. Hermann, R, Manigold, C, Rittinghausen, R, Fritze, D, Scheltler, G: Sequential methotrexate (MTX) and 5-Fluorouracil (FU) in colorectal adenocarcinoma. *Proc AACR/ASCO, 22:*457, 1981.

71. Kemeny, N, Ahmed, T, Michaelson, R, *et al.*: Activity of sequential low dose methotrexate and fluorouracil in advanced colorectal carcinoma: Attempt at correlation with tissue and blood levels of phosphoribosylpyro phosphate. *J Clin Oncol, 2:*311-315, 1984.

72. Kemeny, NE: Personal communication.

73. Ahmed, T, Kemeny, N, Michaelson, R, Harper, H: Phase II trial of bisantrene in advanced colorectal carcinoma. *Cancer Treat Ref*, March, 1983.

74. Leichman, L, Fabian, C, O'Bryan, R, *et al.*: Evaluation of 5-FU vs. A phase II drug in metastatic adenocarcinoma of the large bowel. Southwest Oncology Group (SWOG), Study 7940. *Proc ASCO, 2:*120, 1983.

75. Klopp, CT, Alford, TC, Baternan, J, *et al.*: Fractionated intraarterial cancer chemotherapy with methyl bis amine hydrochloride: A preliminary report. *Ann Surg, 132:*811-832, 1950.

76. Clarkson, B, Young, CW, Dierich, W, *et al.*: Effects of continuous

hepatic artery infusion of antimetabolites on primary and metastatic cancer of the liver. *Cancer, 15:*472-488, 1962.

77. Brennan, MJ, Talley, RW, Drake, EH, *et al.*: 5-Fluorouracil treatment of liver metastases by continuous hepatic artery infusion via Couinaud catheter. *Ann Surg, 158:*405-419, 1963.

78. Sullivan, RD, Zurek, WZ: Chemotherapy for liver cancers by protracted ambulatory infusion. *JAMA, 194:*481-486, 1965.

79. Watkins, E, Khazei, AM, Nahra, KS: Surgical basis for arterial infusion chemotherapy of disseminated carcinoma of the liver.

80. Buroker, T, Sawson, M, Correa, J, *et al.*: Hepatic artery infusion of 5-FUDR after prior systemic 5-Fluorouracil. *Cancer Treat Ref, 60:*1277-1279, 1976.

81. Niederhuber, JE, Ensminger, W, Gyves, J, Thrall, J, Walker, S, Cozzi, E: Regional chemotherapy of colorectal carcinoma metastatic to the liver. *Cancer, 53:*1336-1343, 1984.

82. Oberfield, NA: Intraarterial hepatic infusion chemotherapy in metastatic liver cancer. *Semin Oncol, 10:*206-214, 1983.

83. Kemeny, N, Daly, J, Oderman, P: Hepatic artery pump infusion: Toxicity and results in patients with metastatic colorectal carcinoma. *J Clin Oncol, 2:*595-600, 1984.

84. Johnson, LP, Wasserman, PB, Rivkin, LP: FUDR hepatic arterial infusions via an implantable pump for treatment of hepatic disease. *Proc ASCO, 2:*119, 1983.

85. Hodgson, WJ, Mittelman, A, Ahmed, T, Friedland, ML: Combined intrahepatic chemotherapy and surgical debulking for metastatic adenocarcinoma of the liver. *Proc ASCO, 3:*141, 1984.

86. Berger, M: Update on intra-arterial hepatic infusion for metastatic colorectal cancer in a community hospital setting. *Proc ASCO, 3:*136, 1984.

87. Patt, Y, Boddie, A, Soskie, M: Exploration of various floxuridine doses for hepatic arterial infusion through infusaid pump. *Proc ASCO, 3:*137, 1984.

88. Kaneshiro, CA, Kasimis, BS, Moran, E, *et al.*: High dose hepatic artery infusion (HAI) of FUDR: Good tolerance of a systematic dose modification. *Proc ASCO, 3:*139, 1984.

89. Cohen, F, Steinbaum, F, Alpert, J, *et al.*: Treatment of liver metastases from colon cancer using an implantable electronically programmable intrahepatic arterial infusion pump. *Proc ASCO, 3:*139, 1984.

90. Balch, CM, Urist, MM, McGregor, ML: Continuous regional chemotherapy for metastatic colorectal cancer using a totally implantable infusion pump. *Am J Surg, 145:*285, 1983.

91. Levin, B, Karl, R, DuBrow, R, *et al.*: Regional hepatic chemotherapy for metastatic cancer with an implanted drug infusion system. *Clin Res, 30:*783, 1982.

92. Barone, RM, Byfield, JE, Goldfarb, PB, *et al.*: Intra-arterial chemotherapy using an implantable infusion pump and liver irradiation for hepatic metastases. *Cancer, 50:*850-862, 1982.

93. Weiss, GR, Garnick, MB, Osteen, RT, *et al.*: Long term hepatic arterial infusion of 5-Fluorodeoxyuridine for liver metastases using an implantable infusion pump. *J Clin Oncol, 1:*337–344, 1983.

94. Cohen, AM, Greenfield, A, Wood, WC: Treatment of hepatic artery chemotherapy using an implantable drug pump. *Cancer, 51:*2013–2019, 1983.

95. Kemeny, MM, Battifora, H, Blaney, DW, *et al.*: Sclerosing cholangitis after continuous hepatic artery infusion with FUDR. *Ann Surg, 202:*176–181, 1985.

96. Johnson, LP, Rivkin, SE: The implanted pump in metastatic colorectal cancer of the liver. Risk vs. Benefit. *Am J Surg, 149:*595–598, 1985.

97. Schwartz, SI, Torres, LS, McCune, CS: Assessment of treatment of intrahepatic malignancies using chemotherapy in an implantable pump. *Ann Surg, 201:*560–567, 1985.

CHITTI MOORTHY, M.D.
RAMON KAUL, M.D.
DATTATREUYUDU NORI, M.D.

CHAPTER 13

Role of Radiation Therapy in Primary and Metastatic Liver Malignancies

RADIATION TOLERANCE OF NORMAL LIVER

The majority of liver tumors (both primary and metastatic) are far advanced at the time of presentation, involving both lobes and presenting in multiple foci thus making them unresectable. Currently available chemotherapeutic agents have consistently failed to show response rates over 15–25%. The experience with hepatic radiation for primary liver tumors shows occasional successes, but no consistent long term responses or improved survivals. Radiation for hepatic metastases has shown encouraging results with significant palliation of distressing signs and symptoms.

To understand the scope and the limitations of successful therapy with radiation to the liver, it is imperative to have a clear understanding of the limitations imposed by the radiation tolerance of normal liver, and also other adjacent dose constraining radiosensitive normal tissues that cannot be excluded from the hepatic radiation field due to their anatomical location, sheltered by liver acting like an umbrella (e.g., kidneys TTD 5/5 is 2,000 rads, TTD 50/5 is 250 rads at 200r/fx, 5 fx/wk).

Historically, an initial misconseption of hepatic radioresistance as stated by Ellinger in 1945 was based on extremely high doses of radiation (tens of thousands of roentgens) reported to be required to produce clinicopathologic hepatic disease in experimental animals (8) and the rarity of clinical cases of hepatic disease in humans at erythema doses (8, 44). Though the syndrome of radiation hepatitis was described by Ingold, *et al.* in 1964, the first report of an effect of irradiation on the human liver was by Case and Warthin in 1924 who described inflammation of the bile duct epithelium with little change in the blood vessels or hepatic cells in three patients treated with radiation for gastric carcinoma (7).

In 1942 Warren (50) reported a review of results from animal work and stated "one could draw no definite conclusions as to the sensitivity of human liver to irradiation." He also described no correlation between the dose of radiation and the degree of hepatic injury.

Brick (5) in 1955 reported necrosis of liver as the most common finding and fibrosis in 3 cases out of 9 autopsies on radiated liver specimens which received more than 5,000 rads to the left lobe of the liver. The Memorial Series (40) (36 cases) and the Stanford Series (23) (40 cases) treating whole liver at 1,000 rads per week observed 3 cases of radiation hepatitis occurring at 3,500 rads and 1 at 3,000 rads. Kaplan and Bagshaw (24) reported 2 cases of radiation hepatitis at doses between 2,500–3,000 rads (Table 1). In the Stanford Series criteria employed in the diagnosis of radiation hepatitis included significant liver function alterations and a needle biopsy of the liver showing radiation induced liver changes.

With the information available in the literature, some authors suggest maximum dose ranges for whole liver radiation depending on whether radiation is given alone or in combination with chemotherapy, and whether the intent is prophylactic or treatment of the involved organ. For the uninvolved organ maximum dosage

TABLE 1
RADIATION HEPATITIS; INCIDENCE vs. DOSE
Memorial Series (40) and Stanford Series (23)

Dose in Rads	Incidence of Radiation Hepatitis		
	Ingold, et al. (Stanford)		Phillips & Murikami (Memorial)
3000	11.0%	(1/9)	0/9
3000–3500	22.2%	(2/9)	1/11
3500–4000	38.8%*	(7/18)	0/6
4000	75.0%†	(3/4)	
Totals	32.5%	(13/40)	1/36

* 1 death at 3850 rads, 2 cases of persistent damage at 3900 rads and 3975

† 2 patients died at 4000 rads and 5100 rads

None of the cases of either portal or persistent radiation hepatitis have occurred at or below 3500 rads.

is 3,000–3,500 rads in 3½ weeks (Ingold, *et al.*) (23), 3,000 rads in 2 weeks according to Whitley (52), 2,500 rads in 10 fractions in 2 weeks along with 5 FUDR (Webber) (51) and 1,500–2,400 rads in 5–8 fractions when used with 5-FU, and Adriamycin (Friedman) (17).

ROLE OF EXTERNAL RADIATION (XRT) IN PRIMARY HEPATIC MALIGNANCIES

Primary hepatocellular carcinoma (hepatoma) is a major cause of cancer deaths in Asia and Africa, though it is an uncommon malignancy in the United States. Its management continues to baffle the surgeons, radiation oncologists and medical oncologists alike. The criteria for treating primary liver cancer revolves about several prognostic factors. First, the general condition of the patient and his metabolic status especially the liver function status. Second, the degree of involvement of the liver: i.e., whether unilobar or bilobar, single focus or multicentric presentation. Third, the presence of distant metastases. Extensive liver tumor or distant metastases, jaundice, hypoalbuminemia, ascites, varices, portal hypertension, hypersplenism, poor performance status, adenocarcinoma histology constitute unfavorable prognostic factors (17). Patients with some of these poor prognostic factors are poor risk surgical candidates, and have poor tolerance to radiation and chemotherapy.

The independent reports on hepatic lobectomy by Lortat-Jacobs and Robert (32) in France and Quattlebaum (43) in the United States two decades ago sparked lively interest in the hepatoma management. Since then, some long term survivors were reported in the literature after successful curative resection of localized tumors. At present, the treatment of choice for early hepatoma confined to one lobe is complete surgical excision. Nevertheless, the majority of hepatic tumors are unsuitable for surgical extirpation due to bilobar involvement, multicentric origin, and adjacent organ involvement and distant spread. While objective responses have been seen after chemotherapy, there has been no significant increase in the length of survival. The management in the majority of these patients has been palliative. The role of radiation has also remained palliative in view of the constraints against delivering high tumoricidal radiation doses, imposed by the limits of liver tolerance and limits of tolerance to radiation of other normal tissues.

Ariel in 1956 claimed symptomatic response lasting from 9 months to 50 months in 5 of 10 patients (Table 2) with primary liver cell cancer treated with XRT! On the other hand, in 1954, Cohen and colleagues (6) in Johannesburg treated 9 patients with primary liver cancer with 220kv radiation through 2 or more large fields of 20x20 cm given tissue dose (calculated at the center of the liver) of 2,500–4,000 rads in 5–19 days. One patient died shortly after treatment and eight survived from 3–34 weeks.

TABLE 2
PRIMARY HEPATOMAS: SURVIVAL DATA
IN POST-RADIATION RESPONDERS AND NON-RESPONDERS*

Age/Sex	Disease Extent	Survival Duration	Remarks
RESPONDERS			
30 yr. F	Bilobar	4 yrs. & 8 mos.	Decrease in size of the mass, sense well being
30 yr. F	Right lobe	4 yrs. & 7mos.	Prolonged symptom control, mass smaller & moveable
48 yr. F	Bilobar	4 yrs.	Marked response, relief of all symptoms, recurrence treated with repeat XRT, good response
25 yr. F	Right lobe	1 yr. & 4 mos.	Marked shrinkage of mets, Mets to OS pubis also responded well
27 yr. F	Extensive bilobar	9 mos.	Jaundice subsided, appetite improved, sense of well being. No control of ascites
NON-RESPONDERS			
14 yr. F	Bilobar	1 yr.	Marked ascites
35 yr. F	Bilobar	4 mos.	Poor tolerance to therapy - metabolically poor
50 yr. M		4 mos.	Hematemasis
41 yr. F	Bilobar	3 mos.	No response
40 yr. M	Right lobe	2–5 mos.	No beneficial response

Responders had average survival duration of 3–5 years.
Non–responders had average survival duration of 5 months.

Modified from Ariel, IM and Pack, G.

Autopsies showed disappearance of all liver tissue (radiation hepatectomy). The patients died of liver failure. However, accurate documentation by means of CT scanning may allow more focused radiation to be given, thus keeping side-effects to a liver, perhaps already damaged by cirrhosis, to a minimum (46).

In 1960 Phillips and Murikami (40) reported the results of radiation with ortho-voltage treatment to a tumor dose of 2,000–3,000 rads. No response was noted under 2,000 rads. In their 22 patients who received approximately 3,000 rads in 3 weeks, regression was achieved in 14 cases (64%) with marked response in 9 cases (40%). Half of the patients had excellent symptomatic relief, and an additional 5 patients had partial symptomatic relief. Average survival duration was one year with two long term survivors at 36 months and 45 months.

In 1966 the Primary Liver Cancer Research Unit (12–15) (PLCRU) was founded and the clinical trials were conducted in South Africa. Fifteen of 19 patients were treated by abdominal trunk bridge technique consisting of 3 fields each, measuring 20x20 cm using 240 kv maximum self rectified unit. A skin dose of 4,000 rads yielded a whole liver dose of 3,200 rads. Twenty-seven of 59 patients were treated with Co 60 using two large fields for a dose of 1,200 rads in 4 fractions in 17 days to 4,500 rads in 15 fractions in 41 days. Median total dose was 3,600 rads in 31 days. The median survivals showed no improvement over deep x-ray therapy (78 days to 120 days).

El-Domeiri, *et al.* in 1971 published a series of 137 patients from Memorial Sloan Kettering Cancer Center over a period of 20 years (10). One hundred five (76%) patients were unresectable. All were untreated and died within 6 months. The patients who received radiation (30% of the total) survived longer than 6 months.

Based on the results of responses and toxicity, a radiation dose schedule consisting of 2,500 rads in 2½ weeks to 3,000 rads in 3-4 weeks delivered through multiple portals (AP–PA and right lateral portal when indicated) may be well tolerated. A boost dose of 400–500 rads to a small field over the gross residual tumor may be indicated depending upon the size of the tumor and prior or concomitant therapy. There is not enough accumulated experience with radiation on partially resected and regenerating liver tissue, therefore caution is advocated in these situations.

Due to the lack of consistently significant survival enhancement despite encouraging loco-regional disease responses to radiation there is a growing trend to combine chemotherapy and radiation in an attempt to achieve loco-regional tumor control by R.T. (which would mean less tumor burden for chemotherapy) and also take advantage of possible potentiating effect of chemotherapy to aid in radiosensitization. Friedman and his co-workers in the Northern California Oncology Group (NCOG) (18) compared intrahepatic arterial doxorubicin and 5-FU with whole liver radiation therapy (300 rads/dxx7) in 13 patients. Objective regression was seen in 6 for up to 15 months; 5 had stable disease for up to 7 months; 11 of the 13 also had symptomatic improvement. NCOG recently conducted a three arm randomized study of R.T. alone vs. R.T. and chemotherapy (18) (Table 3). The toxicity with gastritis and anemia were acute toxic effects. Significant leukopenia or thrombocytopenia were not encountered. There was no documented incidence of radiation hepatitis or nephritis.

TABLE 3
PRIMARY HEPATOMA
COMBINATION CHEMOTHERAPY PLUS RADIATION
(INTRA-ARTERIAL vs. INTRAVENOUS INFUSION)*

Chemo	Whole Liver Radiation	Partial Responders
Adria + 1A 5-FU + MMC	300 r/dx 7 = 2100 r	1/8 (12.5%)
Adria + IV 5-FU + MMC	300 r/dx 7 = 2100 r	6/12 (50%)
	300 r/dx 7 = 2100 r	0/10

Friedman, et al. (17, 20)

Primary Liver Tumors in Infancy and Childhood

Surgical resection is again the choice of treatment for resectable localized tumors. Thirty to 50% of these tumors are localized to liver and are amenable for resection. The reported 5 year survival rate in Foster's series was 30% (16). Though long term survivals are not frequently reported with combination chemotherapy and radiation regimens, limited palliation and prolongation of life from 12-24 months can be achieved in some patients (48).

In this group appropriate utilization of aggressive combined modality therapy may reduce loco-regional failures and improve survival rates. These modalities include surgery for localized resectable tumors; postoperative radiation and adjuvant chemotherapy for multicentric disease, positive surgical margins, bilobar involvement, and direct extension to adjacent viscera. For locally advanced disease at presentation, debulking chemotherapy and/or radiation followed by surgical resection in patients who demonstrate tumor reduction to resectable degree documented by CT scan may be a logical approach.

ROLE OF EXTERNAL RADIATION
FOR HEPATIC METASTASES

Although surgical resection may benefit a select group of patients with solitary or a minimal number of lesions confined to one lobe the proportion of patients eligible for such a procedure is low. Bleeding was a major problem of surgical resection with an expected 25% operative mortality rate (29). Thus, palliation of symptoms in most of these patients requires modest doses of radiation, usually delivered to the entire organ. Factors that influence the treatment of metastatic liver cancer are: 1) The ability to control the primary tumor. 2) Time of appearance of the metastases whether before, during or after the diagnosis and treatment of the primary tumor. 3) The gross characteristics of the growth whether nodules (solitary or multiple) or diffuse infiltration. 4) The extent of the liver involvement whether one lobe or more than one lobe. Metastases seldom break through the liver capsule and extend to contiguous structures. 5) The biologic effect of the metastases; certain metastatic growths within the liver (carcinoid tumor) may occupy large segments of the liver without appreciably damaging the remainder of the hepatic structure or function, whereas others will have a profound effect adversely affecting the liver. 6) The blood supply to the metastasis. 7) Metabolic status of the patient. Ascites is usually an ominous sign. Prolonged severe jaundice is an unfavorable factor. 8) The condition of the remaining normal liver, e.g., cirrhosis. 9) The histological type of the primary tumor markedly influences the degree of response to therapy. Lymphomatous infiltration, leukemias, neuroblastomas, seminomatous testicular tumors respond well to radiation. Squamous cancers from bronchus and cervix may respond fairly well. Adenocarcinoma (stomach, rectum, pancreas, breast) may show poor response.

Case and Warthin in 1921 were the first to report the use of radiation in the palliative management of hepatic metastases (7). Later Phillips and Karnofsky (41) in 1954 reported the results of roentgen therapy of hepatic metastases in a series of 36 patients treated with 2,000-3,750 rads in 8-22 days at 250 rad fractions. Seventy-two percent of the patients achieved pain relief and 47% had improvement in the liver function tests. The documented radiation liver damage was found in one patient who received 3,500 rads whole liver radiation. One patient who had both kidneys included in the radiation therapy field died of radiation nephritis. Prasad and colleagues (42) claim 95% symptomatic improvement in patients who completed therapy (19 of 20) and 70% improvement when all patients in the series are included (19 of 27 patients, 2,500 rad in 3-3½ weeks). Improvement in ascites was noticed in 50% (4 of 8) and in bilirubin levels in 28% (2 of 7). There was no significant improvement in survivals compared to untreated group. Average survival was 4 months. From the Netherlands in 1975, Turek-Mai Scheider and Kazem (33) reported an overall response rate of over 90% of 11 patients who received 150 r/day (6 patients received 2,500 rads in 3 weeks and 5 patients between 1,200-2,000 rads total doses). Six of 6 patients who received 2,500 rads and 2 of 5 patients who received less than 2,000 rads showed good response (72%) described as complete symptom relief, normalization or substantial improvement of LFT's and liver scans. Additionally, 2 patients who received 1,200 and 1,600 rads had moderate response described as partial symptom relief, improvement of LFT's and reduction in size of metastases on liver scans. No evidence of radiation hepatitis was noticed at autopsy. The results from this study seem to indicate significant palliation can be achieved between 1,800-2,500 rads.

JCRT series reported (in 1978 by Sherman, Weichselbaum, *et al.*) (47) a review of 55 patients who were treated with approximately 2,400 rads to the whole liver at 300 rad daily dose. Thirty-one patients received concomitant chemotherapy and 14 were prior chemotherapy failures. Sixty-four percent had massive liver involvement and 92% were adenocarcinoma metastatic to the liver. There was 89% response with 44% showing excellent response, 90% pain relief, decreased liver size and improvement in liver function tests. The median survival was 9 months for the excellent response group and 2.5 months for non-responders (4.5 months for overall group). Palliation of symptoms lasted for the duration of the patients' survival thus indicating a high palliative index. There were no cases of radiation hepatitis. The common side effects were nausea and vomiting.

The median survival of patients having an excellent response to radiation was comparable to that of patients having regional arterial chemotherapy. The overall complication rate of those patients completing therapy was 12%. RTOG carried out a multi-institutional pilot study of palliative radiation for hepatic metastases and the results were reported in 1981 by Borgett, Gelber, Brady, *et al.* (4). From May 1976 to July 1980, 109 patients from 20 institutions were analyzed. (Solitary liver metastases received 3,040 rads in 19 fractions or 3,000 rads in 15 fractions followed by an optional 2,000/rad 10 fractions boost to residual disease. Those with solitary hepatic metastases plus other sites of metastases or with multiple hepatic metastases received 3,000 rads/15 fractions, 2,560 rad/16 fractions, 2,000 rad/10 fractions, or 2,100 rad/7 fractions.) Pain relief was observed in 55%, LFT, bilirubin, SGOT, alkaline phosphatase improvement in 40%; palpable liver mass reduction in 49%, improvement in performance status in 25% and weakness, fatigue improvement in 19%. There were no documented cases of radiation induced hepatitis, nephritis or pneumonitis. Pain relief occurred within 2 weeks in 77% of the responders. The response rates were more frequent for patients with severe symptoms than for those whose symptoms were initially mild. Improvement in patients with mild, moderate and severe pain was seen in 27%, 64% and 70% respectively. Ambulatory patients responded better. Primary site, extent of metastases and treatment regimen did not significantly affect the pain relief. This study seems to suggest that whole liver radiation can be given quickly so that prolonged hospitalization with all associated psychological and economic hardships may be avoided. Radiation is also a relatively safe way to treat metastatic hormone–secreting tumors since the hormone spillage associated with acute injury, as in embolization or anesthesia, does not occur (49).

External Radiation with Hypoxic Cell Sensitizer (Misonidazole) for Liver Metastases

A Phase II RTOG Study (30), utilizing Misonidazole (1.5 gr/m^2 daily dose) as radiation sensitizer plus whole liver radiation of 2,100 rads, reported pain relief (76%), improved Karnofsky status (58%), alkaline phosphatase level reduction (42%), bilirubin level reduction (60%) and hepatic size reduction (32%) (Table 4). A prospective randomized study of hepatic radiation and Misonidazole vs. hepatic irradiation alone is presently being done by the RTOG.

TABLE 4
HEPATIC METASTASES
MISONIDAZOLE plus RADIATION.
ASSESSMENT OF PALLIATION RESPONSE

Presentation	Relief/Improvement		Complete Improvement	% Worsened
Signs/Symptoms				
Abdominal pain	17/23	(74%)	65%	8%
Nausea/vomiting	6/10	(60%)	60%	15%
Abdominal distention	8/15	(53%)	40%	10%
Jaundice	1/6	(17%)	17%	15%
Ascites	3/5	(60%)	60%	12%
Anorexia	8/22	(36%)	36%	15%
Weakness/fatigue	8/23	(35%)	30%	32%
Fever/night sweats	5/6	(83%)	83%	12%
Liver size		(32%)		
Liver Function				
Alkaline phosphatase		(42%)		
Bilirubin levels		(60%)		
Performance Status		(58%)		

1. These responses were assessments at the 4th week.
2. The symptom complex relief lasted most of the patients remaining life span. Palliation index 88% in patients with minimal symptoms and 72% in patients with marked symptoms.
3. No significant additional morbidity from the sensitizer and no evidence of radiation induced hepatic damage.

Combined (Chemotherapy and Radiation) Treatment Approach for Hepatic Metastasis

Some of the recent trials in management of liver metastases are aimed at enhancing the response through intravenous and intra-arterial chemotherapy along with radiation. Freidman, Cassidy and colleagues (18, 19) reported 43% improvement in liver size. (Utilizing 1,500–2,100 rad at 300 rad/fx + concomitant 5-FU and Adriamycin.) Almost all patients achieved pain relief and improved liver function tests. Toxicity included nausea, fever, moderate WBC and platelet count suppression, but no documented hepatic injury. Table 5 briefly outlines some of the recent clinical results of combined approach therapy.

TABLE 5
HEPATIC METASTASES
COMBINED RADIATION AND INTRA-ARTERIAL CHEMOTHERAPY

Radiation Schedule	Chemo Schedule	Response		Authors References
		No.	%	
1500-2100r, 300/d/1-2 wk	5-FU, 10 mg/kg/d Total dose 2660-8000 mg	10/21	48%	Friedman, Cassidy *et al.* (19, 20)
	Adria, 2.5-10 mg/kg/d Total dose 21-85 mg			
2500-3000r, 250-300/d/2 wk	5-FU, mg/d or FUDR 0.5 mg/kg/d during radiation	10/16	62%	Lokich, Kinsella *et al.* (31)
2500 r, 250/d/2wk	FUDR - 25 mg/d, 300-500 mg/d	13/25	54%	Weber Solderberg** *et al.* (51)
300r/250r/d/2wk	5-FU, 6-10 mg/kg/day	7/10	70%	Barone, Byfield* *et al.* (3)

(49/85 = 58% overall response)

*Colon primaries metastatic to liver
**Median survival in responders was 11 months (Weber, *et al.*) (51).

Radiation Technique

The radiation dose of 2,500–3,000 rads are given at 200–300 rad fractions to the whole liver utilizing AP–PA fields, the size of the field determined by the palpation and the liver scan. A right kidney block is used at 1,800–2,000 rads. This should be a full kidney block if the IVP indicates that the liver covers the entire kidney. Sometimes an upper pole block is sufficient on its own. A third field may be added through the right lateral direction to avoid kidneys. Field size should be reduced and tailored to match the reduction in liver size in response to radiation, or a boost field is added as needed (Figure 13.1).

RADIOISOTOPE THERAPY IN HEPATIC MALIGNANCY

Efforts have been made to produce palliation and control of hepatic malignancy through high local radiation dose delivered by the introduction of radioactive isotopes through percutaneous, intravenous, hepatic intra–arterial or superior mesenteric arterial routes. Studies have been conducted utilizing Yttrium 90 (Y–90) colloidal and chromic phosphate (P–32, CrPO4), or colloidal gold (Au 198). The concept of selective localization and primary hepatic radiation injury to the central veins of the liver lobules and the tendency of the early foci of Hodgkin's disease of the liver to develop in the region of the periportal triad and peripheral sinusoids, have provided the clue for possible effective irradiation of the foci with internally deposited radioactive particulate material. This permits a dose gradient which is expected to be minimal in the central vein region and maximal in periportal triad and periphery of the liver lobule, in the region of maximal uptake by the Kupffer cells. (This dose gradient may afford a significant degree of protection to the radiosensitive elements of the central veins at tumoricidal doses of Hodgkin's disease.)

Intravenous Au–198 studies were initiated at Stanford in 1965. There appeared to be some response in lymphomas, but hematopoietic depression became a serious problem. The technique was discontinued in 1972.

Yttrium–90 is a pure beta emitter (0.9367 MEV energy) with 64.2 hours half life and 3.86 days average life (64.2.693). The isotope is firmly bound to resin microspheres of 15 microns in diameter. Therefore, they may not pass through the capillaries. It

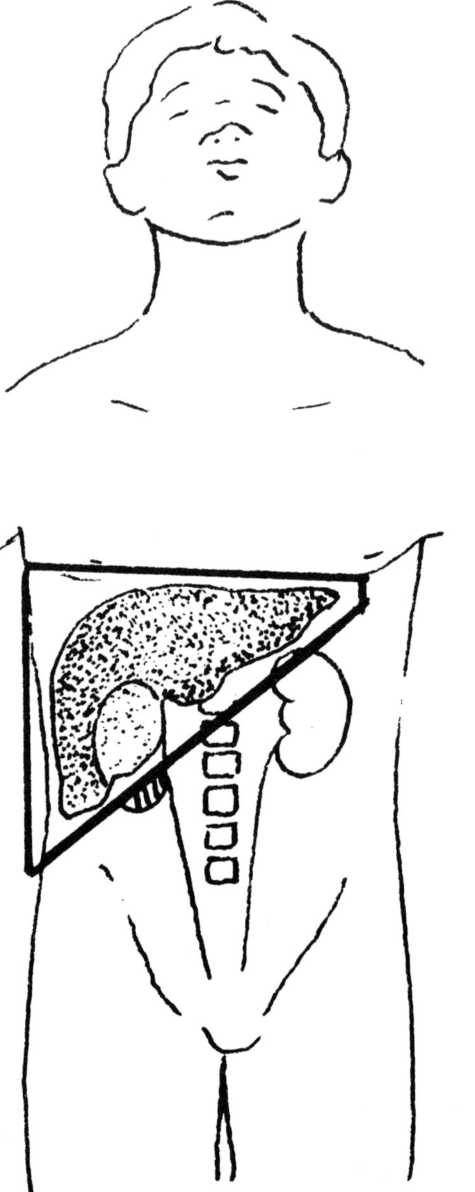

Figure 13.1. Radiation field arrangement for hepatic radiotherapy.

has low specific gravity so that the microspheres stay in suspension in 10% dextran. The dosimietry (34) is based on the estimated weight of liver in grams which is determined by the body weight or body surface area and by the extent of liver enlargement. Assuming uniform distribution of the isotope within the liver the absorbed dose for each gram of tissue is 182 rads/milicurie of the isotope. The quantity of isotope required is calculated using the formula:

$$\text{isotope in microcuries} = \frac{\text{desired dose (rads) x organ weight (grams)}}{182}$$

Rationale

Once infused into the hepatic arterial supply, Y-90 microspheres travel through the blood stream and lodge in the end capillaries of the hepatic parenchyma. This enables four times more concentraion of Y-90 in vascular tumors than in normal liver — a gradient essential for higher therapeutic ratio.

Procedure

The Y-90 microsphere isotope suspension is thoroughly homogenized by using a magnetic homogenizer or by rapid agitation of the vial prior to withdrawal of the isotope into the lead shielded syringe. (The isotope is produced, tested for sterility and calibrated at Medical Research Foundation, Atlanta, GA.) The isotope suspension is then injected through the cannulated hepatic artery or remote catheter cannulization of the hepatic artery. Concomitant use of vasoconstrictor agents can further increase the differential uptake in the tumor compared with the normal liver.

Results

The distribution and localization of the isotope was assessed by Bremsstrahlung scans. Ariel and Padula (1) treated 65 patients (100-150 mci YT 90 on day 1 plus 15 day continuous intra-arterial 5-FU at 1 G/day) and claim 60% subjective response, 40% objective response and a median survival of over 13 months. Toxicity was limited to nausea, vomiting, diarrhea and stomatitis. Grady (12) reported a 68% objective tumor regression and 4 of 25 long term survivors (21). Mantravadi, Strigos, *et al.* (34, 35) utilized percutaneous catheterization of liver via the transfemoral arterial route. Of 15 patients in the series, 9 had enlarged liver prior to treatment, 3 showed reduction in liver size, 2 had no change and 4 had progression of hepatomegaly (Figures 13.2, 13.3, and 13.4). The results of these studies appear to identify a select group of patients with liver metastases who may benefit from Y-90 therapy. These patients had a well vascularized tumor, no extrahepatic disease, a Karnofsky performance of 70% or above and the primary site was in the colon or stomach.

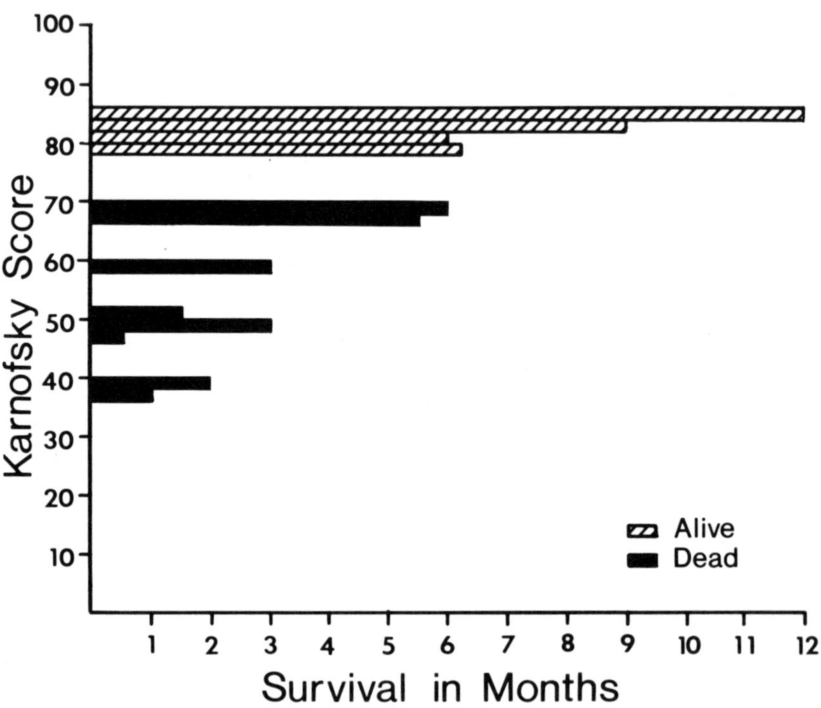

Figure 13.2. Treatment results of intra-arterial Yttrium-90 as related to the general condition of the patient expressed as a Karnofsky score. (Reproduced by kind permission of Rao Mantravadi, M.D., Chicago, Illinois.)

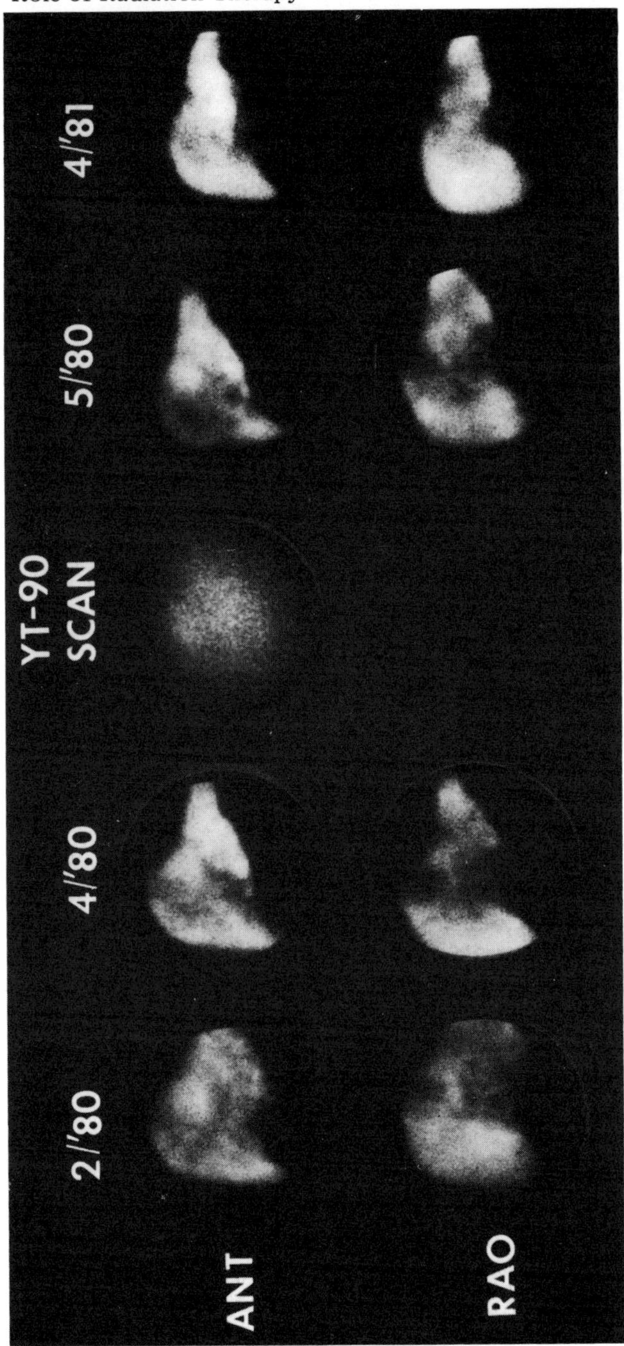

Figure 13.3. Serial liver scans of a patient with hepatoma treated with Yttrium–90. The patient is now a 4–year survivor. (Reproduced by kind permission of Rao Mantravadi, M.D., Chicago, Illinois.)

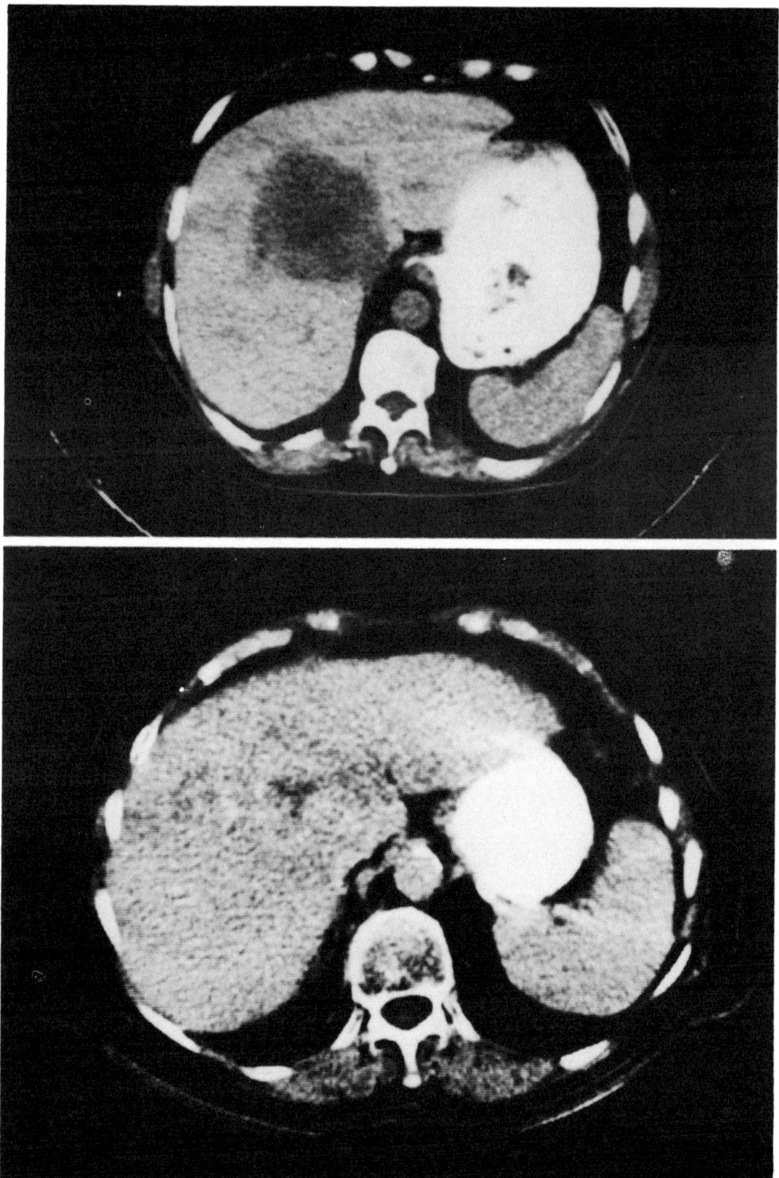

Figure 13.4. Pre- and post-treatment CT scans after therapy with Yttrium-90. Note the near total disappearance of the tumor mass 9 months following treatment. (Reproduced by kind permission of Rao Mantravadi, M.D., Chicago, Illinois.)

Radioactive Chromic Phosphate (P-32)

P-32 chromic phosphate in colloidal form has a particle size of 0.5-1.5 and a physical half life of 14.3 days. It decays into Sr-32 by emitting a beta particle (maximum energy of 1.71 MEV, mean energy pf .695 MEV), with a maximum range of 8 mm and an average range of 2 mm in tissue. There is sufficient Bremsstrahlung radiation for imaging and evaluation of isotope localization (Figure 13.5).

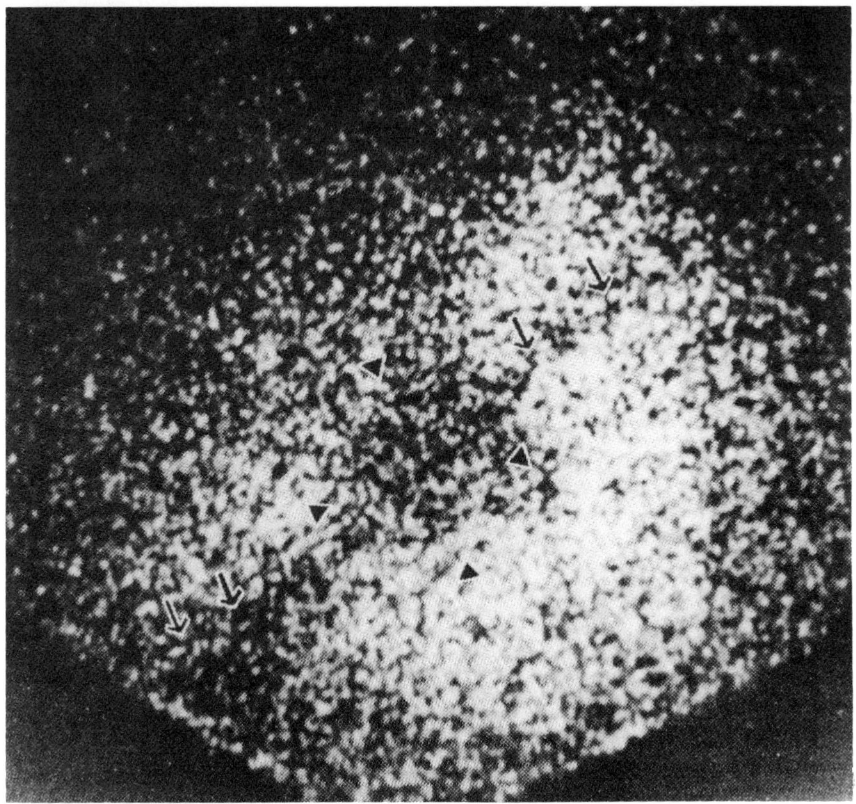

Figure 13.5. Bremsstrahlung scan of the liver following P-32 infusion. The 5 x 5 cm lead marker corresponds to a central defect shown by arrowheads and the arrows show the subcostal plane. (Reproduced by kind permission of the Radiological Society of North America from *Radiology, 148:*555-559, 1983.)

Intra-arterial injection of this isotope offers the advantages of accessibility, homogenous isotope distribution, and decreased uptake by other organs particularly the bone marrow and spleen. Mantravadi, Spigo, *et al.* (35) recently reported their work in progress utilizing elective superior mesenteric intra-arterial P-32 for prevention of liver metastases in high risk colorectal cancers postoperatively. There are several reasons for such therapy. First, following resection of the primary tumor, liver metastases constitute the only site of distant spread in 39% of patients. Second, if the tumor and the draining lymph nodes were completely resected, then treatment failure involving the liver represents micro metastases. These might have been present at surgery and would represent a low tumor burden more likely to respond to treatment. Third, intra-arterial P-32 with its high concentration in liver, with its dose differential (tumor vs. normal tissue) would offer higher therapeutic potential. The dose of P-32 required was calculated by the formula:

$$\text{dose (Mci)} = \frac{\text{desired dose (rads x organ weight in grams)}}{730}$$

because the absorbed dose for each gram of liver tissue was calculated as 730 rad/Mci (197GY/MBq).

The dose selected by these authors was 4,500 rad liver dose over the life of the isotope. Once the isotope is injected through the selectively catheterized superior mesenteric artery, it readily passes through the wall of small bowel into the superior mesenteric vein and then into the portal vein (Figures 13.6 and 13.7). Then the colloid particles reaching liver are phago-cytozed by the Kupffer cells. The isotope is expected to pass the same route that colon carcinoma cells would take during hematogenous spread. Twenty-three patients (35) were treated in this fashion between July 1982 and July 1983 and to date indicate no untoward reactions or evidence of radiation hepatic injury. Of the patients, 3 died (1 with myocardial infarction, 2 with local recurrence, but had no metastases in the liver). At surgery only 2 patients had isolated liver metastases and these were resected. The rest of the patients had no documented metastases prior to the therapy.

None of the 23 patients treated on P-32 so far developed any evidence of liver metastases. Though the preliminary results seem very impressive longer follow up may shed some light on the prophylactic potential of this simple technique.

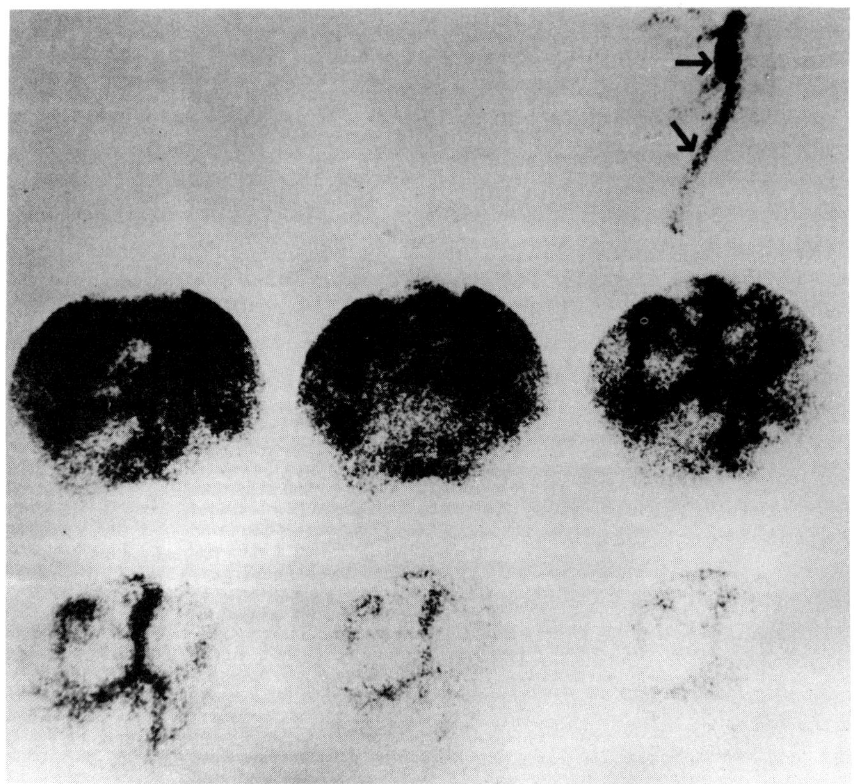

Figure 13.6. Superior mesenteric radionuclide angiogram with TC-99m sulfur colloid. Each frame represents a 10-second acquisition. The arrows demonstrate the superior mesenteric artery. (Reproduced by kind permission of the Radiological Society of North America from *Radiology, 148:*555, 1983.)

RADIO-LABELED ANTIBODY THERAPY

Radio-labeled I-131 Antibody (IgG) can be selectively targeted to tumor associated antigens in malignant tissue. Clinical studies were under way with this unique method in management of liver tumors. The tumor effective (27, 36, 37, 38, 39) half life of I-131 Antibody in hepatoma is 3-3.5 days. It has been estimated that the hepatoma tumor dose per administered cycle of I-131 antibody to be 1,100 rads and 1-1.5 rad of total body irradiation for every milicurie of I-131 Antibody administered (27).

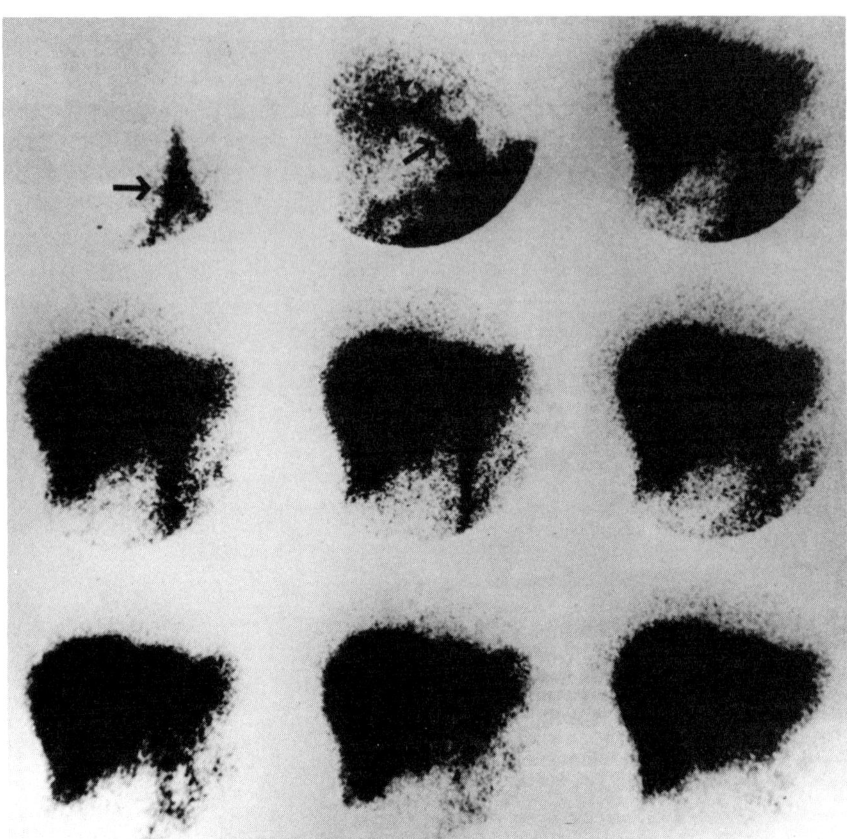

Figure 13.7. Superior mesenteric radionuclide venogram with TC-99m sulfur colloid. Note the rapid transit through the venous system, with subsequent localization in the liver but not in the spleen. The arrows show a superior mesenteric vein and the arrowheads the portal vein. (Reproduced by kind permission of the Radiological Society of North America from *Radiology*, *148:*555, 1983.)

Recently, a Phase I-II Study of Isotope immunoglobulin was conducted (37-157 Mci of I-131 labeled antibody) in 18 patients. The dose limiting factor was the development of thrombocytopenia due to TB I of free circulating radio-labeled antibody (9). Liver function studies revealed transient elevation in 72% of the patients due to acute radiation effects. An objective antitumor response was noticed in 6 of 9 patients (Figure 13.8). This study

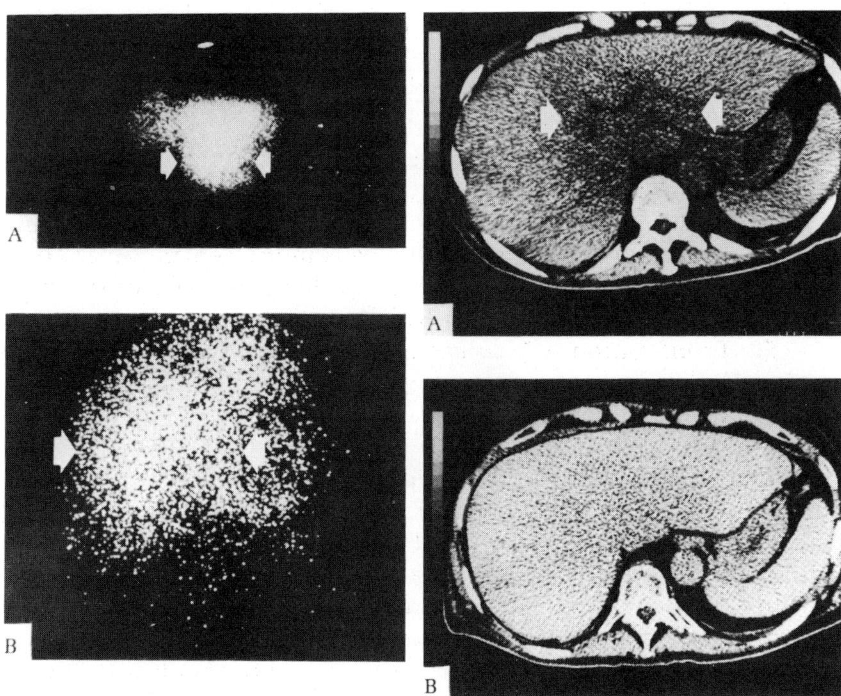

Figure 13.8. The left side of this illustration shows in A the technicium scan of a patient with a hepatoma with a small region of normal liver as demonstrated by the arrows. The radio-immunoglobulin scan B of the same patient showing the malignant tumor in the area of the arrows after administration of I-131 Antiferratin IgG (rabbit). The right hand side of the illustration shows the computerized axial tomograph of the same patient's liver with marked tumor involvement shown by the Arrows A. The same tomographic cut is then taken from the patient following radio-labeled antibody B. (Reproduced by kind permission of *Comprehensive Therapy, 10:*9-10, 1984.)

suggests that the dose administered can be reduced. The specific activity (isotope-antibody ratio) can be increased and isotope labeled antibody can be fractionated.

RADIATION INJURY TO LIVER

The radiation dose schedules for hepatic tolerance/injury were discussed in the early part of this chapter and here we will consider the radiation induced hepatic lesion (acute and chronic), its pathology, pathophysiology, clinical syndrome, and clinical implications. Histiologically (23, 44) the acute radiation effects, (2 weeks-6 months post radiation) demonstrate:

1. Centrilobular hemorrhage.
2. Dilatation of hepatic sinusoids around central veins (sinusoidal congestion).
3. Proliferation of endothelial cells in the centrilobular zone.
4. Atrophy and degeneration of liver cells (necrosis with lipochrome pigment in Kupffer cells).
5. Proliferation of collagen-forming cells in the centrilobular zone.
6. Lack of inflammatory infiltrates around the necrotic hepatocytes.

The changes in acute radiation hepatitis can be distinguished from other hepatic injury. Viral hepatitis demonstrates ballooning degeneration with associated cell mediated immune lymphocytic infiltrates and patchy micro-focal hepatic cell death. Portal vein thrombosis does not show dilation and stasis of pericentral sinusoids. Chemotherapy induced liver injury shows fatty or hydropic degeneration of hepatocytes with inter and intracellular cholestasis, portal lymphoplasmacytic infiltrates and piecemeal necrosis (35).

Clinically, the patient may have rapid weight gain, ascites and smooth non-nodular hepatomegaly. Liver function test impairment may be shown by slightly elevated SGOT, BSP, bilirubin and alkaline phosphatase levels. The TC-99 liver scan may reveal a characteristic sharply demarcated zone of photon deficient area corresponding to the radiation portal (Figure 13.9). The CT scan (25) images also may reveal similar low attenuation sharply demarcated zones with divergence. The subsequent regeneration of hepatic tissue may show improvement in this defect (Figure 13.10).

The chronic phase of radiation hepatitis (6 months or more post radiation) (44, 45) represents the progression of acute injury to the central vein, sinusoids and hepatic cells. Histopathologically the chronic phase reveals (28, 45) lobular distortion, severe narrowing in central veins, pericentral sclerosis, portal fibrosis and absence of vasculitis, thrombo-occlusive or intimal proliferative changes in hepatic arteries (Figure 13.11). The lesion resembles "cardiac" type of cirrhosis dominated by centrilobular scarring (28).

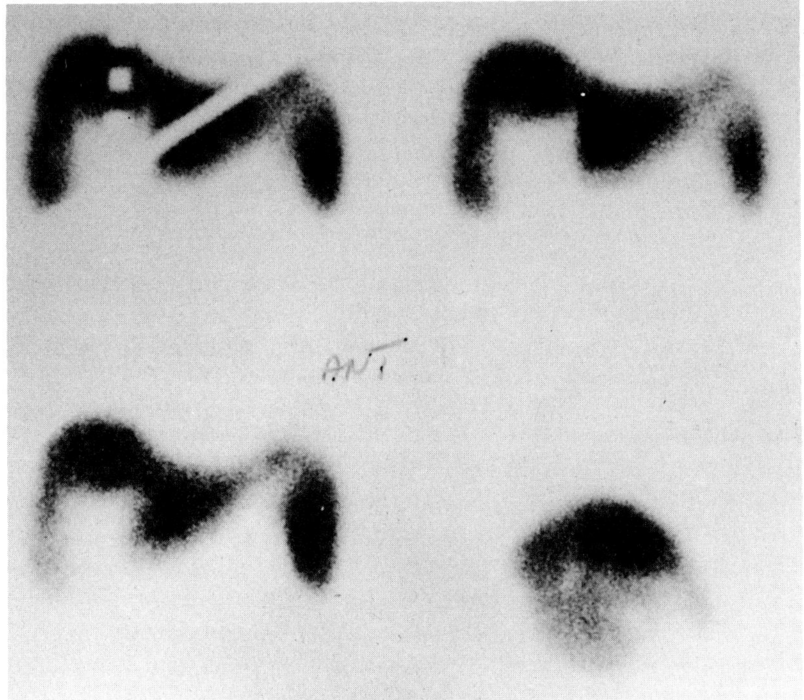

Figure 13.9. Radiation changes in the liver shown in the nuclear scan.

The tests for hepatocyte function usually are near normal since the hepatocytes are not isolated from blood flow although the sclerotic and fibro proliferative central vein changes produce a picture of veno-occlusive disease. The clinical manifestation is that of ascites, esophageal varices, hypersplenism (retrograde transmission of hepatic hypertension to the portal system) (28), and normal or slight elevations in liver function tests including bilirubin, BSP, alkaline phosphatase, SGOT and LDH.

The information through clinical studies thus indicates that the TTD 5/5 (tolerance dose for 5% radiation hepatitis) is 3,000 rads and TTD 50/5, (the tolerance dose for 50% incidence of radiation hepatitis) is 4,000 rads at 200 rad fractions given conventionally.

When the liver is radiated through a moving strip technique (stripfield whole abdominal R.T.) the radiation hepatic changes can be seen at 2,000 rads. Autopsy studies (Lewin and Millis) (28)

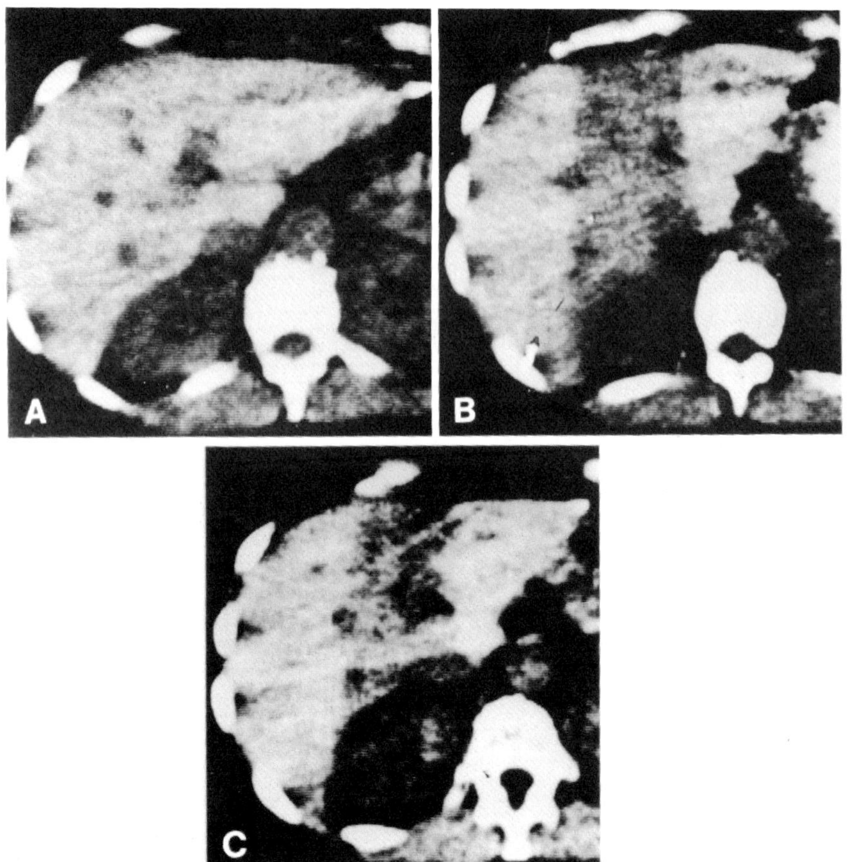

Figure 13.10. CT scan of the liver (A) before irradiation treatment with normal parenchyma but possible dilatation of the intrahepatic bile ducts. The (B) illustrations show repeat examination immediately after irradiation treatment. The CT scan now shows a sharply demarcated zone of low attenuation with slightly divergent borders corresponding to the field of treatment. The (C) illustration shows the repeat examination 5 weeks after irradiation. CT scan shows that the borders are more irregular probably due to regeneration of hepatic tissue. (Reproduced by kind permission of A. Kolbenstadt, M.D., Oslo, Norway from *Radiology, 135:*391, 1980.)

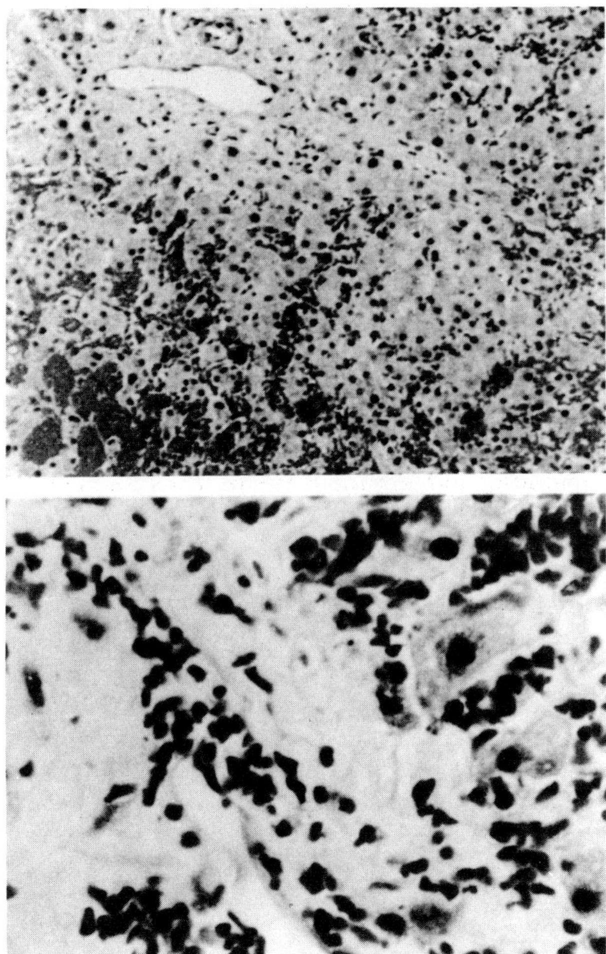

Figure 13.11. Histopathology of acute radiation changes in radiation injury. The top illustration is microscopic low power and the bottom is microscopic high power. (Reproduced by kind permission of the American College of Radiology from *Radiation Oncology*, 1975.)

report that the radiation doses were similar for acute and chronic radiation hepatitis. Similar dose disease relationships seem to apply in children (10, 11), though thrombocytopenia at 2,000–2,500 rads and abnormal liver scans at 1,200–2,500 rads were reported (28).

SUMMARY AND FUTURE DEVELOPMENTS

The large quantity of blood circulating through the liver would probably tempt one to speculate that a good radiation response of liver tumors occurs in the well oxygenated liver tumor bed. But, the normal liver is evidently not a radioresistant organ, its radiosensitivity exceeded perhaps only by the kidney, bone marrow, lymphoid and germinal tissue, thus hampering the curative attempts through radiation for aggressive hepatic malignancies demanding higher tumoricidal doses than the liver tolerance doses. Palliative doses of radiation probably can be delivered for inoperable liver tumors provided the liver is not too badly damaged by the tumor, there is no nutritional deficiency or associated disease, prior chemo sensitization has not taken place and provided the patient is not metabolically impoverished. Efforts must be made to maintain a good hepatic metabolic state since the starved liver cells suffer greater radiation injury.

Whole liver radiation of 2,500 rads to 3,000 rads, given at conventional fractionation schedules appear to be well tolerated and offer significant palliation. Similar doses of whole liver radiation may also offer benefit to primary liver tumors and a reduced field gross tumor boost may be considered allowing for the prior chemotherapy, surgery, and the metabolic status of the patient. Aggressive multimodal approaches with surgery, radiation (preop and postop and chemotherapy, debulking, or adjuvant) are under investigation and may provide improvement in survivals.

Recent developments of radio–labeled antibody therapy, intra–arterial radioisotope therapy (P–32 and Y–90) offer logical approaches towards this goal and have shown encouraging results. Prophylactic treatment of liver in patients at high risk for liver metastases (e.g., with P–32 in intra–arterial therapy for locally advanced colorectal carcinomas, pancreatic cancer, etc.) should receive significant attention in future clinical studies and may provide significant survival advantages.

REFERENCES

1. Ariel, IM, Padula, G: Treatment of symptomatic cancer to the liver from primary colon and rectal cancer by the intra-arterial administration of chemotherapy and radioactive isotopes. *J Surg Oncol, 10:*327-336, 1978.

2. Ariel, IM, Pack, G: Palliative treatment of inoperable cancer of the liver, biliary system and pancreas. In: *Neoplasms of the Pancreas, Biliary System and Liver,* Chapter 22, pp. 447-490, 1962.

3. Barone, RM, Byfield, JE, Frankel, S: Combination of infusional 5-FU and radiation therapy for the treatment of metastatic carcinoma of the colon to the liver. *Dis Colon Rectum, 22:*376-382, 1972.

4. Borgett, BB, *et al.*: Palliation of hepatic metastases: Results of RTOG Pilot Study. *Rad Oncol Biol Phys, I:*587-591, 1981.

5. Brick, IB: Late effects of million volt irradiation on gastrointestinal tract AMA. *Arch Int Med, 96:*26-31, 1955.

6. Cohen, L, Shapiro, ME, *et al.: Brit J Radiol, 27:*402-406, 1954.

7. Case, JT, Warthin, AS: Occurrence of hepatic lesions in the patients treated by intensive deep roentgen radiation. *Am Roentgenol Radium Ther, 12:*27-46, 1924.

8. Ellinger, F: Response of liver to irradiation. *Radiology, 44:*241, 1945.

9. Ettinger, DS, Order, DE, Wharam, MD, *et al.*: Phase I-II study of isotopic immunoglobulin therapy for primary liver cancer. *Cancer Treat Rep, 66:*289-297, 1982.

10. El Domieri, AA, Huvos, AG, Goldsmith, HS, *et al.*: Primary malignant tumors of the liver. *Cancer, 27:*7, 1971.

11. Fellows, DE, Jr., Kawter, GF, Teft, N: Hepatic effects following abdominal irradiation in children, detection by Au 198 scan and confirmation by histologic examination. *Am J Roentegnol, 103:*422, 1968.

12. Falkson, G, Feddes, EW: *British Med J, 4:*454, 1968.

13. Falkson, G, Van Eden, *et al.: Cancer, 33:*1207-1209, 1974.

14. Falkson, G, Falkson, HC: *Cancer Chemother Rep, 36:*77-85, 1965.

15. Falkson, G, Falkson, HC: *Cancer Chemother Rep, 49:*31-46, 1965.

16. Foster, JH: Survival after liver resection for cancer. *Cancer, 26:*493, 1970.

17. Friedman, MA, Volverding, PA, Cassidy, MJ, *et al.*: Therapy for hepatocellular cancer with intrahepatic arterial adriamycin and 5-FU combined with whole liver irradiation: An NCOG Study. *Cancer Treat Rep, 63:*1885, 1979.

18. Friedman, MA, Volverding, PA, *et al.*: Hepatic radiation plus multiple drug intra-arterial chemotherapy for patients with liver tumors. Abstract: Proc of ASTR. *Rad Oncol Biol Phys, 5:Suppl 2:*117-117, 1979.

19. Friedman, MA. Cassidy, MJ, Levine, M, *et al.*: Combined modality therapy of hepatic metastases. *Cancer, 44:*906-913, 1979.

20. Friedman, MA: Primary hepatocellular cancer — present results and future prospects. *Int J Rad Oncol Biol Phys, 9:*1841-1850, 1983.

21. Grady, ED: Internal radiation therapy for hepatic cancer. *Dis Colon Rectum, 22:*371, 1979.

22. Herbsman, H, Gardner, B, *et al.*: Treatment of hepatic metastases with combination of hepatic artery infusion chemotherapy and external radiation therapy. *Surg, Gynecol, Obstet, 147:*13–17, 1978.

23. Ingold, JA, Reed, GB, Kaplan, HS, *et al.*: Radiation hepatitis. *Am J Roentgenol, 93:*200–208, 1965.

24. Kaplan, HS, Bagshaw, MA: Radiation hepatitis: Possible prevention by combined isotopic and external radiotherapy. *Radiology, 91:*1214, 1968.

25. Kolbenstvedt, A, Kjolseth, I, *et al.*: Post irradiation changes of liver demonstrated by computerized tomography. *Radiology, 135:*391, 1980.

26. Kraut, JW, Kaplan, HS, Bagshaw, M: Combined fractionated isotopic and external irradiation of liver in Hodgkin's disease. *Cancer, 30:*39–46, 1972.

27. Leichner, PK, Klein, JL, Garrison, Jr., *et al.*: Dosimetry of I-131 labeled antiferritin in hepatoma, a model for radio-immunoglobulin dosimetry. *Int J Rad Oncol Biol Phys, 7:*323–333, 1981.

28. Lewin, K, Millis, RR: Human radiation hepatitis, a morphological study with emphasis on the late changes. *Arch Pathol, 96:*21, 1966.

29. Liu, TY: Primary cancer of the liver: Quadrennial review. *Scand J Gastro Enterol, (Suppl) 6:*223–241, 1970.

30. Liebel, SA, Order, DE, Rominger, CJ, *et al.*: Palliation of liver metastases with combined hepatic radiation and misonidazole: Results of RTOG Phase I-II Study. *Cancer Clin Trials, 4:*285–293, 1981.

31. Lokich, J, Kinsella, T, Perr, J, *et al.*: Concomitant hepatic irradiation and intra-arterial fluorinated pyrimidine therapy: Correlation of liver scan liver function tests and plasma CEA with tumor response. *Cancer, 48:*2569–2574, 1981.

32. Lortat-Jacobs, JL, Robert, HG: Hepatectomie Droite Reglee. *Presse Med, 60:*549, 1952.

33. Maischeider, MT, Kazem, I: Palliative irradiation of liver metastases. *JAMA, 232:*625–627, 1975.

34. Mantravadi, RVP, *et al.*: Intra-arterial Yttrium-90 in the treatment of hepatic malignancy. *Radiology, 142:*783–786, 1982.

35. Mantravadi, RVP, Dimitrios, G, Spigos, *et al.*: Intra-arterial chromic phosphate for prevention of postoperative liver metastases in high risk colorectal cancer patients. *Radiology, 148:*555–559, 1983.

36. Order, SE, Klein, JA, Ettinger, D, *et al.*: A Phase I-II study of radio-labeled antibody integrated in the treatment of primary hepatic malignancies. *Int J Rad Oncol Biol Phys, 6:*703–710, 1980.

37. Order, SE: Monoclonal antibody-potential role in radiation therapy and oncology. *Int J Rad Oncol Biol Phys, 8:*1193–1201, 1982.

38. Order, SE, Klein, JL, Leichner, P, *et al.*: Radio-labeled antibodies in the treatment of liver malignancies. In: *Gastrointestinal Cancer,* Levin and Riddel (Eds.). North Holland: Elsevier (to be published).

39. Order, SE: Radioimmunoglobulin therapy of cancer. In: *Comprehensive Therapy,* 1984: 10 (1): pp. 9–18.

40. Phillips, R, Murikami, K: Primary neoplasms of liver: Results of radiation therapy. *Cancer, 13:*716, 1960.

41. Phillips, R, Karnofsky, DA, *et al.*: Roentgen therapy of hepatic metastases. *Am J Roentgenol Radium Ther Nucl Med, 71:*826, 1954.

42. Prasad, B, *et al.*: Irradiation of hepatic metastases. *Int J Rad Oncol Biol Phys, 2:*129-132, 1977.

43. Quattelbaum, JK: Massive resection of the liver. *Ann Surg, 137:*787, 1953.

44. *Radiation Biology and Radiation Pathology Syllabus.* Published by American College of Radiology, Chicago, Illinois, 1975.

45. Reed, GB, Cox, AG, Jr.: The human liver after radiation injury: A form of veno occlusive disease. *Am J Pathol, 148:*597, 1966.

46. Rostock, RA, Fishman, EK, Order, SE: CT scanning for radiation therapy treatment planning of hepatoma. *Int J Rad Oncol Biol Phys, 11:* 1413-1418, 1985.

47. Sherman, DM, Weischelbaum, R, Order, SE, *et al.*: Palliation of hepatic metastases. *Cancer, 41:*2013, 1978.

48. Shiu, MG, Fortner, J: Current management of hepatic tumors. *Surg, Gynecol, Obstet, 140:*1-7, 1975.

49. Tochner, ZA, Kinsella, TJ, Glatstein, E: Hepatic irradiation in the management of metastatic hormone-secreting tumors. *Cancer, 56:*20-24, 1985.

50. Warren, S: Effects of radiation on normal tissues. IV. Effects of radiation on gastrointestinal tract including salivary glands, liver and pancreas. *Arch Pathol 34:*749, 1942.

51. Weber, BM, Solderberg, CH, *et al.*: Combined treatment of hepatic metastases. *Cancer, 42:*1087-1095, 1978.

52. Whitley, HW, Stearns, MW, Jr., *et al.*: Radiation therapy in the palliative management of patients with recurrent cancer of the rectum and colon. *Surg Clin N Am, 49:*381, 1969.

W. JOHN B. HODGSON, M.D.

CHAPTER 14

Management of Liver Tumors

INTRODUCTION

Every year, 30,000 patients in the United States develop metastases to the liver from colorectal cancer. This represents the largest group of hepatic metastatic digestive diseases. In addition, there are 13,400 cases of primary cancer of the liver and biliary passages (1).

The median survival time for all patients with liver tumors is in the region of 4-5 months and in the more fortunate group, those with colorectal metastases, it is in the region of 6-7 months. Symptomatic patients survive for a shorter period of time but the asymptomatic patients may survive as long as two years (2, 3)

It is our feeling that no liver cancer should be left untreated, even if the patient does not have symptoms. Lack of symptoms is not an indication for therapeutic nihilism but is an indication that treatment is more likely to be successful in tumors caught at an early stage. That is why the American Cancer Society advises screening for colorectal cancer and the Japanese screen for esophagogastric cancers.

VASCULAR DYNAMICS

Although an understanding of liver tumor vascularity and its morphology and dynamics is not mandatory for the management of liver tumors, it does help to clarify the rationale behind many of our therapeutic approaches. Experimental work indicated that in the earlier stages tumor cells were nourished by diffusion from the surrounding normal liver vessels. When the tumor became larger than 1 mm in diameter, single vessels were shown to be encircling these implants and with further growth multiple vessels appeared to be involved. These vessels were randomly derived from either arterial or portal sites. There was free mixing of the two circulations but eventually the arterial circulation became predominant (4, 5).

Even in larger liver tumors with well developed vascularity and a well developed encircling plexus from the arterial circulation, there was always a minor portal component. This may be sufficient to sustain the tumor until a collateral arterial circulation can develop following hepatic artery ligation. Such collateralization has been seen in as little as 4 days (6).

Another interesting finding is that in the apparently avascular centers of tumors, highly abnormal vessels are present which may, under certain circumstances, be perfused. The tumor vessels are abnormal in animal models and angiography in patients has demonstrated the same findings, showing that contrast material tends to move through the tumors more slowly than would be the case with normal vessels. There are also multiple abnormal arterio-venous shunts which allow earlier venous filling than would be the case in normal tissue (7).

However, studies of vascular dynamics have indicated that arterial perfusion of a tumor is actually greater than the arterial perfusion of the liver. Interestingly, the perfusion through the portal system of a tumor may be the same as that of normal liver (8).

Therefore, if the portal vein was also ligated to the appropriate lobe, then a higher tumor kill ratio would result. In patients, unilateral devascularization has been used successfully with minimal side effects and atrophy of the ligated lobe with its tumor (9).

Studies are continuing with vaso-active drugs to determine their effect on tumor vessels but so far the results have been inconsistent and there can be few conclusions drawn (10).

Similarly, it is difficult to quantify the effect of changes in permeability of the tumor vessels. However, it is speculated that an increase in permeability associated with the development of vascular stasis and an ultimate cessation of flow to tumors may be partly responsible for the favorable therapeutic effect of hyperthermia (11).

SCREENING
(tumor markers)

With these thoughts in mind, the first major step in the management of any liver tumor is to find it. In order to do this, the informed physician has to search for the tumor if relative success in management is to be achieved.

Screening for primary tumors of the liver in high risk patients, such as those who are HBsAg positive and in patients with some forms of cirrhosis, especially the macronodular variety, may be of benefit. Periodic measurements of serum alpha-fetoprotein levels are made. Positive results above 500 ng/ml strongly suggest hepatoma and if these can be resected at an early stage 50–75% long-term survival may be achieved (12, 13, 14).

In addition, it must be remembered that alpha feto-protein levels may be normal in the sugbroup of fibrolamellar hepatocellular carcinomas but the carcinoembryonic antigen (CEA) may be raised. As this tumor apparently metastasizes late and occurs in young people, it should be aggressively resected (15, 16). Secondary liver tumors are vastly more common in America and the most widely used tumor marker is the CEA. Periodic levels are obtained because one measurement on its own will not give an accurate answer. But the finding of a progressive rise of the CEA level is strongly suggestive of the development of metastatic tumor. Indeed, it is important to note that nearly half the patients who have been followed and then subjected to second-look laparotomy on the basis of rising CEA levels have had resectable tumors (17). Waiting for the tumor to show itself will not have such a happy outcome.

Liver function tests have not been helpful in early detection of hepatic neoplasms and we do not recommend general screening using this approach. The finding of elevated liver enzymes and serum alkaline phosphatase is usually an indication of severe and extensive disease. The presence of normal liver function studies does not rule out tumor.

NON-INVASIVE RADIOLOGY

Of course, it is rather difficult to persuade patients to have a second-look operation on the off-chance that we may find tumor. In addition to the CEA and alpha-fetoprotein levels, it is recommended that a cheap screening non-invasive test is also done at intervals when following this type of patient. The radionuclide liver scan is cheap and easy to carry out although it is not very specific. However, it does have the useful function of raising the suspicion of the presence of tumor. In fact, some studies have demonstrated that the liver scans may be specific enough to detect tumors in the liver in 87% of the patients (18). More accurate information may be obtained by computer enhancement but this is not yet widely available (19). A negative study should not be regarded as a clearance to the patient, especially in the presence of a rising CEA. Further studies should be carried out under these circumstances.

Ultrasonography, in good hands, can detect 94% of liver tumors (20). But it is important that the ultrasonographer is technically excellent in order to achieve these results. The less dedicated ultrasonographers, particularly in a screening situation, should be expected to miss a good number of liver tumors.

A far more expensive way of examining the patient for the suspicion of tumor is the computerized transaxial tomography but again, if this is done as a routine and no specific effort is made to closely examine the liver, poor quality pictures can be obtained and tumors can be missed. An interested and helpful radiologist is mandatory in the management of patients in these techniques and as indicated in the chapter in CT scanning, for a very accurate detection of tumors down to half a centimeter in size, we recommend infusion of the superior mesenteric artery and then the scan is done during the portal phase (21, 22).

INVASIVE RADIOLOGY

Angiography on its own is not recommended as a screening procedure but it is a major part of the preoperative workup of patients with liver tumors.

For the surgeon, the arteriogram is critical for determining the type of tumor, extent of spread, resectability and variation of vascular anatomy.

Patients who present with symptoms and in whom initial screening demonstrates tumors in the liver do need continuing examination and follow-through in order for a diagnosis to be made. Although the arteriogram is very invasive, it is actually more controlled than, for example, a percutaneous liver biopsy. This can be a disaster in hemangiomas or hemangio-sarcomas.

The angiogram can sometimes actually help in the diagnosis of focal nodular hyperplasia and, like the liver cell adenoma, there are large dilated arteries surrounding the tumor but the neovascularity is not so dense in the adenoma as in focal nodular hyperplasia. In particular, the main hepatic artery is routinely dilated in the adenoma (23).

The cavernous hemangioma is the most common benign tumor of the liver and can be diagnosed by CT scanning when sequential filling from the outside will be seen. The angiographic appearance is of a very vascular lesion with unremarkable blood vessels with the arteries showing normal tapering. The hallmark of these lesions is their prolonged blush or opacification which may last up to 20 seconds (24).

Regenerating nodules may also be mistaken for tumors but they have a vascularity which is similar to surrounding liver. Although the feeding vessels within the regenerating nodule may be tortuous, no actual tumor vascularity is seen. The branches are more normal than would otherwise be the case (25).

Hepatomas can be diagnosed because the blood filled spaces in the trabeculae are filled solely with arterial blood whereas in the normal liver the sinusoids are mostly filled by portal blood. There is much arterio-venous shunting and there is portal and hepatic vein invasion (26).

Cholangio-carcinomas are difficult to diagnose angiographically (27).

Metastases to the liver range from hyper to hypovascular. All metastases appear as filling defects on the portal phase since all are predominantly supplied by hepatic arterial branches. This helps in the diagnosis of these tumors when the CT scan is carried out after perfusion of the superior mesenteric artery (28).

Angiography demonstrates that only about half the patients have classic vascular anatomy consisting of right and left hepatic branches supplying right and left lobes of the liver. There is a significant group of 14% in which the entire right hepatic artery may be replaced by the superior mesenteric artery (29). In general, the blood supply may originate through one vessel, two vessels or three entirely separate vessels to the liver. Then the angiographer can help the surgeon in the placement of a pump, for example, by embolizing the smaller arteries so that a catheter can subsequently be placed to supply the liver through the major arteries (30). Similarly, the gastroduodenal artery can be embolized to prevent flow of chemotherapeutic agents away from the liver.

When this embolization of single vessels is done, infarction does not occur. In fact the angiographer can observe immediate change in the dye pattern in the liver whereby one side can be fully perfused from the other side after embolization of a major branch in a matter of minutes.

Obviously, changing from diagnostic to therapeutic management of the patient angiographically involves a great deal of skill but it is possible to even place the catheter for intra-arterial hepatic chemotherapy percutaneously when a skilled interventional radiologist is on hand (31).

There is much evidence that direct embolization into the tumor itself may be a very effective way of carrying out management of these cancers (32).

Larger arteries can rapidly re-establish blood flow via collaterals following embolization. This is much more difficult when embolization is carried out at the arteriolar or pre-capillary level (31). Then small particulate matter such as Gelfoam or Ivalon or newer agents such as Cyanoacrylate, or absolute alcohol, are used (33).

One of the complications of embolization, and hence, infarction, is superimposed infection. We find that pain, fever, tenderness, white blood cell elevation, and abnormal biochemical values of liver function and even gas bubbles on abdominal x-ray occur routinely. But all of these may be produced by non-septic infarction of the tumor and actual abscess formation in our hands has not been a major problem (34).

The patients are carefully watched and treated with antibiotics before embolization and also for about a week afterwards. When their symptoms begin to subside, it is normal for them to be able to be discharged from the hospital or to go onto the next phase of treatment.

CLASSIFICATION

We prefer to use embolization as part of our multidisciplinary approach, dependent on our classification of a particular patient's tumor.

The completion of the x-ray studies will allow us to stage the patient and to identify the anatomy. Staging is important because a single tumor, much discussed in the literature, is a rarity. In our series, these tumors probably represent about 5-10% of tumors at the most (35). Management of single tumors is very straightforward but the management of the more common and more extensive disease is much more involved.

The history and physical examination will give many of the clues necessary to diagnose the type of liver tumor. Screening tests help confirm this. We prefer to make the definitive diagnosis by excision or open biopsy.

Accurate positioning of the tumors in the liver is important for adequate treatment and sizing is necessary for staging. Stages I to IV demonstrate increasing tumor load (3, 36). The subset "a" indicates that the major vascular structures of the liver are involved with the tumor, even if this tumor is small. Unresectability will obviously affect the outcome of the patient.

Factors in addition to diagnosis and staging need to be identified. The determination of Child's classification (37) has indicated that those with poor classifications cannot complete their treatments as their liver reserve is insufficient. On the other hand, patients with apparently extensive tumor who can be classified by Child's system as A, will usually tolerate very aggressive treatment and do well. Similarly, performance status clearly correlates with outcome.

Hence, a patient with a good Child's classification, a good performance status and a moderate amount of tumor is clearly going to do well with most aggressive treatment and we have been delighted to see that our expectations have been fulfilled with, for example, survivals in the region of 4 years and more in patients with bilateral metastases to the liver.

ANATOMY

The most important point to remember about the anatomy of the liver is that the right side only extends to a line drawn between the gall bladder and the inferior vena cava whereas the liver tissue to the left of this line is all left lobe. The reason for this arrangement is that the portal vein and hepatic artery actually run into the left medial segment but divide to supply the liver, either side of the gall bladder, separately.

From the surgical viewpoint, however, the venous drainage is of paramount importance since it is situated posteriorly in the liver and there is no relationship to the lobe supplied by the hepatic artery and portal vein. Recent studies have indicated that the variation in the venous drainage may be as great as the variation in hepatic artery supply to the liver (38).

Knowledge of the peritoneal attachments in the liver will help the surgeon to approach the posterior aspect and to identify venous anatomy during the early part of the resection, thus enhancing safety.

The knowledge that there can be collaterals arising in the embryological pathways in portal venous obstruction (39) will help in the management of centrally located tumors.

Knowledge that the hepatic arteries are not end arteries but that there is a potential extensive collateral circulation help in the management of a patient by hepatic artery ligation or embolization (40, 41).

Knowledge of the biliary anatomy helps avoid injury to these ducts. Resection of bile duct tumors is feasible since it is possible to develop planes between them and the portal veins (42). Also, arteries which may traverse the area can be divided with impunity as collaterals will develop from other areas with extreme rapidity.

Subsegmental anatomy (43) is increasing in importance with the realization that, particularly in cirrhotic livers, preservation of as much non-tumorous liver as possible leads to results which are very acceptable because of the low early mortality (44).

HEPATIC ARTERY LIGATION

Hepatic artery ligation in the patient who does not have cirrhosis is a safe procedure. Indeed, even in some patients with cirrhosis, sequential embolization of the hepatic artery branches has been carried out with minimal morbidity (32). The dogma of danger with hepatic artery ligation can be dropped. It is not necessary to spend time re-anastomosing arteries in the porta hepatis in order to try and guarantee blood flow to both lobes. The liver is quite capable of developing an arterial blood supply through one hepatic artery branch or even through the hepatic peritoneal ligaments (40). Further, we have found that even the complication of ischemic cholecystitis is a rarity in hepatic artery ligation.

As regards tumor management, hepatic artery ligation does not prolong survival but can result in considerable symptomatic improvement over the short term. There may be a diminution of tumor size so that in a few weeks, resection may become possible in previously unresectable patients (45, 46, 47).

Like hepatic artery ligation, hepatic de-arterialization does not appear to extend survival in patients with hepatic tumors, and as it has a 10% mortality, it is no longer being recommended (47).

Transient occlusion of the hepatic artery is an interesting adjunct and has been carried out because there is such rapid re-vascularization of hepatic tumors. The idea is that re-vascularization will be less likely to occur if the surgeon determines when arterial flow is to continue to the liver and when it is going to be shut off (48).

Hepatic artery ligation is of benefit in Stage IIa, III or IIIa patients in whom lengthy survival should not be expected in any case. Median survivals of up to 8 months have been achieved. There does appear to be definite benefit in patients with carcinoid syndrome from ligation of the hepatic artery alone.

PORTAL VEIN LIGATION

Portal vein ligation has generally been used in the management of lacerations of the portal vein and not as a method of tumor treatment. However, in those instances where it has been used for the management of tumors, such as patients with near normal hepatic function from the residual liver tissue and no coagulopathy, unilateral ligation of the portal vein can result in a median survival time of 10 months (9).

TECHNIQUES OF INTRAHEPATIC CHEMOTHERAPY

Placement of catheters for intrahepatic chemotherapy has been refined over recent years and many of the earlier technical problems have now been solved. The main reason for this is the use of silastic catheters which are soft and do not migrate or block the hepatic artery. Also, catheters placed subcutaneously have a low rate of infection.

For this reason, it has been possible to give chemotherapy almost continuously. Methods in vogue include placement of an infusion port with a catheter guaranteeing access directly to the liver. A special Huber needle is used for connection to a continuously acting pump which may be portable. Alternatively a totally implantable but much more expensive system can be used, such as the Infusaid pump, which only needs to be refilled once every two weeks. This pump will continue to give about 3 cc of a chemotherapeutic agent every day and is a very acceptable system to the patients (49, 50, 51).

The main problems which occur with intrahepatic chemotherapy are the development of peptic ulceration due to failure

to appreciate aberrant gastric or duodenal vessels during placement of the catheter or the simple development of collateralization despite ligation of the vessels (52).

At this time the reported results of continuous intrahepatic
treatment vary with between 50–80% response rates and it is still
questionable as to whether or not survival is enhanced (53).

However, some patients unquestionably do have a considerable survival time and live long enough to develop chemical
hepatitis and biliary sclerosis (54, 55).

HEPATIC RESECTIONS

Surgeons learning the technique of hepatic resection should
commence with simple procedures such as wedge resections and
then expand to well established methods of lobectomies. A left
lateral segmentectomy is easier to perform than a left hemihepatectomy which is easier to perform than a right hemihepatectomy.
Trisegmentectomies are difficult procedures (56). They are also
associated with significant postoperative problems and in all cases
when this much liver has been removed, the patient develops
jaundice and low albumin levels and may even suffer from hypoglycemia (57).

Techniques such as the ultrasonic scalpel do help in making
the actual procedure of resection safer in that the intrahepatic
blood vessels can be clamped before division so that blood loss is
reduced. The less ischemic damage that occurs to a liver during a
procedure the better, as a more even postoperative course results
(58).

A good knowledge of anatomy is, therefore, essential and
careful control of blood vessels before division, whether extrahepatic or intrahepatic is mandatory.

The expected mortality of liver surgery these days should be
no more than 5–8%. Similarly, morbidity should be minimal.
Massive resections are not required for minimal disease and it is
now frequently possible to remove several tumors from both sides
of the liver during one operative session (59–64).

The results of these more aggressive resectional approaches to
liver surgery are that more patients are surviving for longer periods
of time and probably, for all resections, a survival rate of 5 years
in the order of 25% is possible and this is the same survival rate as
patients with Duke's C cases of colorectal carcinoma. In our insti-

tution, even in patients with bilateral disease, after resection, we are able to obtain survivals into the third and fourth postoperative years.

PRE AND POSTOPERATIVE MANAGEMENT

Physiological monitoring before, during and after the operation, with the aggressive use of the Swan–Ganz catheter, has been demonstrated to reduce surgical morbidity and mortality. Even for patients over the age of 70, mortality rates for surgery in general can be halved with careful monitoring (65).

CHEMOTHERAPY

It is generally accepted that a weekly bolus of 5–FU intravenously in the management of colorectal liver metastases has no effect on survival and the response rate is only about 15% (66, 67).

When a 5–day loading schedule is instituted before the weekly bolus of 5–FU is given, then a 20% remission rate can be obtained (68, 69).

Continuous intrahepatic chemotherapy appears to have a response rate in the order of 40% and with continuous systemic chemotherapy is probably slightly less than this. However, in considering the cases involved, the extent of tumor has a critical role to play in survival time. Those with less than 20% involvement of the liver have a median survival of 13.5 months whereas those with more than 60% involvement have only a median survival of about 6 months. This does not seem to be affected by the chemotherapeutic agent (70).

Other agents have been used and combinations have been used but there are no clear advantages over 5–FU (71).

In patients with hepatomas, doxorubicin does appear to have a satisfactory response rate in the region of 25% (72). The response to systemic 5–FU is minimal but does seem to improve remarkably when given via the hepatic artery to a rate of 43% (73). An interesting approach was used when a one-year survival rate of 24% was obtained when arterial chemoembolization with Mitomycin C microcapsules was performed in unresectable patients (74).

RADIOTHERAPY

This is normally reserved for symptomatic patients with unresectable liver tumors and in combination with chemotherapy significant palliation may be achieved (75). Studies have indicated that the response may be random and that the use of radiotherapy associated with chemotherapy may not confer significant benefits (76). However, if a patient does respond, it is most likely to be in an individual not previously treated.

Responses can be gratifying. We have seen patients with massively involved and large livers demonstrate shrinkage of the liver and tumor; ascites may disappear; swelling of the legs fade; the patient becomes comfortable once again. Survival may not be enhanced by very much but on the other hand, it is possible that it becomes measured in months instead of weeks in the responders.

The important point about managing a patient with radiotherapy is to carefully fractionate the radiation dosage and to limit the maximum amount provided to 2,500 to 3,000 rads (77).

SUGGESTED PROTOCOL

In Figure 14.1, our protocol is listed. This protocol provides a scheme of treatment for patients with all stages of tumor involvement of the liver. In this, we believe that we do not abandon the patient if they do not fit into a simple protocol; we can tailor the treatment for each individual patient depending on their stage of the disease; we can move from one form of treatment to the next should their stage worsen; we have combined several modalities where one would be insufficient for that stage of the patient's disease.

Our algorythm can only be used when the patient's physician has diagnosed the liver tumor. As indicated at the beginning of this capter, the level of suspicion must be high as there are many cases awaiting diagnosis.

Confirmation of the liver tumor and accurate staging is done by sophisticated radiological techniques and we rely heavily on CT scanning and angiography.

The solitary lesions are separated from multiple lesions. Usually solitary lesions will be Stage I which is less than 25% involvement of the liver and will be resectable (58–64). However, sometimes because of the position of the lesion, it is unresectable

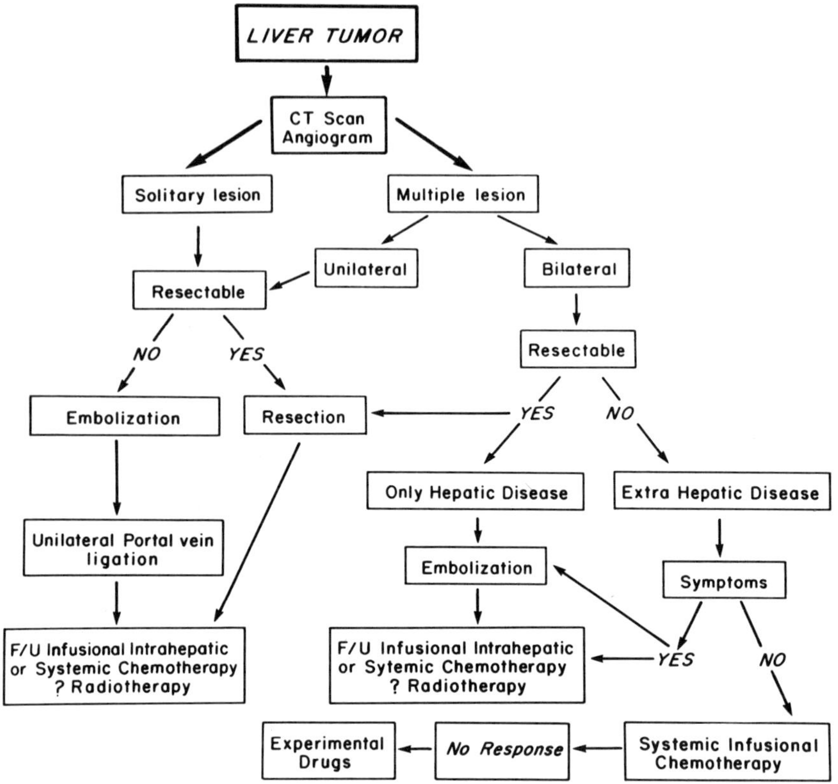

Figure 14.1 Protocol for total management of liver tumors, dependent on staging.

and then is Stage Ia. Then we would proceed to possible embolization of the tumor if the angiographer could direct the catheter
into the supplying arterial branch of the tumor (30–32). We would
then proceed to a unilateral portal vein ligation on the side to
which the tumor is biased (9). Finally we would also add a catheter for intra–arterial hepatic chemotherapy. This chemotherapy
would be supplied using an Infusaid pump or an external pump
(49–55).

In patients with multiple lesions, the staging will depend on
the volume of tumor (3, 36). In patients with unilobar disease, the
most likely categorization would be between 25% and 75%
involvement or Stage II. If the major draining veins of the liver

were not involved, then such lesions would be resectable by lobectomy. As in solitary lesions, after resection, chemotherapy would be given and probably systemically in this situation (69). However, if the tumors were not resectable, then we would proceed to embolization of the affected lobe plus unilateral portal vein ligation plus infusional intrahepatic arterial chemotherapy.

Where the disease was more advanced and a patient would have more than 75% involvement of the liver as in Stage III but did not have involvement of the draining veins in the liver, consideration would be given as to resection but this would only be carried out if residual liver tissue could be preserved. Alternatively, embolization of the main tumor bulk could be done followed by unilateral portal vein ligation and intrahepatic chemotherapy. Note that in patients with stiff livers, the intrahepatic catheter can be placed in the portal system.

In patients of Stage IIa and Stage IIIa who were suffering from bilateral disease, clearly resection is not possible and so appropriate measures such as local wedge resection may still be offered together with embolization and unilateral portal vein ligation together with intrahepatic chemotherapy via a pump. Radiotherapy is sometimes helpful in this situation (74, 75, 76).

In patients with Stage IV disease, the first line of attack is to resect the extrahepatic disease and if this is possible, the patient can be re-staged. However, if it is not possible to resect the extrahepatic disease then our approach is to use systemic infusional chemotherapy, using a port and an external pump. When there is no response to this line of treatment, we would then try experimental drugs providing the patient still had a reasonable performance status. In this same line, we may occasionally embolize symptomatic lesions.

CONCLUSIONS

With this comprehensive approach, a wide range of patients can be treated and much significant palliation can be obtained. Those patients who have enhanced survival do so as outpatients and the quality of their life is usually very satisfactory. In this way, because we have covered all the range of disease, we are able to return patients to their environment so that they may continue to contribute to society.

REFERENCES

1. Silverberg, E: Cancer Statistics, 1985. *CA, 35:*19-35, 1985.

2. Foster, JH, Berman, MM: Solid liver tumors. *Major Probl Clin Surg, 22:*62-104, 1977.

3. Taylor, I: Colorectal liver metastases: To treat or not to treat. *Br J Surg, 72:*511-516, 1985.

4. Ackerman, NB: The blood supply of experimental liver metastases. IV. Changes in vascularity with increasing tumor growth. *Surgery, 75:*589-596, 1974.

5. Breedis, C, Young, G: The blood supply of neoplasms in the liver. *Am J Path, 30:*969-985, 1954.

6. Bengmark, S, Rosengren, K: Angiographic study of the collateral circulation to the liver after ligation of the hepatic artery in man. *Am J Surg, 119:*620-624, 1970.

7. Ackerman, NB, Hechmer, PA: The blood supply of experimental liver metastases. V. Increased tumor perfusion with epinephrine. *Am J Surg, 140:*625-631, 1980.

8. Ackerman, NB, Hechmer, PA, Makohon, S: Failure of histamine type mediators to enhance vascular permeability in experimental liver metastases. *Surg, Gynecol, Obstet, 151:*647-651, 1980.

9. Honjo, I, Suzuki, T, Ozawa, K, *et al.*: Ligation of a branch of the portal vein for carcinoma of the liver. *Am J Surg, 130:*296-302, 1975.

10. Peterson, HI, Altsten, M, Skolnik, G, Karlsson, L: Influence of a prostaglandin synthesis inhibitor and of thrombocytopenia on tumor blood flow and tumor vascular permeability. Experimental studies in the rat. *Anticancer Res, 5:*253-257, 1985.

11. LeFor, AT, Makohon, S, Ackerman, NB: The effects of hyperthermia on vascular permeability in experimental liver metastases. *J Surg Oncol, 28:*297-300, 1985.

12. Fortner, JG, Maclean, BJ, Kim, DK, *et al.*: The 70s evolution in liver surgery for cancer. *Cancer, 47:*2162-2166, 1981.

13. Adson, MA, Farnell, MB: Hepatobiliary cancer - surgical considerations. *Mayo Clin Proc, 56:*686-699, 1981.

14. Furukawa, R, Tajima, H, Nakata, K, *et al.*: Clinical significance of serum alpha feto-protein in patients with liver cirrhosis. *Tumour Biol, 5:*327-338, 1984.

15. Craig, JR, Peters, RL, Edmonson, HA, Omata, M: Fibrolamellar carcinoma of the liver: A tumor of adolescence and young adults with distinct clinicopathological features. *Cancer, 46:*372-379, 1980.

16. Teitelbaum, DH, Tuttle, S, Carey, LC, Clausen, KS: Fibrolamellar carcinoma of the liver. Review of three cases and the presentation of a characteristic set of tumor markers defining this tumor. *Ann Surg, 202:*36-41, 1985.

17. Attiyeh, FF, Stearns, MW, Jr.: Second-look laparotomy based on CEA elevations in colorectal cancer. *Cancer, 47:*2119-2125, 1981.

18. Kim, DK, McSweeney, J, Yeh, SDJ, Fortner, JG: Tumors of the liver as demonstrated by angiography, scan and laparotomy. *Surg, Gynecol, Obstet, 141:*409-410, 1975.

19. Strauss, LG, Clorius, JH, Frank, T, van Kaick, G: Single photon emission computerized tomography (SPECT) for estimates of liver and spleen volume. *J Nucl Med, 25:*81-85, 1984.

20. Smith, IE, Taylor, KHW, McCready, VR, *et al.*: A comparison of Grey-scale ultrasound with other methods for the detection of liver metastases from breast carcinoma. *Clin Oncol, 2:*47-53, 1976.

21. Clark, RA, Matsui, O: CT of liver tumors. *Semin Roentgenol, 18:* 148-162, 1983.

22. Matsui, O, Kadoya, M, Suzuki, M, *et al.*: Work in progress: Dynamic sequential computed tomography during arterial portography in the detection of hepatic neoplasms. *Radiol, 146:*721-727, 1983.

23. Casarella, WJ, Knowles, DM, Wolff, M, Johnson, PM: Focal nodular hyperplasia and liver cell adenoma. Radiologic and pathologic differentiation. *Am J Roentgenol, 131:*393-402, 1978.

24. McLoughlin, MJ: Angiography in cavernous hemangioma of the liver. *Am J Roentgenol, 113:*50-55, 1971.

25. Rabinowitz, JG, Kinkabwala, M, Ulreich, S: Macro-regenerating nodule in cirrhotic liver. *Am J Roentgenol, 121:*401-411, 1974.

26. Okuda, K, Obata, H, Jinnouchi, S, *et al.*: Angiographic assessment of gross anatomy of hepatocellular carcinoma: Comparison of celiac angiograms and liver pathology in 100 cases. *Radiol, 123:*21-29, 1977.

27. Reuter, SR, Redman, HC, Bookstein, JJ: Angiography in carcinoma of the biliary tract. *Brit J Radiol, 44:*636-641, 1971.

28. Reuter, SR, Redman, HC: *Gastrointestinal Angiography*, Second Edition. Philadelphia: W.B. Saunders, 1977.

29. Ruzicka, FF, Jr., Rankin, RS: Normal arterial anatomy of the abdominal viscera. *CRC Crit Rev Diagn Imaging, 9:*337-385, 1977.

30. Chuang, VP, Wallace, S: Hepatic arterial redistribution for intraarterial infusion of hepatic neoplasms. *Radiol 135:*295-299, 1980.

31. Clouse, ME, Lee, RGL, Duszlak, ES, *et al.*: Peripheral hepatic artery embolization for primary and secondary hepatic neoplasms. *Radiol, 147:* 407-411, 1983.

32. Chuang, VP, Wallace, S, Soo, C-S, *et al.*: Therapeutic Ivalon embolization of hepatic tumors. *Am J Roentgenol, 138:*289-294, 1982.

33. Ellman, BA, Green, CE, Eigenbrodt, E, *et al.*: Renal infarction with absolute alcohol. *Invest Radiol, 15:*318-322, 1980.

34. Rankin, RN: Gas formation after renal tumor embolization without abscess. A benign occurrence. *Radiol, 130:*317-320, 1979.

35. Lockich, JJ: Primary and metastatic liver cancer. *Semin Oncol, 10:* 227-250, 1983.

36. Pettaval, J, Leyvraz, S, Douglas, P: The necessity for staging liver metastases and standardizing treatment response criteria. The case of second-

aries of colorectal origin. In: *Liver Metastases*, Van de Velde, CJH, Sugarbaker, PH (Eds.). Amsterdam: Martinus Nijhoff, 1984, pp. 358-367.

37. Child, CG, Turcotte, JG: Surgery and portal hypertension. In: *The Liver and Portal Hypertension*, Child, CG (Ed.). Philadelphia: WB Saunders, 1964, p. 50.

38. Nakamura, S, Tsuzuki, T: Surgical anatomy of the hepatic veins and the inferior vena cava. *Surg, Gynecol, Obstet, 152:*43-50, 1981.

39. DelGuercio, LRM, Hodgson, WJB, Morgan, JC, *et al.*: Splenic artery and coronary vein occlusion for bleeding esophageal varices. *World J Surg, 8:* 680-687, 1984.

40. Mays, ET, Wheeler, CS: Demonstration of collateral arterial flow after interruption of hepatic arteries in man. *N Eng J Med, 290:*993-996, 1974.

41. Kennedy, PA, Madding, GF: Surgical anatomy of the liver. *Surg Clin N Am, 57:*233-244, 1977.

42. Evander, A, Fredlund, P, Hoevels, J, *et al.*: Evaluation of aggressive surgery for carcinoma of the extrahepatic bile ducts. *Ann Surg, 191:*23-29, 1980.

43. Couinaud, C, Le Foie: *Études Anatomiques et Chirurgicals*. Paris: Masson et Cie, 1957.

44. Nagasue, N, Yukaya, H, Ogawa, Y, *et al.*: Hepatic resection in the treatment of hepatocellular carcinoma: Report of 60 cases. *Br J Surg, 72:* 292-295, 1985.

45. Bengmark, S, Brix, M, Borgisson, B, *et al.*: Treatment of hepatic tumors. *Digestion, 3:*309-317, 1970.

46. Mays, ET: Vascular occlusion. *Surg Clin N Am, 57:*291-323, 1977.

47. Lee, Y-TN: Non-systemic treatment of metastatic tumors of the liver - a review. *Med Pediat Oncol, 4:*185-203, 1978.

48. Bengmark, S, Fredlund, PE: Temporary dearterialization combined with intra-arterial infusion of oncolytic drugs in the treatment of liver tumors. In: *Progress in Clinical Cancer, VII*, Ariel, IM (Ed.). New York: Grune and Stratton, 1978, p. 207.

49. Buchwald, H, Grage, TB, Vassilopoulos, PP, *et al.*: Intra-arterial infusion chemotherapy for hepatic carcinoma using a totally implantable infusion pump. *Cancer, 45:*866-869, 1980.

50. Balch, CN, Urist, MM, McGregor, ML: Continuous regional chemotherapy for metastatic colorectal cancer using a totally implantable infusion pump. *Am J Surg, 145:*285-290, 1983.

51. Cohen, AM, Kaufman, SD, Wood, WC, Greenfield, AJ: Regional hepatic chemotherapy using an implantable drug infusion pump. *Am J Surg, 145:*529-532, 1983.

52. Daly, JM, Kemeny, N, Oderman, P, Botet, J: Long-term hepatic arterial infusion chemotherapy. *Arch Surg, 119:*936-941, 1984.

53. Schwartz, SI, Jones, LS, McCune, CS: Assessment of treatment of intrahepatic malignancies using chemotherapy via an implantable pump. *Ann Surg, 201:*560-567, 1985.

54. Kemeny, MM, Battifora, H, Blayney, DW, *et al.*: Sclerosing cholangitis after continuous hepatic artery infusion with FUDR. *Ann Surg, 202:*176-181, 1985.

55. Johnson, LP, Rivkin, SE: The implanted pump in metastatic colorectal cancer of the liver. Risk versus benefit. *Am J Surg, 149:*595-598, 1985.

56. Starzl, TE, Bell, RH, Beart, RW, Putnam, CW: Hepatic trisegmentectomy and other liver resections. *Surg, Gynecol, Obstet, 141:*429-437, 1975.

57. Coppa, GF, Eng, K, Ranson, JH, *et al.*: Hepatic resection for metastatic colon and rectal cancer. An evaluation of preoperative and postoperative factors. *Ann Surg, 202:*203-208, 1985.

58. Hodgson, WJB, DelDuercio, LRM: Preliminary experience in liver surgery using the ultrasonic scalpel. *Surgery, 95:*230-234, 1984.

59. Kortz, WJ, Meyers, WC, Hanks, JB, *et al.*: Hepatic resection for metastatic cancer. *Ann Surg, 199:*182-186, 1984.

60. Fortner, JG, Silva, JS, Golbey, RB, *et al.*: Multi-variate analysis of a personal series of 247 consecutive patients with liver metastases. I. Treatment by hepatic resection. *Ann Surg, 199:*306-316, 1984.

61. Adson, MA, Van Heerden, JA, Adson, MH, *et al.*: Resection of hepatic metastases from colorectal cancer. *Arch Surg, 119:*647-650, 1984.

62. Tomas-de la Vega, JE, Donahue, EJ, Doolas, A, *et al.*: A 10-year experience with hepatic resection. *Surg, Gynecol, Obstet, 159:*223-228, 1984.

63. Cady, B, McDermott, WV: Major hepatic resection for metachronous metastases from colon cancer. *Ann Surg, 201:*204-209, 1985.

64. August, DA, Sugarbaker, PH, Ottow, RT, *et al.*: Hepatic resection of colorectal metastases: Influence of clinical factors and adjuvant intraperitoneal 5-Fluorouracil via Tenckhoff catheter on survival. *Ann Surg, 201:*210-218, 1985.

65. Savino, JA, DelGuercio, LRM: Preoperative assessment of high risk surgical patients. *Surg Clin N Am, 65:*763-791, 1985.

66. Sugarbaker, PH, McDonald, JS, Gunderson, LL: Colorectal cancer. In: *Cancer, Principles and Practice of Oncology*, DeVita, VT, Jr., Hellman, S, Rosenberg, SA (Eds.). Philadelphia: JP Lippincott, 1982, pp. 643-723.

67. Moertel, CG, Fleming, TR, Creagan, ET, *et al.*: High dose vitamin C versus placebo in the treatment of patients with advanced cancer who have had no prior chemotherapy. *N Eng J Med, 312:*137-141, 1985.

68. Brennan, MJ, Talley, RW, San Diego, EL, *et al.*: Critical analysis of 594 cancer patients treated with 5-Fluorouracil. In: *Proc Internat Sympos Chemotherap Cancer*, Plattner, PA (Ed.). New York: Elsevier, 1964, pp. 118-150.

69. Grage, TB, Vassilopoulos, P, Shingleton, WW, *et al.*: Results of a prospectively randomized study of hepatic artery infusion with 5-Fluorouracil versus intravenous 5-Fluorouracil in patients with hepatic metastases from colorectal cancer: A Central Oncology Group Study. *Surgery, 86:*550-555, 1979.

70. Kemeny, N, Daly, J. Oderman, P. *et al.*: Hepatic artery pump infusion: Toxicity and results in patients with metastatic colorectal carcinoma.

J Clin Oncol, 2:595-600, 1984.

71. Kemeny, N, Yagoda, A, Braun, D: Metastatic colorectal carcinoma: A prospective randomized trial of methyl CCNU, 5-Fluorouracil (5-FU), and Vincristine (MOF) versus MOF plus Streptozotocin (MOF STREP). *Cancer,* 51:20-25, 1983.

72. Ramming, KP: The effectiveness of hepatic artery infusion in treatment of primary hepatobiliary tumors. *Semin Oncol,* 10:199-205, 1983.

73. Reed, M, Vaitkevicius, V, Al Sarraf, M, *et al.*: The practicality of chronic hepatic artery infusion therapy of primary and metastatic hepatic malignancies: Ten year results of 124 patients on a prospective protocol. *Cancer,* 47:402-409, 1981.

74. Ohnishi, K, Tsuchiya, S, Nakayama, T, *et al.*: Arterial chemoembolization of hepatocellular carcinoma with Mitomycin C microcapsule. *Radiology,* 152:51-55, 1984.

75. Byfield, JE, Barone, RM, Frankel, SS, *et al.*: Treatment with continued intra-arterial FUDR infusion and whole liver radiation for colon carcinoma metastatic to the liver. *Am J Clin Oncol,* 7:319-325, 1984.

76. Borgelt, BB, Gelber, R, Brady, LW, *et al.*: The palliation of hepatic metastases: Results of the radiation therapy oncology group pilot study. *Int J Radiol Oncol Biol Phys,* 7:587-591, 1981.

77. Thomas, P: Radiotherapy in the treatment of liver metastases. In: *Liver Metastases,* Van de Velde, CJH, Sugarbaker, PH (Eds.). Amsterdam: Martinus Nijhoff, 1984, pp. 206-213.

Index